OFFICE MANAGEMENT OF

SPORTS INJURIES &

ATHLETIC PROBLEMS

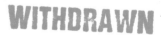

MORRIS B. MELLION, MD

EDITOR

Associate Professor
Departments of Family Practice
Orthopaedic Surgery and Rehabilitation (Sports Medicine)
University of Nebraska Medical Center
Associate Professor
School of Health, Physical Education and Recreation
University of Nebraska at Omaha
Omaha, Nebraska

HANLEY & BELFUS, INC. / Philadelphia
The C.V. Mosby Company / St. Louis • Toronto • London

Publisher: HANLEY & BELFUS, INC.
                    210 S. 13th Street
                    Philadelphia, PA 19107

North American and worldwide sales and distribution:
                    THE C.V. MOSBY COMPANY
                    11830 Westline Industrial Drive
                    St. Louis, MO 63146

In Canada: THE C.V. MOSBY COMPANY
                    5240 Finch Avenue East
                    Unit 1
                    Scarborough, Ontario M1S 4P2

OFFICE MANAGEMENT OF SPORTS INJURIES AND ATHLETIC PROBLEMS
ISBN 0-932883-08-7

Last digit is the print number: 9 8 7 6 5 4 3 2 1

DEDICATION

To Irene, Rosie, and Frank,

who make it all worthwhile.

CONTENTS

CONTRIBUTORS

ROSEMARY AGOSTINI, MD
Family Practice and Sports Medicine, Virginia Mason Hospital Sports Medicine Center, Seattle, Washington; Fellow, Cleveland Clinic, Cleveland, Ohio

LOREN H. AMUNDSON, MD
Professor of Family Medicine, University of South Dakota School of Medicine; Active Medical Staff, McKennan and Sioux Valley Hospitals, Sioux Falls, South Dakota

KRIS BERG, EdD
Professor and Director of Exercise Physiology and Fitness Center, School of Health, Physical Education and Recreation, University of Nebraska at Omaha, Omaha, Nebraska

RICHARD B. BIRRER, MD, MPH
Associate Professor, Family Practice, State University of New York—Downstate Medical Center, Brooklyn, New York; Chairman, Department of Family Medicine, Geisinger Medical Center, Danville, Pennsylvania

DENISE FANDEL, MS, ATC
Instructor, Department of Health, Physical Education, and Recreation; Head Athletic Trainer, and Instructor, School of Health, Physical Education, and Recreation, University of Nebraska at Omaha; Omaha, Nebraska

WALTER B. FRANZ, III, MD
Department of Family Practice, Mayo Clinic, Rochester, Minnesota

ANN C. GRANDJEAN, MS, RD
Associate Director, Swanson Center for Nutrition, Inc., Omaha, Nebraska; Chief Nutrition Consultant, U.S. Olympic Committee;

Instructor, Sports Medicine Program, Orthopaedic Surgery and Rehabilitation Department, University of Nebraska Medical Center, Omaha, Nebraska

BRIAN C. HALPERN, MD
Sports Medicine Physician and Educator, Sports Medicine Princeton, Princeton, New Jersey

JIMMY H. HARA, MD
Associate Clinical Professor, Division of Family Medicine, University of California, Los Angeles, School of Medicine; Assistant Chief of Service and Residency Director, Department of Family Practice, Kaiser-Permanente Los Angeles, Los Angeles, California

RON D. HALD, RPT, ATC
Sports Physical Therapist, Sports Rehabilitation Center, University of Nebraska Medical Center, Omaha, Nebraska

JEFFREY W. HILL, MD
Assistant Professor of Family Practice, University of Nebraska Medical Center, Omaha, Nebraska; Medical Director, Bicycle Ride Across Nebraska

TIM P. HUSTON, MD
Team Physician, Saddleback College, Mission Viejo, California

WALTER W. HUURMAN, MD
Associate Professor of Orthopaedic Surgery and Rehabilitation, and Assistant Professor of Pediatrics; Director of Children's Orthopaedics, Department of Orthopaedic Surgery and Rehabilitation, and Department of Pediatrics, University of Nebraska Medical Center; Vice-Chief of Staff, University of Nebraska Hospital, Omaha, Nebraska

ROGER H. KOBAYASHI, MD
Associate Professor of Pediatrics, Pathology and Medical Microbiology, University of Nebraska Medical Center, Omaha, Nebraska

MORRIS B. MELLION, MD
Associate Professor, Departments of Family Practice, and Orthopaedic Surgery and Rehabilitation (Sports Medicine), University of Nebraska Medical Center; Associate Professor, School of Health, Physical Education and Recreation, University of Nebraska at Omaha, Omaha, Nebraska; Team Physician, University of Nebraska at Omaha; Chairman, Committee on Health Education, American Academy of Family Physicians

MARK E. MCKINNEY, PHD
Associate Professor and Director, Division of Preventive Medicine, Department of Family Practice, University of Nebraska Medical Center, Omaha, Nebraska

JAMES C. PUFFER, MD
Associate Professor and Chief, Division of Family Medicine, University of California, Los Angeles, School of Medicine, Los Angeles, California; Chairman, Medical Services Committee, United States Olympic Committee Sports Medicine Council; Head Physician, 1988 United States Summer Olympic Team.

WM MACMILLAN RODNEY, MD
Associate Professor of Family Medicine, University of California, Irvine, Irvine, California; chairman, Medical Services Committee, United States Olympic Committee Sports Medicine Council; Head Physician, 1988 United States Summer Olympic Team

GUY L. SHELTON, BS, RPT, ATC
Senior Sports Physical Therapist, Sports Rehabilitation Center; Clinical Instructor, Department of Orthopaedic Surgery and Rehabilitation; Clinical Instructor, Division of Physical Therapy Education; University of Nebraska Medical Center, Omaha, Nebraska

W. MICHAEL WALSH, MD
Associate Professor of Orthopaedic Surgery and Rehabilitation, and Director, Sports Medicine Program, Department of Orthopaedic Surgery and Rehabilitation, University of Nebraska Medical Center, Omaha, Nebraska

FRANK G. YANOWITZ, MD
Associate Professor of Medicine, University of Utah School of Medicine; Medical Director, The Fitness Institute, Latter-Day Saints Hospital, Salt Lake City, Utah

PREFACE

Although sports medicine has historical roots that date back to the ancient Greek Olympics, it is also a very young area of medicine in the modern sense. The term "sports medicine" was probably coined at the 1928 San Moritz Winter Olympics, when 33 team physicians from 11 nations met and formed a committee to plan the First International Congress of Sports Medicine, to be held that summer at the Amsterdam Summer Olympics. The first book using the term "sports medicine" in its title was published in German in 1932, but the term was not used in the title of an English-language book until 30 years later.

Sports medicine has not been a specific medical discipline such as general surgery or cardiology or family practice. It has been an area of interest and concentration for physicians, other health care professionals, researchers, and educators in a wide variety of disciplines.

Ideally, sports medicine is practiced by a "team" consisting of athlete, physician, and coach, each of whom has a support system to draw upon (Fig. 1). For the athlete, the support system consists primarily of family, with friends and teammates also playing nurturing roles. The coach is backed up by the administration of the school, team, or league. The physician can draw upon two major support groups. For clinical support, the physician may turn to specialist colleagues, physical therapists, nutritionists, sports psychologists, podiatrists, and health educators. For a better understanding of the performance capabilities of the athlete, the physician may turn to medical researchers, exercise physiologists, kinesiologists, and a variety of physical educators and other researchers.

The athletic trainer plays a special role on the sports medicine team, since he or she is in an ideal position to maintain open and free communication with athlete, physician, and coach alike. The athletic trainer is therapist and counsellor for the athlete, advisor and friend to the coach, and eyes and ears for the physician. The importance of the athletic trainer as a key member of the sports medicine team has become so obvious in high level competition that it is now becoming clear that every high school should have an athletic trainer on its staff.

In spite of the fact that the ideal delivery of health care to the athlete would take place in a team or school facility, such as an athletic training room, the vast majority of sports medicine is practiced in the physician's office. The editor has surveyed family physicians in Nebraska to determine the sports medicine content of their practices; 216 responded. One hundred forty-one (65%) perform "organized team or league physical examinations" for school sports or community leagues, and 200 (93%) routinely perform preparticipation physical examinations in their offices for their own patients participating in school or community league sports. Ninety-seven (45%) of the family physicians responding indicated that they serve as team physicians in one or more sports, with 76 of these indicating that they are team physicians for both male and female sports teams.[1] These data only begin to suggest the depth of involvement in sports medicine of the practicing family physician, pediatrician, general internist, and general practitioner.

It is axiomatic that, in order to supervise the health care of athletes, the physician practicing sports medicine must function as a generalist. There are many specialists and subspecialists with strong interests in the care of the athlete, but their success in the long run will depend on their being versatile

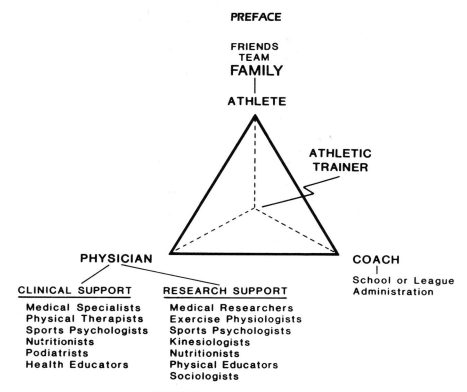

FIGURE 1. The Sports Medicine Team.

enough to take the generalist approach, which is so important for the athlete's physical and emotional well-being.

This book is written for the office-based physician, generalist and specialist alike, who finds that he or she is caring for competitive or recreational athletes. It focuses on the issues, injuries, and medical problems faced by people of all ages who incorporate athletics as a part of their basic life-style. It is not meant to be a comprehensive, encyclopedic reference but rather a readable, informative text for the practicing physician, resident, and medical student. Many sections are orthopedically oriented in order to deal with the common overuse problems in athletic injuries, but these sections are not designed to go into surgical management or fracture reduction in any depth.

Two chapters deserve special mention. "Tracking Problems of the Kneecap," by Dr. W. Michael Walsh, is a separate chapter with its own identity because it is the editor's belief that, while these problems are one of the most commonly encountered groups of musculoskeletal syndromes, they are also the most commonly misdiagnosed and inadequately treated. "Bicycle Injuries: Prevention, Diagnosis, and Management," by Drs. Jeffrey W. Hill and Morris B. Mellion, is included because most bicycle injuries and overuse syndromes require that the physican have a reasonably in-depth undrstanding of the mechanics and fit of the modern bicycle in order to provide proper diagnosis and treatment.

REFERENCE

1. Mellion MB: The sports medicine content of family practice. J Fam Pract 21:473-474; 1985

Acknowledgments

I would like to express my personal thanks to the many people who made both obvious and subtle contributions to the development of this book.

Dr. Robert L. Bass, Chairman, and Dr. Michael A. Sitorius, Vicechairman, of the Department of Family Practice at the University of Nebraska Medical Center have provided the opportunity for me to teach and write about sports medicine as it is practiced by the family physician. I am grateful to them and to my family physican faculty colleagues for the support which I have received while editing and partly writing this book.

Dr. John Connolly, Chairman of the Department of Orthopaedic Surgery and Rehabilitation, and Dr. W. Michael Walsh, Director of the Sports Medicine Program at the University of Nebraska Medical Center, have provided me a faculty position in sports medicine, a clinical population to treat and learn from, and continuous encouragement.

Mr. Bobby E. Thompson, Ms. Connie J. Claussen, and Mr. Donald Leahy, Athletic Directors, Ms. Denise M. Fandel and Mr. Wayne F. Wagner, Head Athletic Trainers, and the entire coaching staff of the University of Nebraska at Omaha have provided the opportunity for me to work as team physician with an excellent group of college athletes competing in a variety of men's and women's sports.

Dr. Richard B. Flynn, Dean of the College of Education, and Dr. Michael Stewart, Director of the School of Health, Physical Education, and Recreation at the University of Nebraska at Omaha, have provided the opportunity for me to teach a semester-long course on sports medicine each year. The challenge of organizing my thoughts into a curriculum and then presenting it to a bright group of exercise science graduate students and undergraduate majors has been a great impetus to my own studying and writing.

Special thanks is due to Dr. John A. Feagin, past president of the American Orthopaedic Society for Sports Medicine, who encouraged me to make the transition from private practice to academic family practice and sports medicine, and who suggested to Dr. Walsh that he recruit me into the Sports Medicine Program at the University of Nebraska Medical Center.

A word of thanks is also due to the publishers, Hanley and Belfus, Inc., who encouraged me to create this textbook.

Special thanks go to Ms. Mary Walsh Jones and Ms. Janis M. Church-Bruner for devoting seemingly endless hours to working and reworking the manuscript.

I want to thank Mr. William J. Wassom, graphics designer of the Department of Biomedical Communications at the University of Nebraska Medical Center, for the excellent illustrations he provided in the chapters I authored and co-authored.

Finally, I want to express my deepest appreciation to a very talented group of sports medicine colleagues, the authors and co-authors who made this book possible. It was a wonderful treat to work with these bright, articulate men and women.

MORRIS B. MELLION, M.D.

Omaha, Nebraska

1 The Preparticipation Physical Examination

JIMMY H. HARA, M.D.
JAMES C. PUFFER, M.D.

Primary care physicians are frequently called upon to perform preparticipation examinations for hopeful youngsters and determined adults seeking to participate in organized sports or vigorous physical activity. Indeed, it has been estimated that well over one million man-hours are consumed annually in examining over six million youth,[28] and the number of adults seeking evaluation prior to initiating exercise programs is increasing annually.

Given this information, it should be no surprise that many are beginning to question the benefit and cost effectiveness of such examinations.[24,29] A study of 763 adolescent athletes by Risser[24] uncovered significant problems in only 16 athletes; two were subsequently disqualified and one received treatment prior to participation. The cost of identifying these three adolescents was estimated to be $4537 per athlete.

Are these examinations really worth the time and effort that are required to do them properly? Certainly Garrick sums up the frustration of many who conduct such evaluations annually for young athletes when he states, "The pre-participation examination is much like the elephant being examined by blind men—it appears differently depending upon how it is approached. To the school administrator it fulfills the school's legal and insurance requirements. To the coach it is theoretically a means of beginning the season with athletes who have some common level of health and fitness. To the idealist it may be a means of attempting to prevent injuries. To the physician it should be an opportunity to uncover 'treatable' conditions or conditions that will interfere with or be worsened by athletic participation. In reality, it is probably an annual period of frustration, unkept office appointments, and frantic phone calls the day before the first turnout."[10]

Despite its drawbacks, the preparticipation evaluation has its merits if viewed in the proper context. If conducted in a rigorous and comprehensive fashion, with proper emphasis placed on its format, scope, frequency and content, the examination can serve as a valuable foundation for the provision of care by either the team physician or primary care physician.[22]

FORMAT OF THE EXAMINATION

The preparticipation examination has traditionally been performed in the primary care physician's office. Alternatively, through prearrangement, the physician may choose to participate in an en masse screening in a school gymnasium, community activity center, or, less preferably, in a locker room.[9] Garrick has long advocated the group examination concept as a high volume, expedient, low-cost medical evaluation.[10,17] When properly done, these assessments are accomplished in a station-by-station fashion, carefully designed to ensure privacy and performed by a variety of personnel, including primary care physicians, orthopedists, athletic trainers, and physician extenders.[10,21] A recent study in the pediatric literature indicates that the station approach of Garrick was superior to examinations conducted by private physicians in their offices in the ability to identify significant abnormalities.[9] However, many would hasten to add that mustering the needed individuals and coordinating schedules to permit such group endeavors become increasingly difficult year by year outside of academic institutions.

Runyun has long championed the primary care physician's private office as the ideal setting for the preparticipation examination.[27] Philosophically, this approach would fall into line with the American Cancer Society and the International Working Group for Colorectal Cancer and their tenet that the manpower resources as currently distributed in the United States dictate a need to deliver important screening services at the site of regular primary care delivery. The family physician, because of his longstanding relationship with the athlete, his thorough knowledge of the medical history and previous injuries, and his awareness of the athlete's level of physical maturity, can create the best environment in which this examination can be conducted.[21]

Based upon individual circumstances and community resources, the primary care physician must decide which of the above arrangements is best suited to meet the needs of the ever increasing numbers of would-be athletes requiring such services.

SCOPE, FREQUENCY, AND CONTENT OF EXAMINATION

Controversy still persists as to the scope of the preparticipation physical examination. Some have contended that this represents a rare opportunity to provide comprehensive care; we believe that most are now inclined to agree with Rice when he states, "The sports physical is not intended to be a substitute for routine periodic comprehensive health screening or the relationship between the family physician or pediatrican with his patient."[23]

The preparticipation examination should provide the opportunity for the physician to conduct a rigorous and thorough evaluation of the potential athlete's ability to participate without undue risk. It must be sport-specific and should accomplish the following objectives:[21,22]

1. Determination of general health
2. Assessment of cardiovascular fitness
3. Evaluation of pre-existing injuries
4. Assessment of size and maturation
5. Restriction of activity or disqualification from specific activity when contrain-

dicated by physical limitation or disease that would preclude safe participation
6. Recommendations for appropriate activity when participation has been restricted
7. Establishment of a comprehensive data base

The ability of the physician or a team of health care providers to perform an examination that adequately fulfills these objectives is largely dependent upon the frequency with which the examination is conducted. Obviously, regulations in many school districts that require that a preparticipation examination prior to participation in *each* sport would preclude an examination that could realistically be expected to be comprehensive.

Optimally, an examination should be conducted every three to four years, with updating of intercedent medical history on an annual basis. The discovery of a new condition or injury would then trigger appropriate evaluation by the physician. This policy is one that has been widely adopted by sports governing bodies, school districts, and the National Collegiate Athletic Association, and that recommends that the examination be conducted at the time of initial entry of an athlete into the sports program, with annual follow-up.[29] Such a policy is cost effective and efficient and guarantees that the athlete will be thoroughly evaluated.

Some school districts and institutions may provide the physician with a specific form for completion. If a form is not provided, the "Athletic Competition Health Screening Form" developed by the Commission on Public Health and Scientific Affairs of the American Academy of Family Physicians is suggested (Fig. 1). These forms are available from the AAFP Order Department in pads of 50 two-part (self-carbon) forms for a nominal fee.

The health history concentrates on prior disease and injuries as well as the cardiovascular and musculoskeletal systems. The importance of a well-taken history or a well-designed history form cannot be emphasized enough; Goldberg and colleagues have found that most disqualifying conditions show up on the history form.[11] The examination itself should focus on identifying poten-

THE AMERICAN ACADEMY OF FAMILY PHYSICIANS

Athletic Competition Health Screening Form

NAME: _____

SCHOOL: _____

AGE: _____ GRADE: _____

DATE OF BIRTH: _____ SEX: _____

Family Physician: _____ Phone: _____

Address: _____

HEALTH HISTORY Parent or guardian Answer "yes" or "no" ONLY	YES	NO
Chronic / Recurrent Illness?		
Hospitalization?		
Surgery Other Than Tonsils?		
Injuries Treated by Physician?		
Current Medications?		
Organs Missing?		
Heat Exhaustion / Stroke?		
Dizziness, Fainting, Convulsions and / or Headaches?		
Knocked Out?		
Concussion?		
Wear Glasses or Contacts?		
Hearing Defects?		
Dental Appliances Bridge / Brace / Cap / Plate?		
Cough / Pain?		
Problems with Blood Pressure, Heart, or Murmurs?		
Problems with Liver, Spleen, Kidney?		
Hernia?		
Recurrent Skin Disease?		
Bone / Joint Injury? Sprain / Dislocation? Injury that Caused a Missed Practice / Event?		
Allergy to Medications? Name:		
Tetanus Booster in the Last 10 Years?		

The Above Information is Current and Correct to the Best of My Knowledge

_____
Signature of
Parent or Guardian

_____
Date

VITALS	SATISFACTORY YES	NO	PHYSICAL EVALUATION COMMENTS	Recommend Follow-Up
Ht				
Wt				
BP ___				
GENERAL				
HEAD				
EYES			ACUITY R L	
ENT				
DENTAL				
CHEST				
HEART				
ABDOMEN				
GENITALIA				
SKIN				
EXTREMITIES BACK, NECK				
ALLERGY				

SUMMARY OF COMMENTS:

SPORTS PARTICIPATION APPROVED   YES _____   NO _____

LIMITATIONS:

_____
Physician Signature

_____
Date

Ⓡ 1984 THE AMERICAN ACADEMY OF FAMILY PHYSICIANS

FIGURE 1. Athletic competition health screening form developed by the Commission on Public Health and Scientific Affairs of the American Academy of Family Physicians. The forms are available from the AAFP Order Department at $5 per pad of 50 two-part (self-carbon) forms. A sample copy is available free on request. Reprinted with permission.

tially disqualifying conditions, with particular attention to cardiovascular and musculoskeletal assessment. The examination of youngsters additionally should include assessment of physical maturity using standard Tanner staging criteria.[32]

Cardiovascular Assessment. Outflow tract obstruction is a major cause of sudden death in young athletes,[18] and therefore a positive response to the question "Have you ever felt dizzy, fainted, nearly or actually passed out while exercising?" should prompt more detailed cardiovascular evaluation. Systolic murmurs are common in athletes, but accentuation of the murmur with a Valsalva should alert the physician to the possibility of asymmetric septal hypertrophy and obstructive hypertrophic cardiomyopathy.[30] Ventricular dysrhythmias that disappear with exercise are generally regarded as benign. Unexplained ventricular ectopy should raise the possibility of cocaine abuse.

Blood pressure measurement is very important. The upper limits of blood pressure accepted as not requiring further evaluation are 130/75 for children 11 years of age and younger, and 140/85 for children 12 and above.[2,33] Systolic hypertension is frequently encountered in populations of young athletes and is usually related to anxiety or in huskier individuals inappropriate blood pressure cuff size.[33]

Musculoskeletal Assessment. The most important component of the preparticipation examination is the orthopedic screening examination; this screening assessment can generally be accomplished in 90–120 seconds.[2]

After observing general habitus, the cervical range of motion should be checked (the patient is asked to look up, then down, over the shoulders, and then to touch his ear lobes to his shouldertips). The trapezii, deltoids, and rotator cuffs are then checked (shoulder shrug against resistance, abduction to 90°, then internal-external rotation of the shoulders). The extensor-supinator wad and the medial-volar complex are then assessed (have the patient supinate then pronate the wrist with elbows held at 90°). Hand function and rotational deformities are assessed by spreading the fingers and then having the patient make a fist. A duck walk is extremely useful in uncovering hip, knee, and ankle problems. Quadriceps function is assessed by knee extension and thigh tightening (watching the vastus lateralis during this maneuver). With the patient stooped over and touching his toes, evaluation for scoliosis and hamstring tension can be accomplished. Toe walking and heel walking will rapidly reveal problems with leg and foot function.

The physician should not spend more than 1½ to 2 minutes on this musculoskeletal assessment; further evaluation is warranted only if abnormalities are uncovered or a prior history of specific injury is elicited.

INJURY PREVENTION

One of the oft-quoted goals of the preparticipation examination, which has remained elusive, is the prevention of injuries. Marshall has contended that injury risk might be predicted by using a multifactorial analysis, including assessments of musculoligamentous flexibility and laxity.[19] Jackson and others believe that assessments of flexibility and laxity are not clinically reliable predictors of injury risk.[15]

Statements are often made that the physician plays a key role in injury prevention by assuring proper pre-season conditioning.[21] This notion is supported by the data of Moretz and Grana, which revealed lower injury rates as the season progressed.[20] Substantial data suggest that re-injury of a previously injured joint represents the most common clinical scenario.[6] If such is the case, then obviously the history and physical should concentrate on areas of prior injury.

Although the sports medicine literature abounds with various test measurements for body composition (skin fold calipers, submersion weights), strength (isokinetic devices), flexibility (sit and reach, goniometry), power (vertical jumping, Jyvskala test), endurance (12 minute run), and balance (stork test, decremental balance beams), there is no compelling evidence that any of these assessments add any clinically useful information that will help the clinician to accurately predict injury. On the other hand, such data when compiled can provide a useful physiologic profile that can be utilized by the physician, athletic trainer, and coach to monitor the effectiveness of training, efficacy of injury-specific rehabilitation, and readiness to return to play after the rehabilitation process has returned the athlete to previously determined baseline status.[22] Additionally, body composition measurements can be extremely helpful in providing the physician with reliable data from which sound recommendations can be made for "making weight" in sports such as wrestling.

CLASSIFICATION OF SPORTS

The American Medical Association and the American Academy of Pediatrics have established guidelines for those criteria disqualifying athletes from participation in sports based upon level of contact.[3,4] Hirsch[13] and Birrer[5] have modified the original AMA-AAP contact/noncontact division into somewhat more intricate but definitely more comprehensive delineations, which have utility for adults as well as children. The American Academy of Pediatrics has more recently modified their classification into a system akin to that devised by Hirsch.[2]

Collision/contact sports as defined by the American Academy of Pediatrics include football, wrestling, hockey, basketball, baseball, soccer, and lacrosse. Both the American Academy of Pediatrics and the American Medical Association have taken official positions in opposition to boxing, and therefore boxing is no longer included among the collision/contact sports. The so-called noncontact sports include tennis, golf, swimming and diving, track and field, and gymnastics. It takes little imagination to envision situations in which some of the noncontact sports (a diver, pole vaulter or pommel horse gymnast, particularly if not adept at their craft) may offer more potential trauma than some of the so-called contact sports (a nonaggressive, lazy, nonsliding baseball outfielder).

Besides identifying collision and contact levels as distinct from noncontact, Hirsch has further factored the level of strenuousness into his classification schema.[14] Birrer has subdivided noncontact sports into endurance type and leisure activities.[5] It is hard to envision a situation wherein a preparticipation physical examination would be necessary for a leisure activity, apart from cardiac or pulmonary rehabilitation, but these examinations are beyond the scope of this chapter. A comparison of the AMA-AAP, modified AAP, Hirsch and Birrer schemata is presented in Table 1.

DISQUALIFYING CONDITIONS

Before discussing specific conditions considered to be contraindications for specific sports activities, a few caveats are in order. First, physicians all too often find it easier to disqualify an athlete from particular activity rather than to indicate to that same individual those endeavors that in fact would be permissible and certainly healthier than no activity at all.[32] Secondly, although the physician has the responsibility of identifying conditions that contraindicate certain sports activities and of notifying the athlete and/or athlete's parents, it is still up to the athlete and/or athlete's parents to make the final decision about participation.[30] In virtually every disqualifying condition, there are now court cases in which athletes and parents have sued to force schools or leagues to permit participation. If parents insist that their children participate in spite of disqualifying conditions, it is appropriate for the school or institution to insist that they sign a legal waiver of responsibility for potential injury.

Conditions that constitute absolute or relative contraindications for specific sports activities are delineated in Table 2. Conditions that contraindicate participation in collision/contact sports fall into six major categories: (1) neurologic, (2) defects in paired systems, (3) organ enlargement, (4) active infections, (5) vertebropelvic defects, and (6) cardiopulmonary disorders.

Neurologic. A large postsurgical cranial defect is an absolute contraindication for collision/contact sports. A recent seizure (within 12 months) contraindicates participation in collision/contact sports and selected noncontact sports (high bar, swimming and diving, rings). A single concussion ("bell-rung") constitutes grounds for sidelin-

TABLE 1.   CLASSIFICATION OF SPORTS

Sport	AMA-AAP		HIRSCH						BIRRER			NEW AAP		
	Contact	Non-contact	Strenuous Collision	Strenuous Contact	Mod. Stren. Contact	Strenuous Non-contact	Mod. Stren. Non-contact	Minimally Strenuous	Collision	Endurance	Leisure	Collision	Contact	Non-contact
Football	x		x						x			x		
Wrestling	x		x						x				x	
Hockey	x		x						x			x		
Lacrosse	x		x						x			x		
Basketball	x			x					x				x	
Soccer	x			x					x				x	
Baseball	x				x				x				x	
Track		x				x				x				x
Field		x				x				x				x
Swimming		x				x				x				x
Diving		x				x				x				x
Gymnastics		x				x				x				x
Tennis		x				x				x				x
Golf*		x					x				x			
Bowling*								x			x			
Archery*								x			x			

*N.B.: Sports listed as "minimally strenuous" or "leisure" rarely require preparticipation physical examinations.

ing a participant from a game or event, two concussions should sideline for a season, and three or more should usually contraindicate participation altogether. It is unfortunately common knowledge that many elite athletes have exceeded this number of concussions and continued their active participation.

Defects in Paired Organ Systems. Absence of vision in one eye or legal blindness in one eye after correction has traditionally been regarded as a contraindication for collision/contact sports. However, this has changed as a result of improvement in protective eye goggles, and many would now permit such athletes to participate with the use of such protective equipment as well as the execution of a waiver from liability by the athlete and/or his parents. Retinal detachment is a contraindication for collision/contact as well as noncontact sports.

Whereas solitary kidney and testicular nondescent have traditionally been regarded as absolute contraindication for collision/contact sports, recent legal actions have supported athletes with these conditions wishing to participate,[30] and recently developed protective equipment has minimized their risk for subsequent injury.

Organ Enlargement. Organ enlargement of the liver, kidney, or spleen are usually deemed to disqualify participation in collision/contact sports. Again, advances in protective gear may change recommendations in this area. Many authorities recommend no collision/contact sports for three to six months following the disappearance of splenomegaly in Epstein-Barr mononucleosis.[2]

Active Infection. Pyelonephritis, septic arthritis, osteomyelitis, pulmonary infections (including tuberculosis), and systemic infections are all absolute contraindications for all sports participation. Similarly, fever itself would also contraindicate participation. Active otitis media is a specific contraindication for swimming and diving.[32] Boils, impetigo, and herpes simplex gladiatorum disqualify participation in collision/contact sports.[2]

Vertebropelvic Defects. Spondylolisthesis with back pain, Legg-Perthes' disease, slipped capital femoral epiphysis, spinal epiphysitis, and the previously mentioned active bone infections constitute absolute contraindications for collision/contact sports.

TABLE 2. DISQUALIFYING CONDITIONS

CONDITION	ABSOLUTE CONTRAINDICATIONS		RELATIVE CONTRAINDICATIONS	
	Contact	Noncontact	Contact	Noncontact
Seizure within past year	X	X[1]		X
Concussions with consciousness loss	X			
Large post-surgical cranial defect	X			X
Solitary functioning eye	X			
Retinal detachment history	X	X		
Congenital glaucoma	X	X		
Pulmonary infection, including tuberculosis	X	X		
Pyelonephritis	X	X		
Bone infection	X	X		
Systemic infection	X	X		
Cardiomegaly	X			X
Aortic or mitral stenosis	X			X
Cyanotic heart disease	X			X
Active myocarditis/pericarditis	X			X
Major visceromegaly (liver, kidneys, spleen)	X			X
Solitary functional kidney	X			X
Testis overlying pubic ramus	X			
Unhealed fracture	X			X
Spondylolisthesis with back pain	X	X		
Painful hip disease	X	X		
Spinal epiphysitis	X	X		
Blood coagulation defect	X			X
Uncontrolled asthma			X	X
Skin infection, including herpes	X[a]		X	X
Active otitis media		X[2]		
Uncontrolled diabetes mellitus			X	X
Recurrent shoulder subluxation			X	X
Uncontrolled hypertension			X	X

[1] = diving, swimming, high bar, and rings
[2] = swimming and diving
[a] = herpes simplex in wrestlers

Asthma. Apart from active pulmonary infections, uncontrolled asthma is only a relative contraindication for sports participation. Exercise-induced bronchospasm does not contraindicate sports participation and, in fact, is often benefited by sports participation. Likewise, asthma is often benefited by sports conditioning, particularly aquatic sports.

Cardiovascular Disorders. Mitral and aortic stenosis, cyanotic heart disease, pulmonary hypertension, and active myopericarditis are all absolute contraindications for collision/contact sports and relative contraindications for noncontact sports. Hypertrophic obstructive cardiomyopathy is frequently a totally unsuspected cause of mortality in athletes.[12,18] Some authors therefore feel strongly that electrocardiographic and/or echocardiographic screening should be mandatory in any patient in whom a systolic murmur is heard, particularly if accentuated by a Valsalva maneuver.[30] Anomalous coronary circulation and recently an intussusception of a coronary artery serve to remind us of our current inability to screen for every potentially lethal condition.[25] A detailed description of commonly encountered cardiac conditions that preclude participation is found in Table 3, and conditions that do not specifically preclude safe participation are found in Table 4.

LABORATORY TESTS

The appropriate laboratory screening for the preparticipation sports examination is

TABLE 3. CARDIAC CONDITIONS CONTRAINDICATING PARTICIPATION IN COMPETITIVE ACTIVITIES

1. Obstructive hypertrophic cardiomyopathy
2. Congenital coronary artery abnormalities
3. Cystic medial necrosis of the aorta (Marfan's syndrome)
4. Pulmonic stenosis with RV pressure greater than 75 mm of mercury
5. Aortic stenosis with a gradient greater than 40 mm of mercury across the valve

controversial.[2,12,31] Even the role of the CBC and routine urinalysis are not settled.[12,31] Obviously, leukocytosis might serve as the only clue as to the existence of an occult infection or may indicate the gravity of obviously poor dental hygiene.[6] Whereas iron deficiency may be common, iron deficiency anemia is probably not common enough to warrant hemoglobin or hematocrit determinations.[2] The American Academy of Pediatrics Committee on Sports Medicine has suggested biochemical assessment of iron status in menstruating females and boys from impoverished environments experiencing unusually rapid growth.[2] Cost is an issue, and whether routine assessments of iron, TIBC, iron saturation, ferritin, or protoporphyrin are truly warranted is controversial. In spite of poor sensitivity, a hematocrit may be the most cost-effective screen in young menstruating females and underweight males.

Proteinuria is not uncommon in healthy youngsters and in one series proved to be the major cause of further medical investigation.[11] However, most instances of proteinuria prove to be nothing more than benign orthostatic proteinuria.[13,14,30] For this reason, a urinalysis is not recommended for routine screening purposes.

Another dilemma is the role of the electrocardiogram and/or echocardiogram. Whereas they obviously play a role in the child with a history of syncope or pre-syncope and those with systolic murmurs accentuated with the Valsalva, their routine use is certainly not clinically warranted. Considerable attention has recently been focused on Marfan's syndrome as a cause of sudden death. A suggested schema for determining which athletes should routinely be screened echocardiographically for this disorder is shown in Table 5. The role for older adults of the electrocardiographic stress test needed for preparticipation clearance for aerobics or jogging is addressed in a separate chapter.

Each physician must decide the extent to which to routinely utilize ancillary laboratory testing based upon such factors as convenience, population served, and economic factors. If he chose to order no tests whatsoever, he would find himself in excellent company.

MISCELLANEOUS CONSIDERATIONS

Age. Apparently healthy individuals can participate in some level of activity well into

TABLE 4. CARDIAC CONDITIONS THAT WOULD NOT SPECIFICALLY CONTRAINDICATE PARTICIPATION

1. Mitral valve prolapse in absence of significant ventricular arrhythmias or severe initial regurgitation
2. Small shunts associated with atrial septal defect (ASD), ventricular septal defect (VSD), or patent ductus arteriosus (PDA)
3. Wolff-Parkinson-White syndrome (WPW) in absence of documented atrial fibrillation with rapid ventricular response
4. Primary ventricular arrhythmias in the absence of underlying coronary, myocardial, or valvular disease

TABLE 5. SUGGESTED SCREENING FORMAT FOR MARFAN'S SYNDROME

Screen all men over 6 feet and all women over 5 feet 10 inches in height with electrocardiogram and slit lamp examination when any two of the following are found:

1. Family history of Marfan's syndrome*
2. Cardiac murmur or midsystolic click
3. Kyphoscoliosis
4. Anterior thoracic deformity
5. Arm span greater than height
6. Upper to lower body ratio more than one standard deviation below the mean
7. Myopia
8. Ectopic lens

*This finding *alone* should prompt further investigation.

their later years; by adulthood, most individuals are well aware of their limitations and at least have the potential of exercising good judgment.[23]

Preadolescent youth have historically been a great concern. Over 20 years ago, Dr. Carl Lendgren warned, "These are the tender years when muscles lack the fibrous toughness needed for protection. Ribs and skulls are too fragile and even skin is tender and easily torn. Judgment, as well as the body, is immature. Broken wrists, legs, and torn ears and lacerated faces in these children represent too high a price to pay for the fun or training they receive."[16] On the other hand, at a recent American Academy of Pediatrics meeting, Dr. William Strong stated that "Parents need not worry about younger children because they don't push themselves."[26] In fact, he feels that the greater risk is with adolescents because peer pressure causes them to endure pain and "putting a pushy adult into the equation could lead to trouble."[26] Other authors have advanced similar warnings about coaches who they feel are exercising "a new form of child abuse."[8] Primary care physicians, particularly family practitioners, are in a unique position to assess the family dynamics and recognize these unhealthy circumstances as they might arise.[21]

Gender. Public Law 92-318 mandates that women shall be given the right to participate in sports and use facilities that are of equal quality as those used by men.[12] Many experts feel that the best interests of girls are served by opportunities exclusively designed for girls.[1,34] Analyzing high school basketball injuries in young men and women, one study found a five-fold greater injury rate in young women early in the season, which they attributed to poorer pre-season conditioning.[20] One could similarly argue that women athletes were pushed inappropriately hard early in the season and that the early season pace should have been slower. Much has been written recently indicating that girls can perform at levels that approximate those of boys when differences in height, weight, and body composition are considered.[5,7]

Handicapped. Individuals with more serious disabilities should probably be encouraged to participate in programs specific-ally designed for their physical and emotional needs; the Special Olympics is well known as an excellent example of a type of program that fosters pride and a sense of achievement in a healthy, dignified manner.

Amputees and those with congenital limb defects are to be judged on the basis of individual merit and not excluded from participation if the sole basis of disqualification is the deficient limb(s).[3,12] A recent female gymnast at California State University at Fullerton achieved national level elite competitive status in spite of a lower limb reduction defect.

Drugs. Would-be athletes and established athletes are not immune from the ills of society at large. The recent deaths of Len Bias and Don Rogers underscore the severity of the situation. The painful and deadly truths of drug and alcohol abuse should be addressed in hopes of diminishing this threat to health and longevity. As mentioned, unexplained ventricular ectopy or episodic hypertension and tachycardia may be a manifestation of a very serious underlying health problem. Anabolic steroids, "blood doping," and other practices engaged in to gain a competitive advantage are likewise an unfortunate fact of life and are discussed in greater detail in a separate chapter.

SUMMARY

The preparticipation sports physical examination is an annual exercise that primary care physicians are called upon to perform. The examination concentrates on a history of prior injury and a careful cardiovascular and musculoskeletal examination. Specific disqualifying conditions are delineated based upon level of contact. Athletes and/or their parents should be apprised when disqualifying condition(s) are found, but once so informed, the final decision to participate still resides with the athlete and/or the athlete's parents. Ideally, the physician should consider himself an active participant in a comprehensive program designed to optimize the performance and guarantee the safety of the athlete. He should be well-equipped to offer appropriate guidance with regard to preseason conditioning, rehabilitation of pre-existing injuries, and correction of remediable conditions. The properly conducted preparticipation examination forms the cornerstone of such care.

REFERENCES

1. American Academy of Pediatrics Committee on Pediatric Aspects of Physical Fitness, Recreation, and Sports: Participation in sports by girls. Pediatrics 55:563, 1975.
2. American Academy of Pediatrics Committee on Sports Medicine: Sports Medicine: Health care for Young Athletes. Evanston, IL, American Academy of Pediatrics, 1983.
3. American Academy of Pediatrics: School health: A Guide for Health Professionals. Evanston, IL, American Academy of Pediatrics, 1977.
4. American Medical Association: Medical Evaluation of the Athlete. Chicago, IL, American Medical Association, 1971.
5. Birrer RB: Sports Medicine for the Primary Care Physician. East Norwalk, CT, Appleton-Century Crofts, 1984.
6. Birrer RB, Wilkerson LA: Sports Medicine I. Kansas City, MO, American Academy of Family Physicians (Monograph Series), 1985.
7. Carlson KM: Fact vs. fiction: women in sports. Female Patient 5:48, 1980.
8. Digott RE: Youth in sports: beware of child abuse. New York Times, Sept. 11, 1977.
9. Du Rant RH, et al: The preparticipation examination of athletes. Am J Dis Child 139:657, 1985.
10. Garrick JG: Sports medicine. Pediatr Clin North Am 24:737, 1977.
11. Goldberg B, et al: Preparticipation sports assessment—an objective evaluation. Pediatrics 66:736, 1980.
12. Hara JH: The school sports physical. In Murphy JT, Rodney WM (eds): The school sports physical and the family physician. Los Angeles, CA, UCLA (Family Health Forum Series), 1980.
13. Hirsch PJ, et al: Check-out for the would-be athlete. Emerg Med 9/30:65, 1980.
14. Hirsch PJ, et al: Preparticipation evaluation for school athletic programs. J Med Soc NJ 78:585, 1981.
15. Jackson DW, et al: Injury prediction in the young athlete. Am J Sports Med 6:6, 1978.
16. Lendgren CV: Boys in contact sports. Med Tribune, Nov. 7, 1964.
17. Linder CW, et al.: Preparticipation health screening of young athletes. Am J Sports Med 9:187, 1981.
18. Maron BJ, et al.: Sudden death in young athletes. Circulation 62:218, 1980.
19. Marshall JL, Tischler HM: Screening for sports. NY State J Med 78:243, 1978.
20. Moretz A, and Grana WA: High school injuries. Phys Sportsmed 6:92, 1978.
21. Puffer JC: Sports medicine and the adolescent. Semin Fam Med 2:201, 1981.
22. Puffer JC: Sports medicine: The preparticipation evaluation. West J Med 137:58–59, 1982.
23. Rice EL: Periodic preparticipation sports examination is advised. Family Practice News 16(12):43, 1986.
24. Risser WL, et al: A cost benefit analysis of preparticipation sports examinations of adolescent athletes. J School Health 55(7):270–73, 1985.
25. Roberts WC, et al: Intussusception of a coronary artery associated with sudden death in a college football player. Am J Cardiol 57:179, 1986.
26. Rogers CC: Strong statements on kids and sports. Phys Sportsmed 13(8):32, 1985.
27. Runyan DK: The preparticipation examination of the young athlete. Clin Pediatr 22:674, 1983.
28. Ryan AJ: Qualifying examinations: a continuing dilemma. Phys Sportsmed 8:10, 1980.
29. Samples P: Preparticipation exams: are they worth the time and trouble? Phys Sportmed 14:180–87, 1986.
30. Smilkstein G: Health evaluation of high school athletes. Phys Sportsmed 9(8):73, 1981.
31. Smith NJ: Medical issues in sports medicine. Pediatrics in Review 2:229, 1981.
32. Steven MB, Smith GN: The preparticipation sports assessment. Fam Practice Recertification 8:68, 1986.
33. Strong WB: Hypertension in sports. Pediatrics 64:693, 1979.
34. Torg BG, Torg JS: Sex and the little league. Phys Sportsmed 2(5):45, 1974.

2 Exercise Prescription and Cardiovascular Fitness Screening

FRANK G. YANOWITZ, M.D.

Public and professional interests in exercise training, physical fitness and wellness have accelerated since the 1960s, creating an immense sports medicine industry with far-reaching economic and health-care implications. Estimates in 1984 suggest that between one-third and one-half of the American population, almost 100 million individuals, are participating in the "fitness boom."[13] Health promotion programs emphasizing physical activity are being enthusiastically advocated for the worksite, the schools and various community settings.[16] Although published studies on exercise training demonstrate favorable effects on cardiovascular risk factors,[18] there remains considerable uncertainty regarding the risk-benefit ratio or cost-effectiveness of adult fitness programs.[32] In fact, some health professionals are beginning to seriously question basic assumptions about the benefits of exercise and are suggesting that the American public has gone overboard in support of fitness.[19]

There is an interesting and reproducible phenomenon in medicine whenever a new therapy is first introduced, later evaluated, and ultimately finds its place in the overall management of patients. Initially there is thought of a panacea as favorable reports, mostly anecdotal, create a wave of enthusiasm from both providers and recipients of the treatment. This is usually followed by a plethora of unfavorable studies, mostly scientific, documenting the side effects or lack of therapeutic benefits, and leads to considerable discouragement in the medical community. Finally, in time, if the therapy truly has merit, health professionals learn safe and effective methods of prescription,

indications and contraindications, and the prevention or management of toxic side effects. The application of exercise training to preventive medicine is no exception to this commonly observed scenario.

This chapter discusses the principles of exercise prescription and screening for exercise programs. Current recommendations and guidelines published by the American College of Sports Medicine (ACSM) are considered, with an emphasis on practical applications of these guidelines for office practitioners.[2] To begin with, however, a brief review of exercise physiology is presented to provide a basis for the principles of exercise training and prescription.

EXERCISE PHYSIOLOGY

Although there are many components to total fitness (Table 1), this chapter is primarily concerned with the prescription of physical activity to improve *cardiorespiratory endurance,* the one fitness component most likely to have an impact on cardiovascular health.[6] The physiologic parameters of cardiorespiratory endurance can be considered from the perspective of the Fick principle, which relates *oxygen uptake* ($\dot{V}O_2$) to the pro-

TABLE 1. COMPONENTS OF TOTAL FITNESS

HEALTH RELATED	SKILL RELATED
1. Cardiorespiratory Endurance	1. Agility
2. Muscular Endurance	2. Balance
3. Muscular Strength	3. Coordination
4. Body Composition	4. Speed
5. Flexibility	5. Power
	6. Reaction Time

duct of *cardiac output* and *arteriovenous oxygen content difference*. Since cardiac output is the product of heart rate and stroke volume, the Fick equation is expressed as follows:

$$\dot{V}O_2 \text{ (mlO}_2/\text{min)} =$$
$$(\text{HR} \times \text{SV}) \times (\text{CaO}_2 - \text{C}\bar{\text{v}}\text{O}_2)$$

where HR is the heart rate (beats/min), SV is the stroke volume (ml/beat), and $\text{CaO}_2 - \text{C}\bar{\text{v}}\text{O}_2$ is the arteriovenous O_2 content difference (ml O_2/ml blood). From this relationship it can be seen that the uptake of O_2 is determined by the *oxygen transport system*, defined by the cardiac output ($\text{HR} \times \text{SV}$) and the arterial O_2 content (CaO_2), and the *utilization* of O_2, which is reflected by the arteriovenous O_2 content difference.

Figure 1 illustrates the various parameters of the Fick equation at rest, during several submaximal workloads, and at maximal exercise in a normal subject before and after exercise training. Oxygen uptake at rest is approximately 3.5 ml/kg/min, which is conveniently called one *metabolic equivalent (MET)*. During an incremental workload exercise protocol, $\dot{V}O_2$ increases linearly with workload until a workload is reached beyond which $\dot{V}O_2$ fails to rise ($\dot{V}O_2$ max). Following exercise training the $\dot{V}O_2$ response to exercise is similar to the pre-training response up to the pre-training $\dot{V}O_2$ max. After training, however, $\dot{V}O_2$ continues to rise, reaching a new plateau at a higher $\dot{V}O_2$ max and corresponding maximal workload.[22]

The gold standard laboratory measure of cardiorespiratory endurance is the maximal oxygen uptake ($\dot{V}O_2$ max).[22] Also known as the *functional aerobic capacity,* $\dot{V}O_2$ max is usually measured or estimated during treadmill or cycle ergometer exercise testing. Estimations of $\dot{V}O_2$ max are made from the maximal workload achieved during exercise testing and are reasonably accurate for routine assessments of functional capacity. Values of $\dot{V}O_2$ max normalized for body weight (ml O_2/kg/min) can be used to classify cardiorespiratory endurance (Table 2).[11]

The magnitude of improvement in $\dot{V}O_2$ max with training tends to vary with age, pre-training $\dot{V}O_2$ max, and the various parameters of the exercise program.[7] In general, it is reasonable to expect a 10–15% increase in

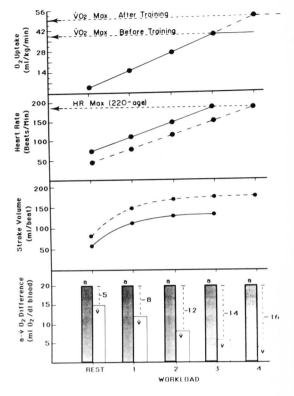

FIGURE 1. Hemodynamic response to incremental work exercise testing before and after training. Solid lines indicate $\dot{V}O_2$, heart rate, and stroke volume responses to progressive exercise before training. Dashed lines represent the after-training responses. The a-$\bar{v}O_2$ difference is represented by the difference in heights of the vertical bars. Workload "3" represents the maximal workload before training; workload "4" is the maximal workload after training.

$\dot{V}O_2$ max after 8–12 weeks of training in healthy individuals.[7] This improvement in aerobic capacity with training is due to both central and peripheral adaptive mechanisms.[7]

At maximal exercise the Fick equation identifies four parameters that are the major determinants of an individual's functional aerobic capacity:

$$\dot{V}O_2 \text{ max} =$$
$$(\text{max HR} \times \text{max SV}) \times$$
$$(\text{max CaO}_2 - \text{min C}\bar{\text{v}}\text{O}_2)$$

TABLE 2.   CLASSIFICATION OF CARDIORESPIRATORY ENDURANCE*

| | $\dot{V}O_2$ Max (ml 02/kg/min) | | | | | | | | | |
| AGE (yrs) | LOW | | FAIR | | AVERAGE | | GOOD | | HIGH | |
	M	W	M	W	M	W	M	W	M	W
20-29	<25	<24	25-33	24-30	34-42	31-37	43-52	38-48	53+	49+
30-39	<23	<20	23-30	20-27	31-38	28-33	39-48	34-44	49+	45+
40-49	<20	<17	20-26	17-23	27-35	24-30	36-44	31-41	45+	42+
50-59	<18	<15	18-24	15-20	25-33	21-27	34-42	28-37	43+	38+
60-69	<16	<13	16-22	13-17	23-30	18-23	31-40	24-34	41+	35+

*M = men, W = women. (Modified from the American Heart Association.[4])

These are (1) the maximal heart rate response to exercise; (2) the maximal stroke volume response to exercise; (3) the maximal arterial O_2 content; and (4) the maximal ability of skeletal muscles to extract O_2, which is indirectly reflected by the *minimal* mixed venous O_2 content. Abnormalities of one or more of these parameters are usually found in people with poor exercise tolerance, dyspnea on exertion, and easy fatigability. In addition, the central and peripheral adaptations to exercise training are reflected by the response of these parameters as one goes from a resting state to maximal exercise.

The heart rate response to exercise before and after training is illustrated in Figure 1. Heart rates increase linearly with O_2 uptake or with workload until a maximal heart rate is reached, which is approximately 220 − age (± 10 beats/min, standard deviation).[4] After exercise training heart rates are lower at rest and at all submaximal workloads, but the maximal heart rate is unchanged.[4]

The lower heart rate response to submaximal exercise with training is also associated with lower systolic blood pressures during exercise. Since the *double product* (HR × systolic BP) is a major determinant of myocardial oxygen consumption,[24] a trained person can perform exercise more efficiently than a sedentary person in so far as cardiac work is concerned. In addition, patients with stable angina pectoris who participate in exercise training programs will generally experience less exertional angina after training, since the myocardial O_2 requirements are less.[27]

The stroke volume response to exercise before and after training is also shown in Figure 1. Unlike the heart rate response, stroke volume increases very modestly during upright exercise and is curvilinear, reaching a maximum at low-to-moderate workloads. This is because ventricular filling during diastole becomes progressively shorter at heart rates above 120/min. After training the stroke volume is greater at rest and throughout exercise. In normal subjects the increased stroke volumes are due to (1) increased ventricular diastolic size (preload), (2) decreased peripheral vascular resistance (afterload), and (3) increased contractility.

Finally, the peripheral adaptations to exercise are illustrated in Figure 1. The arteriovenous O_2 content difference reflects the utilization of O_2 by the various tissues and organ systems of the body. When going from rest to maximal exercise, a progressively greater portion of the cardiac output is redistributed to exercising skeletal muscles, and the extraction of O_2 by the muscle fibers is greatly enhanced. The net result is a progressive widening of the arteriovenous O_2 content difference.

Oxygen extraction by muscle fibers is dependent upon a number of factors, including exercise intensity, capillary density, and aerobic enzyme activity within the muscle mitochondria. Exercise training results in increased density of capillaries around the muscle fibers and increased aerobic enzyme activity in the mitochondria.[29] This allows trained skeletal muscles to extract more O_2 from the arterial blood, further widening the maximal arteriovenous O_2 content difference. Approximately 50% of the increased $\dot{V}O_2$ max with training is accounted for by these peripheral mechanisms.[7] In cardiac patients skeletal muscle adaptations account for most of the improvement in $\dot{V}O_2$ max, since the stroke volume response to exercise is usually compromised by the heart disease.

To summarize the acute and chronic adaptations to exercise, Table 3 illustrates the parameters of the Fick equation at rest (1 MET), during submaximal exercise (8 METs), and at maximal exercise in three hypothetical male subjects. The first subject is sedentary; the second has been training for 6 months; and the third is a world-class long distance runner. For comparative purposes each subject is 25 years old and weighs 70 kg.

At rest all three subjects require 245 ml O_2/ min (3.5 ml/kg/min) with a cardiac output ($\dot{Q}$) of 6.1 L/min and an arteriovenous O_2 content difference of 40 ml/L blood. The subjects differ only in their resting heart rates and stroke volumes. Progressively lower heart rates and larger stroke volumes at rest are the characteristic adaptations to training.

During submaximal exercise (8 METs), each subject's $\dot{V}O_2$ is 2000 ml/min with a cardiac output of 15.6 L/min and an arteriovenous O_2 difference of 128 ml/L blood. Again, the only differences are the lower heart rates and larger stroke volumes in the more trained individuals.

At maximal exercise major differences are found in all parameters except maximal heart rate, which is predominantly age deter- mined. Training is associated with increased $\dot{V}O_2$ max, maximal workload, maximal stroke volume, maximal cardiac output, and maximal arteriovenous O_2 difference. The world class athelete has the largest of these parameters, primarily because of the extent and quality of training, but genetic factors may also play an important role. In addition to the increased maximal workload and $\dot{V}O_2$ max, the chronic adaptations to exercise training enable the more trained individuals to perform submaximal work at a lower cost to the cardiovascular system and a reduced perceived level of effort. This is perhaps the most important physiologic benefit to exercise training.

The preceding discussion is but a brief introduction to cardiovascular exercise physiology in order to illustrate the beneficial adaptations of training, which serve to enhance the functional aerobic capacity and increase the efficiency of the cardiovascular system during work. Readers interested in more indepth reviews of exercise physiology will find an abundant literature on this subject.[3,4,7,28] The next section considers the more practical aspects of screening for aerobic exercise training programs.

CARDIOVASCULAR FITNESS SCREENING

There are two main considerations in screening for cardiovascular fitness pro-

TABLE 3. ACUTE AND CHRONIC ADAPTATIONS TO EXERCISE IN THREE SUBJECTS

	$\dot{V}O_2$* (ml/min)	Workload (METs)	HR (beats/min)	SV (ml/beat)	$\dot{Q}$ (L/min)	$CaO_2 - C\bar{v}O_2$ (mlO$_2$/L)
At Rest						
1. Sedentary	245	1	70	87	6.1	40
2. Trained	245	1	55	110	6.1	40
3. Athlete	245	1	45	136	6.1	40
Submaximal Exercise						
1. Sedentary	2000	8	153	102	15.6	128
2. Trained	2000	8	130	120	15.6	128
3. Athlete	2000	8	106	147	15.6	128
Maximal Exercise						
1. Sedentary	2800	11	195	102	20.0	140
2. Trained	4050	16	195	138	27.0	150
3. Athlete	6300	26	195	200	39.0	160

*$\dot{V}O_2 = (HR \times SV) \times (CaO_2 - C\bar{v}O_2)$

grams. The first is concerned with the evaluation of health status in order to assess the safety of exercise and identify those at high risk for exercise-related complications. The second is to determine a fitness profile that can be used to develop an individualized exercise prescription. Although much of the screening for exercise programs can be done by primary care physicians and their professional staff, some patients may require more careful evaluations by cardiovascular specialists.

Evaluation of Health Status

The American College of Sports Medicine (ACSM) has published revised guidelines for exercise testing and prescription which offer extremely valuable information for health professionals who are evaluating individuals for exercise programs.[2] In particular the guidelines provide explicit recommendations for assessing health status prior to initiating exercise activities. Screening is primarily focused on detecting early coronary heart disease and other cardiac abnormalities that might preclude vigorous unsupervised exercise.

The three major components of the screening evaluation are the medical history, the physical examination, and laboratory tests. From these data a high-risk group can be identified that requires maximal exercise ECG testing.[2] Abnormal responses to exercise testing may identify a much smaller subset of individuals who are in need of more comprehensive cardiovascular studies.

Screening for coronary risk factors (Table 4), especially hypertension, hyperlipidemia and cigarette smoking, has taken on more significance in recent years due to increased professional and public awareness of the potential for primary prevention of atherosclerotic vascular diseases. Because of the widespread prevalence of coronary artery disease, there is also the realization that acute myocardial infarction and sudden death are often the first manifestations of disease, and that these catastrophic events may occur during physical activities.

Table 5 provides a classification of blood pressure categories and recommended follow-up criteria based on initial measure-

TABLE 4. MAJOR CORONARY RISK FACTORS

1. Hypertension
2. Hypercholesterolemia
3. Cigarette smoking
4. Family history of premature atherosclerosis (prior to age 50)
5. Diabetes mellitus
6. Abnormal resting ECG
   Left ventricular hypertrophy
   Old myocardial infarction
   Ischemic ST-T wave changes
   Conduction defects
   Arrhythmias

ments.[25] In adults the diagnosis of hypertension is made "when the average of two or more diastolic BPs on at least two subsequent visits is 90 mm Hg or higher, or when the average of multiple systolic BPs on two or more subsequent visits is consistently greater than 140 mm Hg."[25] The ACSM guidelines recommend exercise testing for individuals over age 35 who have a history of blood pressure readings greater than 145/95.[2] A systematic approach to the management of hypertension beginning with nonpharmacologic therapy and, if needed, stepped-care drug treatment has been published in 1984 by the Joint National Committee on Detection, Evaluation, and Treatment of High Blood Pressure.[25]

The relationship between hyperlipidemia and coronary heart disease, particularly elevated low-density lipoprotein (LDL) cholesterol levels, is firmly established. The published results of the Lipid Research Clinics Coronary Primary Prevention Trial,[20] followed by the NIH Consensus Development Conference on Lowering Blood Cholesterol,[23] have led to revised definitions of moderate and high risk serum cholesterol levels (Table 6). Moderate risk is when the age-adjusted total cholesterol levels are between the 75th and 90th percentiles; high risk is when the levels are above the 90th percentile. Measurements of high density lipoprotein (HDL) cholesterol levels are also helpful in risk assessment because of the inverse relationship between HDL and atherosclerosis.[1] Ratios of total cholesterol to HDL cholesterol above 5.0 are considered to represent increased coronary risk.[2]

The NIH consensus panel recommends

TABLE 5. CLASSIFICATION OF BP AND FOLLOW-UP CRITERIA FOR INITIAL MEASUREMENT*

RANGE (mm Hg)	CATEGORY	RECOMMENDED FOLLOW-UP
Diastolic		
<85	Normal BP	Recheck within 2 yr
85-89	High-normal BP	Recheck within 1 yr
90-104	Mild Hypertension	Confirm within 2 mo
105-114	Moderate hypertension	Evaluate or refer promptly (within 2 wk)
>114	Severe hypertension	Evaluate or refer immediately
Systolic (diastolic <90)		
<140	Normal BP	Recheck within 2 yr
140-159	Borderline isolated systolic hypertension	
>159	Isolated systolic hypertension	
140-199		Confirm within 2 mo
>199		Evaluate or refer promptly (within 2 wk)

*Modified from The 1984 Report of the Joint National Committee on Detection, Evaluation, and Treatment of High Blood Pressure.[25]

that all adults seen by a physician for the first time have blood cholesterol measured.[23] Those in the moderate or high risk categories (Table 6) should be followed up with a fasting lipid profile consisting of total cholesterol, HDL-cholesterol, and triglycerides. Individuals above the 90th percentile risk category in whom secondary forms of hyperlipidemia (eg., thyroid, kidney, or liver disease) have been ruled out should be considered for aggressive dietary management, exercise training, and, if necessary, drug therapy.[1,15] The ACSM recommends exercise testing for those over age 35 who have total cholesterol:HDL cholesterol ratios above 5.0.[2]

TABLE 6. SERUM CHOLESTEROL CONCENTRATIONS ASSOCIATED WITH INCREASED RISK FOR CORONARY ARTERY DISEASE*

AGE (yrs)	SERUM CHOLESTEROL LEVEL (mg/dl)	
	Moderate Risk	*High Risk*
20-29	200-220	>200
30-39	220-240	>240
>39	240-260	>260

*Modified from the NIH Consensus Development Conference.[23]

The other coronary risk factors listed in Table 4 should also be assessed during the screening evaluation. Particular emphasis should be given to cigarette smoking, since this is not only a major risk factor for heart and lung diseases, but smoking is associated with increased cardiovascular mortality.[17] For the health professional working with smokers desiring to improve their cardiovascular fitness, smoking cessation should be given the highest priority of all risk reduction interventions. Although one of the hardest self-destructive behaviors to eliminate, numerous techniques for smoking cessation have been described.[10,12,26,30] It is not enough to simply ask patients to quit smoking. Physicians need to be knowledgeable of the wide variety of smoking cessation strategies for their patients and not give up until a successful strategy has been achieved.

In addition to screening for major coronary risk factors, the health status evaluation should also focus on other abnormalities that might indicate a high risk for exercise complications. The medical history should include a careful review of cardiovascular, pulmonary, and neurologic symptoms. History of alcohol and drug (especially cocaine) abuse should also be sought. Finally, a history of orthopedic problems or arthritis is important to elicit, since these problems might preclude certain types of exercise activities.

In the physical examination particular attention should be given to findings suggestive of cardiovascular, pulmonary, and musculoskeletal abnormalities. It is important to carefully evaluate all heart murmurs, especially systolic murmurs, since hypertrophic cardiomyopathy is probably the leading cause of sudden cardiac death in young athletes.[21] Accentuation of the murmur with standing and during the Valsalva maneuver is characteristic of obstructive cardiomyopathy and differentiates it from innocent murmurs and aortic valvular disease. When in doubt, the patient should be referred for echocardiographic studies.

In older athletes coronary heart disease is the leading cause of exercise-induced sudden death.[31] Studies have shown that over 90% of cases could have been identified as high risk on the basis of coronary risk factors or premonitory symptoms that were ignored or denied by the victims.[31] These data suggest that educating older adults about their risk factors and the warning signs of impending ischemic events is an important prerequisite to implementing a safe exercise program.

The most controversial aspect of the health status evaluation for exercise programs concerns the indications for maximal exercise ECG testing. The ACSM distinguishes three categories of individuals for whom specific recommendations for stress testing have been suggested: (1) apparently healthy individuals, (2) high-risk individuals, and (3) patients with known disease.[2]

Apparently healthy individuals are those without coronary risk factors and without symptoms or findings of disease. In this category those under age 45 may initiate an exercise program without an exercise test providing they follow a well-designed program and are made aware of unusual signs or symptoms that may develop.[2] Maximal exercise testing, however, is suggested for individuals age 45 and above, although the cost-effectiveness of these recommendations has yet to be determined for asymptomatic, low-risk individuals.

The role of exercise testing for high-risk subjects is less controversial since an abnormal response is much more predictive of the subsequent development of primary coronary heart disease events.[5] High risk is defined as the presence of one or more coronary risk factors (Table 4) or symptoms suggestive of disease.[2]

Symptoms of chest pain are especially important because of the widespread prevalence of coronary disease in our population. The medical history will usually suffice to make a differential diagnosis. Patients with typical angina pectoris have the classic presentation of substernal burning or indigestion-like discomfort radiating to the neck or down the inner aspects of the arms; predictably precipitated by exertion or emotional excitement; lasting 3-15 minutes; and promptly (within 1-2 minutes) relieved by rest or sublingual nitroglycerin. Atypical angina pectoris is similar to typical angina but lacks one or two of the typical features (location, duration, quality, precipitating and relieving factors). Nonanginal chest pain lacks three or more of the typical features.

Diamond and Forester,[8] in a classic publication, discuss the applications of probability theory and Bayes' theorem to the diagnosis of coronary artery disease. Table 7, modified from their data, illustrates the probabilities of angiographically significant coronary artery disease based on age, sex, and analysis of chest pain symptoms. Patients with typical angina, especially men, are at such high risk for coronary atherosclerosis that they should be referred for additional studies and more definitive therapy before starting an exercise program. Patients at any age with atypical angina should undergo exercise testing before increasing their exercise activities. Finally, those with non-anginal chest pain should have additional studies, if necessary, to further clarify the etiology of their symptoms. Those over 35 with positive risk factors should undergo exercise testing. Exercise testing is also recommended for asymptomatic individuals over age 35 with positive coronary risk factors.[2]

The final category of individuals who should undergo maximal exercise testing are patients with known cardiovascular, pulmonary, or other chronic diseases such as diabetes mellitus or thyroid, liver, or kidney disease. Patients with coronary artery disease

TABLE 7. PROBABILITY (%) OF CORONARY ARTERY DISEASE ACCORDING TO AGE, SEX, AND SYMPTOMS*

AGE (yrs)	NON-ANGINAL CHEST PAIN		ATYPICAL ANGINA		TYPICAL ANGINA	
	Men	*Women*	*Men*	*Women*	*Men*	*Women*
30-39	5	1	22	4	70	26
40-49	14	3	46	13	87	55
50-59	22	8	59	32	92	79
60-69	28	19	67	54	94	91

*Modified from Diamond and Forrester.[8]

recovering from myocardial infarctions, surgery, or angioplasty procedures are candidates for organized cardiac rehabilitation programs if such programs are available. Otherwise a carefully designed home program with close follow-up, and periodic ECG monitoring, if possible, should be considered.

Table 8 summarizes the current ACSM recommendations for exercise testing as a prerequisite to starting an exercise program.[2] Higher risk individuals include those with one or more coronary risk factors (Table 4) as well as those with symptoms of cardiovascular, pulmonary, or metabolic diseases. Guidelines for exercise test administration and interpretation have been published elsewhere and will not be considered here.[2,9,14]

THE EXERCISE PRESCRIPTION

The term *prescription* implies that a particular dosage is required to achieve specific

TABLE 8. ACSM RECOMMENDATIONS FOR MAXIMAL EXERCISE TESTING PRIOR TO EXERCISE PROGRAM*

CATEGORY	MAXIMAL TEST NEEDED?
Apparently Healthy	
Below age 45	No
45 and above	Yes
Higher Risk	
Below 35, no symptoms	No
35 and above, no symptoms	Yes
Symptoms (any age)	Yes
With disease (any age)	Yes

*Modified from ACSM Guidelines.[2]

therapeutic goals. If the dose is too small there will be an inadequate therapeutic response; if the prescribed dose is exceeded there is increased risk of toxic side effects. Exercise training is clearly a therapeutic intervention that requires careful dosing for some individuals, particularly those at high risk for cardiovascular complications. Even in the healthy population, however, excessive exercise training may lead to a variety of injuries which, although not life-threatening, can have a significant negative impact on continued exercise training.

There are three desirable features to incorporate in a well-designed exercise program: (1) the prescription should be *individualized* according to each person's needs and capabilities; (2) the exercise program should be structured to *improve or maintain functional capacity*; and (3) the exercise activities should be enjoyable to ensure long-term compliance.

The five specific components to be addressed in the design of an exercise prescription are (1) type of exercise, (2) intensity, (3) duration, (4) frequency, and (5) mode of progression. The ACSM has developed explicit recommendations for each of the components that are applicable to all exercise programs designed to enhance cardiorespiratory endurance.[2]

Type of Activity

The major requirements in selecting aerobic exercise activities are that the activities use large muscle groups in rhythmical and dynamic movements for a sustained period of time. As previously stated it is desirable to choose activities that are most likely to be enjoyed or at least lead to more enjoyable activities in the future. Popular forms of exercise include brisk walking, running, hiking, cycling, swimming, rowing, cross-country skiing, rope skipping, aerobic dance, and various recreational games. For the beginning exerciser it is best to choose an initial activity that can be easily sustained without variations in intensity and that does not require a great deal of skill. After 8-12 weeks, with the development of conditioning effects, other more enjoyable activities and recreational games may be substituted, providing they fulfill the requirements of the exercise prescription.

Intensity of Exercise

For cardiovascular conditioning to take place the intensity should exceed approximately 50-60% of functional capacity ($\dot{V}O_2$ max) and, for safety and comfort, not exceed 75-85%.[2] This usually translates to a heart rate training range of 70-85% of maximal heart rate.

Maximal heart rate can be estimated to be 220-age for apparently healthy individuals under age 45 with no coronary risk factors. For older or high-risk individuals a maximal exercise ECG test should be performed to screen for ischemic heart disease and to determine maximal heart rate. All patients with known heart disease or patients taking heart-rate-lowering drugs (beta-blockers, some calcium channel blockers) should also undergo maximal exercise testing in order to determine a safe and effective heart rate training range.

If an exercise test is performed the heart rate training range can be calculated by plotting the straight line relationship between exercise heart rate and exercise intensity measured or estimated in METs or $\dot{V}O_2$. From this linear plot the heart rates associated with a certain percentage of functional capacity, usually 60-75%, can be determined, and this becomes the recommended training range.

Exercise intensity should be checked frequently during a beginning exercise program. This requires some practice in taking one's pulse, usually in the radial or carotid artery locations. Since it is rather difficult to palpate the pulse during exercise, the pulse should be taken for a period of ten seconds immediately after stopping, beginning the count with zero. Multiplying times 6 will give the minute heart rate. If the rate is below the prescribed training range the intensity of exercise should be increased; if the rate is above the range the intensity should be reduced.

After an exercise program has become well established frequent pulse checks may no longer be necessary. The exerciser should be able to associate a certain sense of exertion with the prescribed training range, and that perception then becomes the indicator of the intensity of effort. Most trained individuals know when they are below, within, or above the training heart rate range from their perception of respiration and their overall sense of muscular effort. Once this relative perceived exertion has been learned the need for pulse checks is reduced, although it is recommended that occasional checks be obtained especially when exercising in unusual environmental conditions.

Duration of Exercise

To some extent the duration of an exercise session is inversely related to the intensity of effort for an equivalent training gain. If exercise activities are performed at the upper end of the prescribed heart rate range, the duration can be somewhat shorter. Beginning exercisers, however, should start out with a longer duration and a lower intensity in order to maintain a level of comfort necessary to facilitate enjoyment. The wise adage "train, don't strain" is particularly important to emphasize in the early weeks of an exercise program.

A reasonable beginning program should involve a duration of 15-20 minutes, exclusive of warm-up and cool-down, and an intensity of approximately 50% of functional capacity.[2] Once physiologic adaptations take place, however, the duration and intensity can be increased appropriately. Durations of longer than 60 minutes are usually not necessary for developing or maintaining cardiorespiratory endurance. If symptoms of fatigue persist for one hour or longer after terminating an exercise session, then either intensity, duration, or both were excessive, and the subsequent sessions need to be adjusted accordingly.

It is a good idea for beginning exercisers to keep a log of their exercise training sessions including time of day, heart rate responses, duration, distance, activities, and any unusual symptoms that occurred during or after exercising. Such a diary not only provides a psychological incentive to continuing an exercise program but also facilitates adjustments in training if necessary to improve the overall quality of the program.

Frequency of Exercise

For most healthy adults exercising 3-5 days per week is sufficient.[2] Beginning exercisers may prefer to work out every other day to allow for adequate rest needed to relieve muscle soreness that often accompanies a new program. Some individuals with very low functional capacities (less than 4 METs) may benefit from several 5-10 minute sessions daily at the onset because they may not be able to sustain even a low intensity workout for 15 minutes.

Mode of Progression

A new exercise program can be conceptualized as involving three distinct phases: initial, improvement, and maintenance.[2] The rate of progression through these phases depends upon functional capacity, age, overall health status, and particular needs or goals.

Most sedentary individuals require an initial phase lasting 4-6 weeks. During this period of time it is important to structure the parameters of the exercise prescription to minimize discomfort. This is often a critical period of time for beginning exercisers, since a bad experience at the onset of a program may be detrimental to long-term adherence. A major goal during the transition from a sedentary to an active lifestyle is to develop the exercise habit. This includes not only learning the various exercise activities but also restructuring daily routines to incorporate the exercise sessions. Activities during these initial weeks should include light calisthenics, gentle stretching exercises, and low intensity (40-50% $\dot{V}O_2$ max) aerobic exercise.

Duration should begin at 15-20 minutes per session and gradually increase to 20-30 minutes, keeping the intensity on the low side of the target range.

During the improvement phase (4-6 months) the major physiologic adaptations to exercise training take place. The duration should be increased by about 3-5 minutes per session every few weeks until a total duration is reached (usually 30-60 minutes) which is compatible with one's overall goals. Increases in exercise intensity (i.e., training heart rate) should begin only when the duration of exercise can be sustained for at least 20 minutes, as long as the heart rate remains within the prescribed training range. Again, it is important to stress the need to progress slowly, especially for older or higher risk participants.

At the conclusion of the improvement phase the participant should be at a level of cardiorespiratory fitness that is associated with long-term health benefits and optimal function. The final phase of the exercise program is designed to maintain these physiologic and other health benefits. It is during this phase that individuals may want to redefine their goals, incorporate more enjoyable activities or recreational games into their programs, and participate in competitive events. Also, by this time, the exercise program has become a well-established part of one's overall lifestyle with a high likelihood of long-term adherence. For maintenance of fitness it may not be necessary to exercise as long, frequently, or intensely as during the improvement phase, although a minimum of 3 days per week, 30 minutes per session at the prescribed intensity, is recommended.

The Exercise Session

Regardless of which phase of exercise training, a typical exercise session should be structured to include warm-up, aerobic activities, and cool-down. Some individuals may also incorporate a strength training component if that is of particular interest. The exercise prescription for strength training, however, is not discussed in this chapter. Warm-up should include light calisthenics, stretching, and activities similar to but lower in intensity than the aerobic exercises that have been selected in the exercise prescription. For example, if running is the desired aerobic activity, individuals should walk briskly for 5-10 minutes before beginning to run. Similarly, stationary cyclists should free-wheel for several minutes before increasing the workload on the cycle ergometer. The purpose of the warm-up is to increase flexibility, which may minimize risk for musculoskeletal complications, and to gradually increase the heart rate to the training range. Cool-down activities should follow the reverse sequence as the warm-up. This minimizes venous pooling in the lower extremities and enhances the overall sense of well-being associated with successful completion of the exercise session.

CONCLUSIONS

This chapter has reviewed the principles of exercise prescription and screening for exercise programs. If exercise training is to have favorable cost-benefit effects on cardiovascular risk factors and functional well-being, careful attention must be given by the medical profession to developing the most appropriate exercise prescription for each individual. This is particularly important in the sedentary, middle-aged segment of the population who want to get on the fitness "bandwagon." There is a tendency in our population to enthusiastically rush into new programs without careful preparation or knowledge of the skills required to safely carry out the activities of the program. With the medical profession becoming more involved in providing preventive services and periodic health maintainence, there is now a great opportunity for promoting quality exercise programs that optimize the benefits and minimize the risks.

REFERENCES

1. AHA Special Report: Recommendations for treatment of hyperlipidemia in adults. Circulation 69:1065A, 1984.
2. American College of Sports Medicine: Guidelines For Exercise Testing and Prescription, 3rd ed. Philadelphia, Lea & Febiger, 1986.
3. Astrand P: Quantification of exercise capability and evaluation of physical capacity in man. Prog Cardiovasc Dis 19:51, 1976.
4. Astrand P, Rodahl K: Textbook of Work Physiology, 2nd ed. New York, McGraw-Hill Book Company, 1977.
5. Bruce RA, Hossack KF, DeRouen T, et al: Enhanced risk assessment for primary coronary heart disease events by maximal exercise testing: 10 years experience of Seattle Heart Watch. J Am Coll Cardiol 2:565, 1983.
6. Caspersen CJ, Powell KE, Christenson GM: Physical activity, exercise, and physical fitness: definitions and distinctions for health-related research. Public Health Reports 100:126, 1985.
7. Clausen JP: Effect of physical training on cardiovascular adjustments to exercise in man. Physiol Rev 57:779, 1977.
8. Diamond GA, Forrester JS: Analysis of probability as an aid in diagnosis of coronary artery disease. N Engl J Med 300:1350, 1979.
9. Ellestad MH: Stress Testing: Principles and Practice, 3rd ed. Philadelphia, F.A. Davis Co., 1985.
10. Eraker SA, Becker MH, Strecher VJ, Kirscht JP: Smoking behavior, cessation techniques, and the health decision model. Am J Med 78:817, 1985.
11. Exercise Testing and Training of Apparently Healthy Individuals: A Handbook for Physicians. Dallas, American Heart Association, 1972.
12. Feldman BH: Cigarette smoking as a heart-disease risk factor and methods for smoking cessation. Pract Cardiol 12:164, 1986.
13. The Fitness Boom. Medical World News, July 23, 1984, p. 45.
14. Froelicher VF: Exercise Testing and Training. New York, LeJacq Publishing Inc., 1983.
15. Hoeg JM, Gregg RE, Brewer B: An approach to the management of hyperlipoproteinemia. JAMA 255:512, 1986.
16. Iverson DC, Fielding JE, Crow RS, Christenson GM: The promotion of physical activity in the United States population: The status of programs in medical, worksite, community, and school setting. Public Health Reports 100:212, 1985.
17. Kannel WB: Update on the role of cigarette smoking in coronary artery disease. Am Heart J 101:319, 1981.
18. Kannel WB, Wilson P, Blair SN: Epidemiological assessment of the role of physical activity in development of cardiovascular disease. Am Heart J 104:876, 1985.
19. Legwold G: Are we running from the truth about the risks and benefits of exercise? Phys. Sportsmed 13:136, 1985.
20. Lipid Research Clinics Program: The lipid research clinics coronary primary prevention trial results. JAMA 251:365, 1984.
21. Maron BJ, Roberts WC, McAllister HA, et al: Sudden death in young athletes. Circulation 62:218, 1980.
22. Mitchell JH, Blomqvist G: Maximal oxygen uptake. N Engl J Med 284:1018, 1971.
23. National Institutes of Health Consensus Development Conference: Lowering blood cholesterol to prevent heart disease. JAMA 253:2080, 1986.

24. Nelson RR, Gobel FL, Jorgensen CR, et al: Hemodynamic predictors of myocardial oxygen consumption during static and dynamic exercise. Circulation 50:1179, 1974.

25. The 1984 Report of the Joint National Committee on Detection, Evaluation, and Treatment of High Blood Pressure. Arch Intern Med 144:1045, 1984.

26. The Physician's Guide. How to Help Your Hypertensive Patients Stop Smoking. US Dept of Health and Human Services. NIH Publication No 83-1271, April 1983.

27. Redwood DR, Rosing DR, Epstein SE: Circulatory and symptomatic effects of physical training in patients with coronary-artery disease and angina pectoris. N Engl J Med 286:959, 1972.

28. Rowell LB: Human cardiovascular adjustments to exercise and thermal stress. Physiol Rev 54:75, 1974.

29. Saltin B, Rowell LB: Functional adaptations to physical activity and inactivity. Fed Proc 39:1506, 1980.

30. Sherin K: Smoking cessation: the physician's role. Postgrad Med 72:99, 1982.

31. Simon HB: Sports medicine. *In* Rubenstein E, Federman DD (eds): Scientific American Medicine. New York, Scientific American, Inc., 1985.

32. Siscovick DS, LaPorte RE, Newman JM: The disease-specific benefits and risks of physical activity and exercise. Public Health Reports 100:180, 1985.

3 Sports Nutrition

ANN C. GRANDJEAN, M.S., R.D.

Good nutrition is vital to optimal athletic performance. Unfortunately, however, the daily diet is one subject often neglected as part of the counseling an athlete receives.[74] In addition to the impact on athletic performance, a nutritionally sound diet is essential to both the immediate and future health of the athlete.[15] "There is no area of nutrition where faddism, misconceptions, and ignorance are more obvious than in athletics."[27] A lack of knowledge, coupled with a desire to "win," often leads to practices that are not only contrary to good health but in some cases potentially harmful.

This chapter is designed to review some of the current sports nutrition issues and address some of the questions frequently asked by athletes and their coaches and support staff about nutrition and its relation to sports performance. Carbohydrate loading, precompetition meal, weight loss, weight gain, and vitamin and mineral supplements are discussed.

Without doubt, water is the most important nutrient for the athlete. Unreplaced loss of body water, or hypohydration, can negatively affect athletic performance and the results can be severe. If asked to identify the second most important nutrient for an athlete, most sports nutrition experts would select carbohydrate. Ironically, "making weight," a common practice in athletes, affects carbohydrate status and fluid balance. These interrelationships will also be discussed in this chapter.

AN ADEQUATE DIET

The best diet for any athlete is based on a variety of physiological, sociological, and psychological factors. Athletes come in all shapes, sizes, and ages and both sexes. From the seven-foot-tall basketball player to the four-foot-tall T-ball player, from the 73-pound gymnast to the 350-pound weightlifter, from the little league soccer player to the Olympic swimmer, athletes are a heterogeneous group. These factors, along with the type and intensity of the sport and training program, determine the athlete's nutritional requirements.

A nutritionally adequate diet will provide all the necessary nutrients (carbohydrate, protein, fat, vitamins, minerals, water) plus energy (calories) to meet metabolic needs for optimal functioning of the body.[42] Many coaches, trainers, and athletes are concerned about what constitutes a balanced diet. Just as there are multiple means for achieving any goal, there are numerous dietary patterns that will provide adequate nutrition. Dietary adequacy is determined by quantity and quality. Sufficient quantity (calories) is provided if the athlete is maintaining ideal competitive weight. The number of calories needed depends, for the most part, on body size, age, non-training activity level, and intensity of the training program.

The quality of a diet is determined by the nutrient content. The athlete's nutrient requirement can be met by diverse dietary patterns, any of which can be adequate, provided care is exercised in food selection. Quality can be evaluated using numerous methods ranging in complexity from a check list that grossly determines variety to sophisticated computer dietary analysis programs. The Recommended Dietary Allowances (RDA) are the standards most commonly used for evaluating nutritional quality. Although the National Research Council clearly states that the RDA should be applied to population groups rather than individuals, the RDA remains the standard most frequently used in the United States when evaluating an individual's diet for vitamin and mineral adequacy. When using the RDA, however, one should be aware of its limitations.

As stated by the authors of the RDA:[19]

> The Recommended Dietary Allowances are estimates of acceptable daily nutrient intakes in the sense that the needs of most healthy individuals will be no greater than the RDA. The basis for estimation for Recommended Dietary Allowances is such that if even a specific individual habitually consumes less than the recommended amounts of some nutrients, his/her diet is not necessarily inadequate for those nutrients.
>
> In planning diets, it is usually not possible to supply all the recommended nutrients exactly at the allowance levels. Some nutrients, such as zinc, are in low concentration in the food supply. Therefore to meet the RDA for such nutrients, the RDA for other nutrients will be exceeded. For example, meat and seafood, the best sources of zinc, are also good protein sources. Thus, in meeting the RDA for zinc, the RDA for protein may be exceeded.

In establishing the RDAs the Committee on Dietary Allowances determined the amount of each nutrient that is necessary for health maintenance and added a "margin of safety." The margin of safety reflects our knowledge of individual differences, bioavailability of nutrients, variations in the food supply, and instability of nutrients. Based on these conditions, some individuals' needs can be met when consuming only 20% of the RDA, whereas under another set of conditions 100% would be necessary. However, the values are established so that 100% of the RDA will meet the needs of all healthy people. Even if there was no margin of safety added, one must consider the fact that the "average" requirement is the value equal to 77% of the RDA. Thus, 50% of the population will have their nutritional needs met by consuming 77% of the RDA. A lack of understanding or knowledge regarding this "margin of safety" is one of the factors contributing to overuse of supplements and a misconception of the

RDA. This will be discussed later in this chapter in the section on supplements.

Research has shown that the nutrient intake of some athletes is less than optimal.[11,16,26,46,75] Athletes at highest risk are those competing in the lower weight classes of sports such as boxing and wrestling, and sports such as gymnastics, ballet, and figure-skating where the aesthetics of leanness impacts on the judges. Body size impacts on caloric requirement more than any other single factor. The smaller the athlete, the lower the caloric need. As caloric intake drops below 2000, it becomes increasingly difficult to meet nutrient needs. Whereas a swimmer consuming 4000 calories a day would have to continually make foolish food choices to not meet nutrient requirements, a gymnast maintaining her weight on 1100 calories a day will have difficulty meeting the RDA even if every calorie is "nutrient-packed."

CALORIC INTAKE

Books and articles on nutrition and athletes often contain such statements as:

> The biggest difference in nutrition requirements between the athlete and the nonathlete concerns energy, especially during training or conditioning.[25]

> The unique nutritional requirement of the athlete is his high requirement of energy.[73]

Such statements imply that an athlete automatically has a high caloric requirement because he or she is an athlete. This is not always the case. The energy requirement of an athlete depends on age, gender, height, weight, body composition, type of sport, physical conditioning, clothing worn, playing surface, environment in which the athletic activity takes place, and frequency, intensity and duration of the event or training session.[19,45,53]

Almost any moderate sport can become one of high energy expenditure if it is carried on intensively for long enough. Energy expended riding a bicycle depends on the

TABLE 1. FACTORS AFFECTING THE ENERGY REQUIREMENT OF AN ATHLETE

Age
Gender
Height
Weight
Body Composition
Type of Sport
Physical Conditioning
Clothing Worn
Playing Surface
Environment
Frequency and Intensity of Activity
Duration of Event or Training Session

weight of the cyclist, the speed of the pace, and whether one is cycling uphill, downhill, or on level ground. Table 2 compares approximate caloric expenditures per hour for various activities for two persons, one weighing 205 pounds and the other 125 pounds.

Research on the dietary habits of athletes shows that there is a wide range of energy intake.[15,33] Some sports demand high energy expenditure, but others do not. For example, a competitive runner during a 6-minute mile expends approximately 0.252 kcal/min/kg.[58] On the other hand, a shooter with a small-bore rifle, in a standing position, expends approximately 0.027 kcal/min/kg. Thus a 170 pound runner at a 6-minute pace (6 minutes per mile) will expend approximately 117 calories during that 6 minutes, whereas a shooter of equal weight would expend approximately 13 calories during the same time period.

Without sophisticated equipment, it is difficult, if not impossible, to determine the caloric requirement of any given athlete. However, a frequently received question is, "How many calories should I consume?" The athlete is consuming enough calories if his/her "ideal" body weight is being maintained. However, it must be stressed that it is not uncommon for the "desired" body weight as determined by the athlete or coach to be lower than the "ideal." Chronic dieting and competing at weight levels below ideal weight can impair performance and hinder adequate nutrition intake.

WEIGHT LOSS

Reducing weight to compete in a lower weight classification is a common practice in sports such as wrestling, judo, boxing and weightlifting. Many coaches and athletes believe that training at a heavier weight and dropping weight immediately before competition gives the athlete an advantage. There are no data to support this hypothesis, however; and, in fact, data indicate just the opposite. Many of the techniques used to produce rapid weight loss (fasting, crash diets, dehydration, induced vomiting, laxatives, and diuretics) can endanger an athlete's health and impair performance. Presented with the facts, however, athletes may counter, "Well I dropped 10 pounds in two days and I won!" Your reply... "Your opponent probably dropped twelve, next time you may not be so lucky."

Starvation or extremely low calorie diets (semistarvation) are not recommended for athletes, *ever*. A decrease in performance as reflected by decreases in aerobic power and capacity, speed, coordination, strength and judgment can result from using severely restrictive diets.[2,52] Prolonged fasting or diets that severely restrict calories result in the loss of large amounts of water, electrolytes, minerals, glycogen stores, and lean body mass.[1,2] When glycogen stores are depleted, body protein is used for energy. The amount of protein metabolized during starvation varies greatly among individuals, but if the total daily energy expenditure is 1600 kcal, then approximately 60 grams of protein will be utilized each day.[27] Athletes will find they have more power, endurance, and speed for competition if they maintain their ideal competitive weight throughout the year. The safe level of restriction depends on the athlete's normal intake.

As has been alluded to and will be discussed elsewhere, dehydration can cause decrements in performance. Most of the methods utilized for rapid weight loss result in some degree of hypohydration. Mistakenly, some coaches and athletes think water balance can be achieved if the athlete drinks large volumes of water immediately after weighing in. Research has shown, how-

TABLE 2. APPROXIMATE CALORIES USED PER HOUR

ACTIVITY	205 LB. PERSON	125 LB. PERSON
Archery	420	268
Baseball—infield or outfield	382	234
—pitching	488	299
Basketball—moderate	575	352
—vigorous	807	495
Bicycling—on level, 5.5 mph	409	251
13.0 mph	877	537
Canoeing—4 mph	565	352
Dancing—moderate	341	209
—vigorous	464	284
Fencing—moderate	409	251
—vigorous	837	513
Football	678	416
Golf—twosome	443	271
—foursome	332	203
Handball or hardball—vigorous	797	488
Horseback riding—walk	270	165
—trot	551	338
Motorcycling	297	182
Mountain Climbing	820	503
Rowing—pleasure	409	251
—rowing machine or sculling 20 strokes/min.	1116	684
Running—5.5 mph	887	537
—7 mph	1141	669
—9 mph level	1269	777
—9 mph 2.5% grade	1480	907
—9 mph 4% grade	1564	959
—12 mph	1606	984
—in place 140 count/min.	1993	1222
Skating—moderate	465	285
—vigorous	837	513
Skiing—downhill	789	483
—level, 5 mph	956	586
Soccer	730	447
Squash	849	520
Swimming—backstroke—20 yds./min.	316	194
—40 yds./min.	682	418
—breaststroke—20 yds./min.	392	241
—40 yds./min.	786	482
—butterfly	956	586
—crawl—20 yds./min.	392	241
—50 yds./min.	869	532
—sidestroke	682	418
Tennis—moderate	565	347
—vigorous	797	488
Volleyball—moderate	465	285
—vigorous	797	489
Walking—2 mi./hr.	286	176
—110–120 paces/min.	425	260
—4.5 mph	540	331
—downstairs	544	333
—upstairs	1417	869
Water Skiing	638	391
Wrestling, Judo or Karate	1049	643

ever, that rehydration cannot be achieved and that fluid ingestion is not effective in restoring plasma volume to pre-dehydration levels in four or five hours.[24,80] Since mechanics for controlling water movement between the fluid compartments of the body serve first of all to maintain normal blood volume at the expense of interstitial fluid volume, it is obvious that homeostasis of total fluid volume cannot be achieved in a few hours.

Although the total effects of frequent and excessive weight loss on growth and development are not known, it is the general consensus that such a practice is damaging to growing children. Strauss and colleagues[76] found, in a study on wrestlers, that the dietary restrictions practiced by some wrestlers may adversely affect serum testosterone levels.

Athletes trying to decrease weight obviously want that decrease to be in the form of fat not muscle. The answer is an appropriate decrease in calorie intake with a concomitant increase in energy expenditure. While additional exercise may be possible for those athletes not in heavy training, further increases in caloric expenditure may not be reasonable or desirable for the athlete already training several hours each day. Therefore, dietary restriction becomes the primary method of weight control.

WEIGHT GAIN FOR ATHLETES

The goal in gaining weight is to gain muscle mass, not fat. Muscle mass increases only after a sufficient period of progressive weight training and cannot be increased by simply eating more food or more protein. Monitoring weight gain by using skinfold measurements along with scale weight will indicate the type of body weight being added. The rate of gain and location of added muscle mass will depend on the training program, sex of the athlete, and somatotype of the athlete, as well as other genetic factors.

Athletes engaged in an appropriate weight training program must, however, consume a diet that meets nutrient needs as well as the increased caloric requirement. For some athletes, increasing calorie intake is difficult because increasing the size of meals may cause discomfort, especially if training takes place soon after eating. On the other hand, school, work, and/or training may make adding snacks or additional meals difficult. Again, for most athletes the preferred solution is to increase intake at meals slightly and include two to four snacks a day.

It is impossible to determine exactly the number of calories needed by any one individual to increase muscle mass a given amount. Therefore, the best place to begin is to increase food intake slightly and monitor gains with routine weighings and skinfold measurements. An increase in weight (measured on the scales) with a maintenance or decrease in fat-fold measurements will indicate a gain in muscle, whereas an increase in weight with an increase in fat-fold measurements indicates a gain in fat. Beware, however, that skinfold measurements taken during or immediately after a weightlifting session may be inaccurate due to blood engorgement and edema of the muscle.

PROTEIN

For many years the importance of protein for athletes has been a subject of great controversy. Many athletes and coaches believe that a high protein diet supplies extra energy, enhances athletic performance, and increases muscle mass. There is no evidence, however, that excessive protein improves athletic ability, and as previously stated muscle mass increases only after a significant period of progressive weight training. *Exercise is the single most important factor in increasing the size, strength, and endurance of muscles.*

It appears that protein metabolism during exercise is a multifactorial process altered by numerous stimuli including intensity, duration, and type of exercise as well as training environment, caloric intake, and possibly even gender or age.[57] Although dietary protein does not serve as a major source of energy for most athletes, recent research indicates that the body may depend on protein for an increased percentage of the energy needs in prolonged exercise (greater than two hours in duration).[56,57,66] Evidence is accumulating to indicate that skeletal muscle can oxidize some amino acids, particularly the branched-chain amino acids (leucine, isoleucine, and valine), and that under certain conditions, such as decreased muscle glycogen, total oxidation may become significant. The practicality of this to athletes who chronically engage in prolonged exercise is unknown. It may be that the process of carbohydrate loading provides significant protein sparing effect during prolonged exercise. It is also possible, however, that protein needs may be slightly elevated in individuals engaged in prolonged exercise, particularly when carbohydrate intake is low. Although clearly not as important as either carbohydrate or free fatty acids, protein/amino acids under some conditions may contribute significantly to total exercise calories.

Although definitive data are not available on human protein requirements during training, they do suggest that athletes need approximately 1.0 gm/protein per kilogram body weight and possibly may benefit from up to 2.0 gms during periods of muscle building or training periods of prolonged, intensive exercise. The average American diet should satisfy protein requirements for adult athletes. A protein intake of 2.0 gms/kg body weight will also be adequate for the child or adolescent athlete who is still growing and is engaged in heavy training, provided calorie intake is adequate.

The body's energy needs must be satisfied before its need for growth and repair are met. Protein requirement cannot be considered void of the protein-energy relationship. A decrease in calorie intake increases the protein requirement and vice versa. The higher the caloric intake, the lower the protein requirements (on a gram per kilogram body weight basis), due to the fact that adequate carbohydrate is available for basal metabolism and energy needs so that protein can satisfy growth and maintenance requirement. The energy-protein relationship works in two directions: (1) protein requirements decrease when calories are not a limiting factor and (2) the amount of calories required to maintain body weight decreases when protein is not a limiting factor. This reciprocal relationship must be considered when dietary requirements for either nutrient are assessed.[77] The 19-year-old football player who

is maintaining weight on 4000 calories a day can meet protein requirements with 0.8 gram per kilogram body weight. However, the weight-conscious wrestler or figure skater who is restricting calories will have a higher protein per kilogram body weight requirement. A low energy intake can result in protein oxidation rather than cellular anabolism.

There is great individual variation in protein consumption,[37] and just as athletes with low protein intakes present one concern, excessive protein intake provides another concern. Excessive amounts of protein can cause a gout-like syndrome in susceptible individuals, which, of course, can interfere with performance.

CARBOHYDRATES

Early in the 20th century, research revealed that the most efficient source of energy for humans during exercise was carbohydrate.[18,54,81] Today, athletes, coaches, and trainers are aware of the importance of carbohydrate-rich diets in athletic performance. However, they are not as knowledgeable about the amount, type, and frequency of consumption to enhance performance.

Stored energy is found in the muscle in various compounds. The most "energy packed" compound is adenosine triphosphatase (ATP). However, ATP can be stored in tissue only in limited amounts; thus, other stored energy sources are used to resynthesize ATP. The two major sources of stored energy in the muscle tissue are carbohydrate in the form of muscle glycogen and fat, which is stored as muscle triglycerides. Muscle glycogen is the major source of carbohydrate energy utilized during exercise. Research has shown that low levels of muscle glycogen can impair sports performance[22] and that failure to restore muscle and liver glycogen stores may result in fatigue.[12]

Dietary fat, protein, or carbohydrate can be converted to triglycerides and stored in the muscle. Dietary carbohydrate, however, is necessary to maintain muscle glycogen stores. Thus carbohydrate earns its "second most important" ranking—second only to water.

Athletes participating in sports characterized by brief periods of high energy activity with alternate rest periods, such as football, basketball, swimming, and volleyball, should be able to maintain adequate glycogen stores by consuming 500–600 grams of carbohydrate per day.[20,23] For small athletes such as female gymnasts, who often limit calories to below 1200 daily to maintain desired weight, a carbohydrate intake of 60% of the total calories should be the goal.

Carbohydrate Loading

Carbohydrate loading is the process of manipulating the diet and amount of exercise in an effort to increase glycogen stores in the muscles. This concept first occurred around 1939 when two scientists, Christenson and Hansen,[18] studied the effects of dietary manipulation on man's ability to perform prolonged, hard work. They found that men consuming a high-carbohydrate diet for three days could perform heavy work twice as long as men fed a high-fat diet for the same three days.

What is now referred to as the "classical" technique of carbohydrate loading or muscle glycogen loading was first introduced by Saltin and Hermansen[68] and Bergstrom and colleagues.[12] Carbohydrate loading is based on three assumptions: (1) glycogen is a major substrate during exercise, and depletion of glycogen is a limiting factor for exercise; (2) the amount of glycogen stored in muscle can be increased by dietary manipulation; and (3) increased glycogen storage will enhance performance.

Based on the studies by Saltin, Hermansen, and Bergstrom and colleagues, Astrand,[8] a physiologist, devised a three-phase dietary plan for carbohydrate loading. He proposed that the optimal plan to achieve maximal glycogen storage would be to exercise the same muscles to exhaustion one week before an event. For the following three days, consume a high-protein, high-fat, low-carbohydrate diet. And, during the final phase, consume a carbohydrate-rich diet three days prior to competition. Since that time, a number of studies have been published presenting disadvantages of carbohydrate loading. Hypoglycemia, ketosis, nausea, and fatigue are associated with the low-carbohydrate diet

phase. It is now accepted that the low-carbohydrate intake phase is not necessary. A new "modified" technique designed by Sherman and colleagues[72] increases muscle glycogen stores to levels similar to levels obtained via the "classical" regimen but without the negative side effects. Sherman recommends that athletes consume a mixed diet containing approximately 50% of the kilocalories from carbohydrate rather than a low-carbohydrate diet during the depletion phase. The three days just prior to competition, a diet containing 70% of the calories from carbohydrate is recommended. This dietary regimen must be combined with a depletion-taper sequence of exercise. Seven days prior to the competition the athlete should have a hard workout that is strenuous enough and of adequate duration to deplete glycogen-levels to approximately 25%. Then training should be tapered the rest of the week until the day prior to competition which should be a "rest" day. The depletion-taper sequence of training and the three days of high carbohydrate intake are the key factors.

It must be emphasized that carbohydrate loading is recommended only for endurance athletes such as long-distance runners, cross-country skiers, and road cyclists, who participate in non-stop activities that require 1½ hours or more of intense effort at a high percentage of the VO_2 max. Glycogen loading will not benefit the athlete participating in short-term events, such as sprints, or in sports where the activity may last for a long period of time but the physical effort is characterized by brief periods of high-energy activity (a few seconds to a few minutes) with alternate rest periods, such as football, basketball, wrestling, etc. A more practical concern for these athletes is not the question of carbohydrate loading but rather does their diet contain enough carbohydrate on a day-to-day basis to maintain adequate levels of muscle glycogen for training and workouts. What is this adequate level? Unfortunately research has not yet determined this, but it is most likely an amount between 200–600 gm of carbohydrate per day depending on body size.

Additionally, it must be stressed that the degree of benefit derived from carbohydrate loading even among endurance athletes is individual, and therefore the athlete should determine prior to a major competition the value of this regimen for him/her.

PRECOMPETITION MEAL

Numerous recommendations regarding the precompetition meal appear in sports nutrition publications. Many of these recommendations are empirically based and are not supported by scientific data. The truth is, there is no magic to the food eaten on the day of an event. The primary goal of the precompetition meal is to provide fluid and energy to support the athlete during competition.[41] Physiologically, the most significant consideration is that the meal not interfere with the stresses associated with athletic performance; however, psychological benefits of foods eaten before an event should not be underestimated.

Two major aspects of the precompetition meal that have been investigated are the timing and composition of the meal. Almost every set of guidelines for precompetition meals contains a recommendation on timing. Although there is variation, the most common recommendation is 3 to 4 hours prior to the event. It is postulated that this practice ensures an empty stomach at the time of competition. It must remembered that in addition to the timing of the meal, volume, osmolarity, and chemical composition of the food also influence gastric emptying.[49]

The precompetition meal should be consumed close enough to competition to avoid hunger pangs, diminished concentration, weakness and other symptoms associated with long periods between meals.[48] On the other hand, precompetition emotional stress and anxiety can cause alterations in the gastrointestinal tract resulting in indigestion, nausea and other feelings of discomfort if the precompetition meal is consumed too close to competition time.[79]

Research on the effect of precompetition meals on performance indicates that although consuming either liquid or solid meals as close as 30 minutes prior to performance may cause complaints of stomach and gut distention, it does not have a nega-

tive impact on performance.[5,6,7,9,31] The precompetition meal should consist of foods and beverages the athlete likes, foods that are well tolerated, and foods the athlete generally eats. Having to eat foods one dislikes at a time when nervous tension is high will not enhance performance. The precompetition meal should be moderately high in carbohydrate, minimal in fat, and should be low in bulk.

Diaries can be useful in helping athletes determine their best precompetition meals. Recording the types and amounts of foods eaten, when eaten in relation to competition (e.g., 2 hours prior), and how the athlete felt at the time of the event can serve as a learning tool.

POSTEXERCISE NUTRITION

There are two considerations regarding postexercise nutrition. One is for the athlete involved in multiple-event competition, such as wrestling or tennis tournaments, and track meets. Such multiple-day competitions sometimes leave little time for food consumption. These time constraints, coupled with lack of availability of food or beverages as well as competitive anxiety, may cause the athlete to overlook this important part of a nutritional program. The primary concerns in these situations are fluid status and carbohydrate intake. Frequent small feedings can alleviate the sensations of hunger and provide sources of energy as well as correct for water loss. Foods and beverages the athlete likes taken in small amounts throughout the day can ward off hunger, provide needed calories, help maintain blood glucose levels, and meet fluid needs.

A second concern is nutrition between daily training or practice sessions. As previously mentioned, consuming adequate carbohydrate on a daily basis is necessary to ensure maintenance of adequate muscle glycogen stores. Hard training such as two-a-day workouts can deplete most of the glycogen stored in the muscle. The amount of carbohydrate consumed following exercise is a major factor in the subsequent resynthesis of muscle glycogen after its degradation. Unless sufficient carbohydrate is consumed, muscle glycogen levels will not be normalized on a day-to-day basis between training bouts. A study by Costill, et al.[23] showed that consuming between 150 and 650 grams of carbohydrate per day resulted in proportionately greater amounts of muscle glycogen storage. It appears however that carbohydrate consumption in excess of 600 g/day will not result in proportionately greater levels of muscle glycogen.[20]

Once competition or the workout session is completed for the day, fluids and carbohydrates should be consumed as soon as possible. This is particularly important if the athlete is involved in multiple event competition or heavy daily training sessions. Muscle and liver glycogen stores need to be replaced rapidly so that chronic glycogen depletion does not result. Fluid replacement is extremely important and will be discussed in Chapter 5.

VITAMIN AND MINERAL SUPPLEMENTS

All vitamins needed by the human body can be obtained in adequate amounts by consuming a balanced diet—there is no benefit to taking more. Nevertheless, vitamin and mineral supplements are a multimillion dollar business, and athletes are probably one of the biggest groups of offenders.[79] Surveys of athletes demonstrate that between 54 and 84% use supplements.[11,36,70]

There are many factors that influence athletes in the use of nutrition supplements. One is the attitude that nutrients are "good" and therefore are harmless; the other is the notion that if a little is good, a lot is better. It is common for an athlete consuming five or six different supplements a day to be unaware of the nutrients provided by those supplements. Another factor that contributes to excessive use of supplements is the perception that the RDA are minimum requirements rather than levels estimated to exceed the requirements of healthy individuals. Additionally, dangerously high levels of nutrients are consumed by people because they are unaware of the fact that some nutrients can be toxic or problematic. For example, protein is vital for all growth and maintenance of body tissue, and in fact the term "protein" means "first place." As been previously discussed, protein

has been associated with enhancing athletic performance and increasing muscle mass. However, large amounts of protein or amino acids can cause fluid imbalances, calcium losses, and liver and kidney hypertrophy, suggesting a strain on regulatory mechanisms in these organs.[17,39]

Because many athletes have energy intakes above 4000 calories, the levels of nutrients consumed from food alone are often 200 to 300% of the RDA. With the addition of supplements, the combined food and supplement intake can result in megadoses. Toxicity and adverse effects resulting from high doses have been well documented for several nutrients.[29,59] Figure 1 depicts the fact that vitamin A toxicity is manifest by a variety of symptoms. Although individual variation exists as to the exact dosage and degree of response, there is a similar progression of events that, if allowed to progress, leads to cell death. It is now known that vitamin E is not the innocuous substance it was thought to be for many years, since research has revealed harmful effects of large dosages. A summary of adverse effects of vitamin E is given in Table 3.

The fact that physical performance will deteriorate during prolonged vitamin deficiency is well documented. Various studies on human subjects fed diets deficient in one or more of the water-soluble vitamins have shown deterioration in work performance, decrease in work output, increased fatigue, and increased muscle tenderness. Although the ability to do work is markedly diminished during states of severe vitamin deficiency, once vitamin requirements are met there appears to be no value in consuming additional amounts. Numerous investigations have studied the effects of supplementing nutritionally adequate diets.[4,10,28,44,50,51,65,69,71,78] Supplementation above an adequate diet did not improve work output, muscle strength, resistance to fatigue, recovery, cardiovascular function, endurance capacity, or oxygen consumption. Scientific evidence supports the fact that supplementation of the diet with either single or multi-nutrient preparations does not improve physical performance in athletes consuming a nutritionally adequate diet. However, the psychotherapeutic aspects of supplements cannot be ignored.

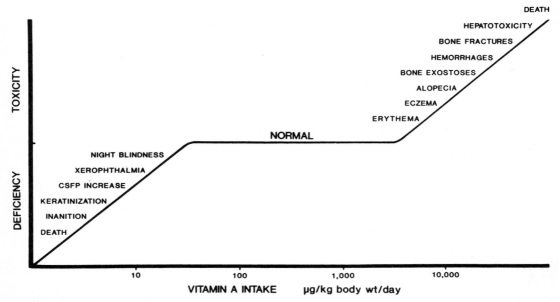

FIGURE 1. This schematic graph depicts the systemic expression of different organ responses to varying levels of vitamin A. (From Miller, D.R. and Hayes, K.C.: Vitamin excesses and toxicity. In Hathcock, J.N. (ed.): Nutritional Toxicity, Vol. 1. New York, Academic Press, 1982, with permission.)

A nutrient by nutrient review of the literature is not practical here. Iron, however, warrants individual attention because of the interest in this mineral shown by many coaches and athletes (especially endurance athletes). Likewise, calcium deserves brief mention because of the incidence of amenorrhea in female athletes and the role of calcium in bone density and therefore stress fractures and healing.

Iron

Iron is present in all cells of the body and plays a key role in numerous biochemical reactions. It plays a vital role in the transport of oxygen (hemoglobin, myoglobin) and in the activation of oxygen (oxidases and oxygenases), and it is present in several enzymes responsible for electron transport (cytochromes). Thus, a deficiency of iron can affect several metabolic functions related to the production of energy. Depressed hemoglobin levels have been associated with impaired oxygen-carrying capacity in the blood and with a decreased maximum aerobic power.[3,30,47,63,64] Understandably, coaches, ath-

letes, and trainers are desirous that athletes achieve optimal iron nutriture.

Unlike other minerals, there is no physiologic regulation of iron metabolism through increased or decreased excretion. The primary control for maintaining adequate levels of iron is the intestinal absorption system, which is influenced in part by the iron status of the individual. The amount of iron absorbed is inversely related to body stores.

The amount of iron absorbed from the diet is dependent on the availability of dietary iron and the behavior of the intestinal mucosa. During digestion, most dietary iron enters a pool of either heme or nonheme.[13] One reason for differences in the amount of food-iron available for absorption relates to the behavior of these two forms of iron by the intestinal mucosa. Each have different pathways of uptake. Heme iron, found in hemoglobin and myoglobin, accounts for 40% of the iron in all animal tissues including meat, liver, fish, and poultry.[60] It is well absorbed, regardless of the dietary composition of a meal.[61] Nonheme iron in the diet comes from plant sources and constitutes the remaining 60% of the iron found in meat. The availabil-

TABLE 3.　POSSIBLE HARMFUL EFFECTS OF HIGH-DOSE VITAMIN E IN HUMANS*

Nausea	Lowered resistance to infections
Diarrhea	
Headache	Risk for women of infertility or spontaneous abortion on dosages above 1,500 IU
Rapid pulse	
Itchy rash	
Extreme fatigue	Suppression of thyroid gland
Muscle weakness	
Blurred vision	Risk to men of sore and enlarged breasts from estrogen-like effect
Inflammation and cracking at corners of mouth	
	Risk of fatty liver development
Serious crisis for persons with high blood pressure	Risk of increased blood fats (triglycerides)
Danger above 150 IU daily to persons with rheumatic heart disease	Increased blood cholesterol
	Creatine in urine, indicating possible muscle damage
Danger to heart patients taking digitalis	Danger to diabetics taking insulin or oral anti-diabetes drug
Increased risk of bleeding for persons low in vitamin K (from long-term antibiotic therapy)	Interference with iron medication used to treat children with iron-deficiency anemia
Risk to vegetarians by blocking conversion of carotenes to vitamin A	Risk of internal bleeding in persons taking anti-clot drugs like warfarin
Increased risk of blood clots, especially in women taking estrogens	

*From Marshall, C.W.: Vitamins and Minerals: Help or Harm? Barrett, S. (ed.): Philadelphia, George F. Stickley Co., 1983.

ity of nonheme iron is generally much less than heme iron and is affected by a variety of substances in the diet. Approximately 23% of the heme iron is absorbed, while only 3 to 8% of nonheme iron is absorbed, depending on the presence of enhancing or inhibiting factors.

Two dietary factors that have consistently been shown to increase nonheme iron availability are meat and ascorbic acid.[38,38A, 62, 67] On the other hand, certain dietary com-

ponents have a profound inhibiting effect on iron absorption. Tea, coffee, soy products, calcium and phosphate salts, eggs, wheat bran, and fiber are inhibitors that have been studied most extensively in humans.[14,38,40,62,67]

Due to the role of iron in sports performance, many athletes, coaches, and trainers believe that iron supplements will maximize performance. Some authors suggest that female athletes consider routine use of iron supplements.[26,40] There is no evidence that the incidence of iron deficiency in the absence of anemia (when measured as plasma ferritin concentration) is higher in female athletes than non-athletes.[26,64] Nor does iron deficiency anemia appear to be any more prevalent in female athletes than non-athletes.[26,64] Although iron supplementation is the accepted treatment for iron deficiency anemia, data do not indicate that supplementation of non-anemic females is of value. Team physicians need to be cognizant that 20-30% of female athletes can be expected to be iron deficient and are therefore at risk of developing anemia. The iron status of female athletes should be determined by a battery of tests (see section on anemia in Chapter 12). Those athletes found to be iron deficient or anemic should receive diet counseling. Supplemental iron may also be indicated. However, routine use of iron supplements by all athletes is not warranted.

Calcium

Most assuredly one of the nutritional controversies of the 1980s that can be expected to continue into the 1990s before being resolved is the question of calcium in prevention and treatment of osteoporosis. What are the long-term effects of amenorrhea in female athletes in relation to both osteoporosis and calcium intake? How do all of these factors affect the occurrence of stress fractures and healing? The answers to these questions are as yet unknown, although there are those with vested interest who recommend increased calcium consumption as the solution. There are no data available to demonstrate that high calcium intakes do in fact help prevent osteoporosis.[32] Several comments must be made, however, on the research conducted to date. One is that the calcium studies for the most part have been balance studies, e.g., measuring intake and output, and have not evaluated whether or not bone density is affected. Secondly the evidence indicating estrogen deficiency as a primary factor in osteoporosis is very strong.

Unfortunately the public is being bombarded with preliminary data and advertising from purveyors of products. The end result in many cases is a misinterpretation of that information. By way of example, this author has encountered women who were taking high levels of calcium supplements because "they are active or are runners" and have read that women participating in vigorous exercise are at risk of osteoporosis. Some of these women were not amenorrheic. In addition, some were also on estrogen therapy, either prescribed as estrogen therapy per se or in the form of oral contraceptive. In some situations, the woman's physician was unaware of the calcium supplementation and the fact that the patient was "double-treating."

Since the susceptible population for osteoporosis in some cases consumes more rather than less calcium than women in general in the United States, epidemiological data do not implicate calcium deficiency as a cause.[43] Until the results of studies currently underway are reported, the approach should be conservative. While on the one hand it is dangerous to ignore the fact that osteoporosis is a disease of affluent Western cultures and therefore diet should be suspected as a factor, the causal dietary factor(s) is unknown. On the other hand, overtreating and resulting complications are a possibility that must be considered.

Water

Water is of primary importance to the athlete. Water is necessary to give structure and form to the body and to provide the aqueous medium in which the functions of the body take place. It is also very important in the regulation of body temperature. During physical exercise great amounts of water may be lost through sweat as the body attempts to maintain normal temperature. Water replacement is of utmost importance to the athlete for optimal performance. This issue is discussed in greater detail in the chapter on "Temperature Control, Heat Illnesses, Fluids, and Safe Exercise in the Heat."

ACKNOWLEDGEMENT. The author wishes to gratefully acknowledge the assistance of Jaime Ruud.

REFERENCES

1. American College of Sports Medicine: Position statement on proper and improper weight loss programs. Med Sci Sports Exerc 15(1):ix, 1983.
2. American College of Sports Medicine: Position stand on weight loss in wrestlers. Med Sci Sports Exerc 8(2):xi, 1976.
3. Anderson, H, Burkve, H: Iron deficiency and muscular work performance. Scand J Clin Lab Invest 25(suppl 114):9–37, 1970.
4. Archdeacon JW, Murlin JR: The effect of thiamin depletion and restoration on muscular efficiency and endurance. J of Nutr 28:241–254, 1944.
5. Asprey GM, Alley LE, Tuttle WW: Effect of eating at various times on subsequent performances in the 440-yard dash and half-mile run. The Research Quarterly 34(3):267–270, 1963a.
6. Asprey GM, Alley LE, Tuttle WW: Effect of eating at various times upon subsequent performances in the one-mile run. The Research Quarterly 35(3):227–230, 1963b.
7. Asprey GM, Alley LE, Tuttle WW: Effect of eating at various times on subsequent performances in the 2-mile run. The Research Quarterly 36:233–236, 1965.
8. Astrand P: Diet and athletic performance. Fed Proc 26:1772–1777, 1967.
9. Ball JR: Effect of eating at various times upon subsequent performances in swimming. The Research Quarterly 33:163–167, 1962.
10. Barnett DW, Conlee RK: The effects of a commercial dietary supplement on human performance. Am J Clin Nutr 40(3):586–590, 1984.
11. Barry A: A nutritional study of Irish athletes. Br J Sports Med 15:99–109, 1981.
12. Bergstrom J, et al: Diet, muscle glycogen and physical performance. Acta Physiol Scand 71:140, 1967.
13. Bjorn-Rasmussen E, Hallberg L, Isaksson B, Arvidsson B: Food iron absorption in man. Application of the two-pool extrinsic tag method to measure heme and non-heme iron absorption from the whole diet. J Clin Nutr 53:247, 1974.
14. Bothwell TH, Charlton KW: Iron deficiency in women. New York: The Nutrition Foundation, 1981.
15. Brotherhood JR: Nutrition and sports performance. Sports Medicine 1:350, 1984.
16. Calabrese LH: Nutritional and medical aspects of gymnastics. Clin Sports Med 4(1):23–30, 1985.

17. Chopra JG, Forbes AL, Habicht JT: Protein in the U.S. diet. J Am Diet Assoc 72:253-258, 1978.

18. Christensen E, Hansen O: Arbeitsfahigkeit and Ernahrung. Skand Arch Physiol 81:160, 1939.

19. Committee on Dietary Allowances, Food and Nutrition Board: Recommended Dietary Allowances, Ed 9. Washington, D.C., National Academy of Sciences, 1980.

20. Costill DL, Blom P, Hermansen, L: Influence of acute exercise and endurance training on muscle glycogen storage. Med Sci Sports Exer 13:90, 1981 (abstract).

21. Costill DL, Bowers R, Branan G, Sparks, K: Muscle glycogen utilization during prolonged exercise on successive days. J Appl Physiol 31:834, 1971.

22. Costill DL: Muscular exhaustion during distance running. Phys Sportsmed 2(10):36-41, 1974.

23. Costill DL, Sherman WM, Fink WJ, et al: The role of dietary carbohydrate in muscle glycogen resynthesis after strenuous running. Am J Clin Nutr 34:1831-1836, 1981.

24. Costill DL, Sparks KE: Rapid fluid replacement following thermal dehydration. J Appl Physiol 34:299-303, 1973.

25. Dardin, E: Nautilus Nutrition Book. Chicago, Contemporary Books, 1981.

26. deWijn JF, Jejongste JL, Mosterd W, Willebrand D: Haemoglobin, packed cell volume, serum iron binding capacity of selected athletes. J Sports Med 11:42-51, 1971.

27. Durnin J, Passmore R: Energy Work and Leisure. London, Heinemann Educational Books Ltd., 1967.

28. Foltz EE, Ivy Ac, Barborka CJ: Influence of components of the vitamin B complex on recovery from fatigue. J of Lab Clin Med 27:1396-1399, 1942.

29. Fumich RM, Essig GW: Hypervitaminosis A: Case report in an adolescent soccer player. Am J Sports Med 11:34, 1983.

30. Gardner GW, Edgerton VR, Senewiratne B, et al: Physical work capacity and metabolic stress in subjects with iron deficiency anemia. Am J Clin Nutr 30:910-917, 1977.

31. Girandola RN, Wisewell RA, Frisch F, et al: Effects of liquid and solid meals and time of feeding on VO$_2$ max. In Fox EL (ed): Report of the Ross Symposium on Nutrient Utilization During Exercise. Columbus, OH, Ross Laboratories, 1983, pp 115-119.

32. Gorden GS, Vaughan C: Calcium and osteoporosis. J Nutr 116(2):319-233, 1986.

33. Grandjean AC: Energy requirements of the athlete. In Andrews F (ed): Food in Contemporary Society—Energy: The Critical Factor. Knoxville, TN, The University of Tennessee, 1982.

34. Grandjean AC: Nutrition for swimmers. Clin Sports Med 5:65, 1986.

35. Grandjean AC: Vitamins, diet and the athlete. In Bertram Zarins (ed): Clin Sports Med 2:105-114, 1983.

36. Grandjean AC: Profile of nutritional beliefs and practices of the elite athlete. In Butts NK, Gushiken TT, Zarins B (eds): The Elite Athlete. New York, Spectrum Publishing, Inc., 1985.

37. Hallberg L: Bioavailability of dietary iron in man. In Darley WJ (ed): Annual Review of Nutrition. Palo Alto, CA, Annual Reviews, Inc., 1981.

38. Hallberg L, and Rossander L: Absorption of iron from Western-type lunch and dinner meals. Am J Clin Nutr 35:502-509, 1982.

38A. Harper AE: Amino acids and nutritional importance. In Toxicants Occurring Naturally in Foods. Washington, D.C., National Academy of Sciences, 1973.

39. Haymes EM: Iron supplementation. In Stull GA, Cureton TK (eds): Encyclopedia of Physical Education, Fitness, and Sports. Salt Lake City, Brighton Publishing Co., 1980.

40. Hecker Al: Nutritional conditioning for athletic performance. Clin Sports Med 3:567, 1984.

41. Hecker AL: Nutritional conditioning and athletic performance. Primary Care 9:545, 1982.

42. Hegstead DM: Calcium and osteoporosis. J Nutr 116:2316-2319, 1986.

43. Henschel A, Taylor HL, Brozek J, et al: Vitamin C and ability to work in hot environments. Am J Trop Med Hyg 24:259-265, 1944.

44. Horstman DH: Nutrition. In Morgan WP (ed): Ergogenic Aids and Muscular Performance. New York, Academic Press, 1972.

45. Houston ME: Diet, training, and sleep: A survey study of elite Canadian swimmers. Can J Appl Sport Science 5:161-163, 1980.

46. Hunding A, Jordal R, Paulev PE: Runners anemia and iron deficiency. Acta Med Scand 216:149-155, 1984.

47. Hutchinson R: Meal habits and their affects on performance. Nutrition Abstract Review 22:283-297, 1985.

48. Kelly KA: Motility of the stomach and gastroduodenal junction. In Johnson LR (ed): Physiology of the Gastrointestinal Tract, Vol. 1. New York, Raven Press, 1981.

49. Keys A: Physical performance in relation to diet. Fed Proc 2:164-187, 1943.

50. Keys A, Henschel AF: Vitamin supplementation of U.S. Army rations in relation to fatigue and ability to do muscular work. J Nutr 23:259-269, 1942.

51. Keys A, Brozek J, Henschel A, et al: The Biology of Human Starvation. Volume I. Minneapolis, The University of Minnesota Press, 1950.

52. Konishif: Exercise Equivalence of Food: Practical Guide for the Overweight. Carbondale, IL: Southern Illinois University Press, 1974.

53. Krough A, Lindhard J: The relative value of fats and carbohydrate as sources of muscular energy. Biochem J 14:290, 1920.

54. Lawrence JD, Bower RC, Riehl WP, Smith JL: Effects of α-tocopherol acetate on the swimming endurance of trained swimmers. Am J Clin Nutr 28:205-208, 1975.

55. Lemon PWR, Nagle FJ: Effects of exercise on protein and amino acid metabolism. Med Sci Sports Exerc 13(3):141-149, 1981.

56. Lemon PWR, Yarosheski KE, Dolny DG: The im-

portance of protein for athletes. Sports Medicine 1:474, 1984.

57. McArdle WD, Katch FI, Katch VL: Exercise Physiology: Energy, Nutrition and Human Performance. Philadelphia, Lea and Febiger, 1981.

58. Miller DR, Hayes KC: Vitamin excess and toxicity. In Hathcock JH (ed): Nutritional Toxicity, Vol. I. New York, Academic Press, 1982.

59. Monson ER, Hallberg L, Layrisse M, et al: Estimation of available dietary iron. Am J Clin Nutr, 31:134–141, 1978.

60. Monson ER, Balintfy JL: Calculating dietary iron bioavailability: refinement and computerization. J of Am Diet Assoc, 80:307–311, 1982.

61. Morck JA, Cook JD: Factors affecting the bioavailability of dietary iron. Cereal Foods World 26:667–671, 1981.

62. Nickerson H, Tipp A: Iron deficiency in adolescent cross-country runners. Phys Sportsmed 11:60–66, 1983.

63. Pate RR, Maguire M, Wyuk JV: Dietary iron supplementation in women athletes, Phys Sportsmed 7:81, 1979.

64. Read MH, McGuffin SL: The effect of B-complex supplementation on endurance performance. J Sports Med Phys Fitness 23(2):178–184, 1983.

65. Refsum HE, Gjessing LR, Stromme SB: Changes in plasma amino acid distribution and urine amino acid excretion during prolonged heavy exercise. Scand J Clin Lab Invest 39:407–413, 1979.

66. Rossander L, Hallberg L, Bjron-Rasmussen E: Absorption of iron from breakfast cereals. Am J Clin Nutr 32:2484, 1979.

67. Saltin B, Hermansen L: Glycogen stores and prolonged severe exercise. In Blix G (ed): Nutrition and Physical Activity. Uppsala, Sweden, Almqvist and Wiksells, 1967.

68. Sharman IM, Down MG, Sen RN: The effects of vitamin E and training on physiological function and athletic performance in adolescent

69. Shephard RJ: Vitamin E and athletic performance. J Sports Med Phys Fitness 23(4):461–470, 1983.

70. Shephard RJ, Campbell R, Pimm P, et al: Vitamin E, exercise, and the recovery from physical activity. Eur J Applied Physiol 33:119–126, 1974.

71. Sherman WM, Costill DL, Fink WJ, Miller JM: Effect of exercise-diet manipulation on muscle glycogen and its subsequent utilization during performance. Int J Sports Med 2:114–118, 1981.

72. Smith NJ: Food for Sport. Palo Alto, CA, Bull Publishing Co., 1976.

73. Smith NJ: Nutrition and athletic performance. In Scott WN, Niconson B, Nicholas JA (eds): Principles of Sports Medicine. Baltimore, Williams and Wilkins, 1984.

74. Steel JE: A nutritional study of Australian Olympic athletes. Med J Aust 2:119, 1970.

75. Strauss RH, Lanese RR, Malarkey WB: Weight loss in amateur wrestlers and its effect on serum testosterone levels. JAMA 254(23):3337, 1985.

76. Torun B, Young VR: Interaction of energy and protein intake in relation to dietary requirements. In Nutrition in Health and Disease and International Development. Symposia from the XII Internal Congress of Nutrition. New York, Allan R. Liss, Inc., 1981, pp 47–56.

77. Watt T, Romet TT, McFarlane I, et al: Vitamin E and oxygen consumption, (letter). Lancet 2:354–355, 1974.

78. Williams MH: Nutritional aspects of human physical and athletic performance. Illinois, Charles C. Thomas, 2nd ed, 1985.

79. Zambraski E, Tipton CM, Tcheng TK, et al: Iowa wrestling study: changes in the urinary profiles of wrestlers prior to and after competition. Med Sci Sports Exerc 7(3):217–220, 1975.

80. Zuntz N: Ueber die Bedeutung der verschiedenen Nahrstoffe als Erzeuger der Muskelfraft. Pfleugers Archives 83:557, 1901.

4 Drugs and Doping in Athletes

JAMES C. PUFFER, M.D.

It was not until the unfortunate death of Danish cyclist Kurt Enemar Jensen at the 1960 Summer Olympic Games in Rome that considerable attention was focused on the mounting problem of drugs and doping in sports. Jensen and two of his teammates had taken amphetamines and Roniacol in the attempt to improve their performance in the 100 kilometer team trials. Although Jensen died, his two teammates were taken to an Italian hospital in critical condition and subsequently survived. This unfortunate incident led to the convention of European sports governing bodies in Janaury 1963 to address the problem of drugs in sport. From this meeting came a definition of doping that was later adopted by the International Doping Conference of the Federation Internationale de Medicine Sportive in Tokyo in October 1964 and the International Olympic Committee (IOC):[6] "Doping is the administration to, or the use by, a competing athlete of any substance foreign to the body or any physiological substance taken in abnormal quantity or by an abnormal route of entry into the body, with the sole intention of increasing in an artificial and unfair manner his performance in competition."

There was no official drug testing program in place at the Tokyo Olympiad in 1964; nevertheless, spot checks of several of the cyclists found them to be receiving unidentified injections before competition. Because many of the athletes refused to cooperate with the International Olympic Committee Medical Commission, a petition was sent to then IOC President, Avery Brundage, deploring the continued use of drugs by Olympic athletes. This resulted in the establishment of a list of banned substances (that included, specifically, sympathomimetic amines, central nervous system stimulants, narcotic an-algesics, antidepressants, and major tranquilizers) and the development of a formal drug testing protocol for use in the 1968 Winter and Summer Olympic Games. Formal drug testing has taken place at every Olympic Games competition since that time, and the results of these formal drug testing procedures are noted in Table 1.

The banned list was subsequently revised to include five major categories of drugs: (1) psychomotor stimulants, (2) anabolic steroids, (3) sympathomimetic amines, (4) miscellaneous central nervous system stimulants, and (5) narcotic analgesics. Prior to the 1984 Olympic Games, caffeine and testosterone were added to the banned list by the IOC. Blood doping, diuretics and beta-blockers were banned following the Los Angeles Olympiad and a new list of doping classes and methods was developed (Table 2). This new classification allowed the IOC to ban pharmacological classes of agents and, unlike the old banned list, provided the flexibility of banning new drugs designed especially for doping purposes. The list also avoids the philosophical problems involved in developing a concrete, operational definition of doping. The IOC interprets the presence of *any* amount of banned substance (with the exception of testosterone and caffeine) in an athlete's urine as sufficient proof that he or she sought an unfair advantage. The most famous application of this principle occurred in 1972 at the Munich Games when swimmer Rick DeMont was stripped of a gold medal when ephedrine was found in his urine. This substance was present in the medication that he had taken to control his asthma; he was unaware that the use of this drug would result in his disqualification. Subsequent discussion of the DeMont case resulted in the IOC later approving specific

TABLE 1. OLYMPIC GAME DOPING RESULTS

	POSITIVE	NO. ATHLETES TESTED
Grenoble, 1968	0	86
Mexico City, 1968	1	668
Sapporo, 1972	1	211
Munich, 1972	7	2079
Montreal, 1976	11*	2061
Lake Placid, 1980	0	N/A
Moscow, 1980	0	2200
Sarajevo, 1984	1†	408
Los Angeles, 1984	11‡	1520

*Eight samples positive for anabolic steroids.
†Positive for anabolic steroid.
‡Ten samples positive for anabolic steroids.

TABLE 2. LIST OF DOPING CLASSES AND METHODS

I.   Doping Classes

   A. Stimulants
     1. Psychomotor stimulants
     2. Sympathomimetic amines
     3. Miscellaneous central nervous system stimulants (including caffeine)
   B. Narcotics
   C. Anabolic steroids
   D. Beta-blockers
   E. Diuretics

II. Doping Methods
   A. Blood doping

III. Classes of Drugs Subject to Certain Restrictions
   A. Alcohol*
   B. Local anesthetics†
   C. Corticosteroids‡

*Not prohibited but levels (breath or blood) may be requested by an international federation.
†Permitted when medically indicated and documented in writing to IOC Medical Commission.
‡Banned except when used topically, via inhalation, locally or intra-articularly and documented in writing to IOC Medical Commission (oral, intravenous and intramuscular use banned).

medications for the control of asthma in Olympic competition. This has resulted in the ability of team physicians to use the aerosolized selective β_2 agonists terbutaline, salbutamol, bitolterol, orciprenaline, and rimiterol for the control of asthma.

PREVALENCE

The prevalence of drug use by athletes has been documented in numerous surveys. The Big Ten Conference conducted a study comparing drug use of male athletes to that of the general student body in 1981.[21] This study found that there was basically little difference in the use of alcohol and marijuana between the two groups (approximately 80% and 20% for each drug respectively); however, 2% of the athletes reported using anabolic steroids, whereas none of the general student body did so. A Canadian study by Clement, investigating drug use among 1687 Olympic athletes in Canada, revealed that 5% used anabolic steroids, 21% were contemplating the use of anabolic steroids, 10% used psychomotor stimulants, 57% used alcohol, 23% used marijuana and 4% used cocaine. A more recent study, completed in 1985 by Anderson and McKeag for the NCAA, investigated drug use by intercollegiate athletes

throughout the United States.[4] A summary of this study is found in Table 3.

From these data, it is apparent that there are probably four major categories of drugs that are used most frequently by athletes: anabolic steroids, stimulants, nonsteroidal anti-inflammatory drugs, and recreational drugs. Of these four categories, the first two are included on the IOC's banned list, whereas the last two are not. Each of these categories will be reviewed in detail. The use of human growth hormone, blood doping, and phosphate/bicarbonate loading, three doping procedures that have recently gained considerable attention, will also be discussed.

ANABOLIC STEROIDS

The use of testosterone or testosterone-like synthetic drugs results in both anabolic and androgenic activity in those using these substances. In other words, they increase protein synthesis, resulting in an increase in muscular bulk, and they also enhance the de-

TABLE 3. DRUG USE BY INTERCOLLEGIATE ATHLETES*

DRUG	PERCENT OF ATHLETES
Alcohol	88%
Amphetamines	8%
Anabolic Steroids	6.5%
Anti-inflammatories	31%
Caffeine	68%
Cocaine	17%
Marijuana	36%

*Adapted from Anderson WA, McKeag DB: The substance use and abuse habits of college student athletes. National Collegiate Athletic Association, June, 1985.

velopment of secondary sexual characteristics in males. In the females, these drugs have masculinizing effects. Anabolic steroids first became available for experimental and therapeutic use in the 1930s and were used extensively during World War II to help restore positive nitrogen balance in victims of starvation.[33] Although these substances have been used for the treatment of refractory anemia, as replacement therapy in hypogonadal males, and in the management of burn victims, there is limited application of these substances for therapeutic purposes at the present time. Nevertheless, they continue to be used by increasing numbers of athletes to enhance muscular strength and power. When used by athletes, they are frequently taken in amounts 10 to 40 times greater than therapeutic doses and are usually used in combination ("stacked") or cycled in a pyramid fashion with other ergogenic substances.[11]

At the cellular level, the anabolic steroids are bound by cytoplasmic proteins and are subsequently transported to the nucleus, where they then activate DNA-dependent RNA polymerase. This results in the subsequent production of messenger RNA, which forms the template for subsequent protein synthesis. Numerous studies have been published supporting both improvement in strength,[5,7,26,48,52] as well as no significant improvement in strength in male athletes.[25,29,33,49] Although there has been con-

siderable confusion in the literature with regard to the benefits of these substances, a recent review by the American College of Sports Medicine on the use of these agents resulted in the following conclusions:[3] (1) Anabolic steroids in the presence of an adequate diet can contribute to increases in body weight and lean mass. (2) The gains in muscular strength achieved through high-intensity exercise and proper diet can occur by increased use of anabolic steroids in some individuals. (3) Anabolic steroids do not increase aerobic power.

Although, after careful review of the literature, this group of experts concluded that the use of these substances may result in the enhancement of muscular strength, it should be noted that use has also been associated with numerous adverse effects, including hepatocellular dysfunction, premature atherosclerosis, decrease in high-density lipoprotein cholesterol levels, oligospermia or azospermia, reduction in testicular size, acne, hair recession and alopecia, premature epiphyseal closure in children, and clitorimegaly and hirsutism in women.[35] A case reported by Overly and colleagues commented on the development of hepatocellular carcinoma in an athlete taking oral anabolic steroids over a prolonged period of time.[37]

A thorough discussion of the use of anabolic and androgenic hormones cannot be complete without mention of the use of testosterone. Prior to the 1984 Olympic Games, testosterone was not on the list of substances banned by the IOC. This was because the qualitative tests that were utilized to detect banned substances could not distinguish exogenous testosterone from naturally occurring testosterone. For these reasons, many athletes avoided detection of anabolic steroids by stopping these substances well before the projected time of drug testing and then switching to injectable testosterone preparations until the time of competition. At the 1980 Moscow Olympic Games, Donike and colleagues independently tested urine specimens (submitted by randomly selected athletes for anabolic steroid testing) for the presence of abnormal quantities of testosterone. They found that as many as two thirds of these samples had quantities of testosterone present that could be considered grossly abnormal and nonphysiologic.[20] As a consequence of these findings, the IOC subsequently decided that in future Olympiads quantitative testing of testosterone would be undertaken.

This quantitative test utilizes the well-known relationship that exists between testosterone and its isomer, epitestosterone. It has been shown that in normal individuals a one-to-one relationship exists between these two molecules. However, when exogenous testosterone is taken, serum testosterone is elevated out of proportion to epitestosterone. The standard utilized for a positive test is a ratio that exceeds 6:1. This technique has been demonstrated to be highly effective in detecting exogenous testosterone usage. Many athletes disqualified in both the 1983 Pan American Games in Caracas, Venezuela and the 1984 Summer Olympic Games had ratios of testosterone to epitestosterone that exceeded this six-to-one standard.

HUMAN GROWTH HORMONE

Because of the effectiveness in detecting anabolic steroids and testosterone with the gas chromatography and mass spectrometry analysis used in these testing procedures, many athletes have now turned to a new hormonal substance in an effort to enhance performance, namely growth hormone. The widespread use of this substance by athletes has further clouded the issue of drug testing, as there is no effective means for reliable testing of exogenous growth hormone at the present time.

It is a well-known fact that human growth hormone is effective in increasing stature of growth hormone–deficient children.[50] Recent evidence has indicated that growth hormone also increases the rate of growth in some short-statured children who are not deficient in growth hormone.[46,51] This has resulted in the spurious thinking by some that providing human growth hormone to otherwise healthy athletes could result in considerable improvement in muscular strength by inducing muscular hypertrophy and hyperplasia, despite the fact that no scientific evidence exists to document this ef-

fect in healthy individuals. It is important to note that most children who are growth-hormone-deficient do not reach a height above the third percentile of the general population when they are treated, and it is unclear whether short-statured children who are not growth-hormone-deficient will eventually become taller adults as a result of the increase in growth rate that they experience after receiving human growth hormone.

While 25 years of experience have indicated that therapeutic replacement of growth hormone is safe for growth-hormone-deficient children, considerable concern has been expressed with regard to the use of this potent metabolic agent in those who are not growth-hormone-deficient.[1,50] While most of the data that exist have been obtained from cohorts in which growth hormone has been used as replacement therapy rather than as a pharmacologic agent, nevertheless several important clinical observations should be noted. Formation of antibodies to growth hormone has been common and hypothyroidism has occurred. Insulin resistance, hyperinsulinism, and impaired glucose tolerance are likely to occur in those using this substance, as may frank diabetes mellitus and hypertension.

Acromegaly is a potential serious side effect in those abusing this substance. It has been estimated that acromegalic patients with growth hormone concentrations in the range of 5–30 ng/ml have production rates of 1.5 to 9 mg/day.[1] At commonly used doses, a 50-kg individual would receive 1 mg/day. Therefore, as little as a twofold increase in dose might result in levels that could cause some of the clinical or biochemical changes noted in acromegaly. Such data should not be taken lightly, bearing in mind that many athletes acquire drugs illegally and self-administer them in doses that commonly exceed pharmacologic ranges.

Finally, reports of iatrogenic Creutzfeldt-Jakob disease associated with human growth hormone therapy are an additional concern.[31] While the production of genetically engineered growth hormone will obviate this problem as it replaces cadaver preparations, strict regulations on the use of the synthetic preparation will result in many athletes continuing to use non-synthetic sources, thereby increasing their potential risk for acquiring this catastrophic neurologic disorder.

STIMULANTS

Historically, stimulants have been well known for their potential use as ergogenic aids. At present, three drugs in this category are most frequently used to enhance performance: amphetamine, cocaine, and caffeine.

Amphetamine

Amphetamines are perhaps the drugs best known by the public to be abused by athletes. Considerable publicity concerning the use of these drugs by professional athletes and the well-publicized suspension of a physician's medical license in conjunction with his role in prescribing amphetamines to addicted players while serving as consulting team physician for the San Diego Chargers have brought these issues to the forefront. There is considerable literature describing the effects of amphetamines on human performance, dating back to the 1950s. Smith and Beecher demonstrated the enhancement of timed trials in selected swimming events.[44] A subsequent study by the same authors demonstrated that athletes using these substances experienced increased feelings of being "revved up" before athletic events, as well as feeling more vigorous, energetic, and alert.[45] A recent report by Chandler demonstrated no substantial improvement in athletic performance with use of amphetamines when selected physiologic components were evaluated.[15] The differences in these two studies most likely can be attributed to the activities that were assessed. Tasks that were sufficiently simple and repetitive as to permit sustained attention and habituation would be predicted to result in evidence of enhanced performance during use of amphetamines, whereas more complicated maneuvers would not. The dose-related relationship of these phenomena are well described by Mandell in his now classic description of the "Sunday syndrome" in professional football players using these substances.[36]

The amphetamines exert a number of physiologic responses, including increases in blood pressure and heart rate, mild bronchodilation, increased metabolic rate, and increases in plasma-free fatty acids. They are known to disrupt thermoregulatory mechanisms and predispose athletes to heat illness. Large doses and long-term use lead to toxic effects and psychological addiction; these effects include restlessness, tremor, dizziness, anxiety, insomnia, provocation of angina pectoris, arrhythmias, convulsions, coma, and cerebral hemorrhage.

Cocaine

Cocaine has gained much exposure recently, not only for its use in professional sports but also as a commonly used recreational drug. This drug acts as a central nervous system stimulant, and for this reason it has been used by many athletes in an effort to enhance performance. Cocaine increases the release and blocks the re-uptake of norepinephrine from neurons in the nervous system; this results in more available epinephrine to bind to receptor sites, causing euphoria, increased speed of peripheral reflexes, and increased blood pressure and heart rate. In the inexperienced user, peripheral reflexes are frequently dyssynchronous, resulting in marked diminishment of performance. This substance has a half-life of approximately 2 to 6 hours, and can be detected in the urine 24 to 36 hours after being taken.

As noted previously, the use of cocaine by athletes is increasing. However, the recent tragic deaths of Maryland basketball star Len Bias and Don Rogers of the Cleveland Browns have underscored precisely how lethal the use of this drug can be. Increased catecholamine levels associated with cocaine used intranasally, intravenously, or by smoking can directly induce ventricular dysrhythmias, coronary vasospasm, vasospasm with thrombosis, and myocardial infarction.[18,28] Any of these events, alone or in combination, can obviously lead to sudden death. A recent report by Isner and colleagues has documented that acute cardiac events and sudden death can occur in the absence of underlying cardiac disease and with doses of the drug that are not massive.[28] Cerebrovascular accidents and rupture of the aorta have also been reported in those using cocaine.[18]

Because this drug is frequently taken by sniffing the substance through the nasal passages, it can result in swelling and congestion of the nasal mucosa as well as ulceration of the nasal septum. Rhinitis, sinusitis, and bronchitis are common side effects in frequent users. Frequent nosebleeds with nasal septum necrosis and ulceration can also be seen in chronic users. As with other stimulants, cocaine use can result in agitation, insomnia, and tremulousness. Toxic psychoses, severe depression, paranoia, and dysphorias have been reported.[18]

Caffeine

Caffeine is a powerful stimulant of the central nervous system and has been used extensively by athletes. It appears abundantly in tea, coffee, and cola drinks and is used frequently by athletes as a stimulant prior to athletic events. Laurin and Letorneau found significant amounts of caffeine in large numbers of urine samples collected from athletes competing in the 1976 Olympic Games in Montreal.[32] A recent study by Ivy and colleagues has demonstrated that caffeine results in increased work output, most likely secondary to increased mobilization of free fatty acids and increased rates of lipid metabolism.[27] Additional research has shown that caffeine ingestion leads to increased power output in skeletal muscle, most likely a result of the direct effect of the drug on mus-

cle contraction secondary to the increase in calcium permeability of the sacroplasmic reticulum.[53] Recent reports from independent investigators, however, have cast some doubt on the ability of caffeine to enhance or prolong work output.[12,14]

Because of the potential for abuse of this substance, the IOC developed quantitative standards for the detection of caffeine in urine for the 1984 Olympic Games. Any athlete who was found to have greater than 15 μg per ml in his or her urine was subject to disqualification. Recently, however, the IOC has lowered this standard to 12 μg/ml. Concern is always raised by athletes as to how much coffee, tea, or cola they can drink without risking subsequent disqualification. Approximately four to eight cups of coffee would need to be consumed to reach disqualifying levels, depending upon the strength of the coffee, the size of the athlete, and the rate of metabolism. Table 4 provides additional information concerning caffeine levels.

Sympathomimetic Amines

This category of drugs has perhaps created the most confusion and furor at international competition at which drug testing has been conducted. The sympathomimetic amines are found in cold remedies, common nasal and ophthalmologic decongestants, and most asthma preparations. The previous controversy surrounding the Rick DeMont case has already been cited, but this unfor-

TABLE 4. CAFFEINE CONTENT OF COMMONLY USED SUBSTANCES

SUBSTANCE	CAFFEINE CONCENTRATION (mg/100 ml)	CAFFEINE LEVEL* (μg/ml)
Coffee	55–85	1.5–3 (one cup)
Tea	55–85	1.5–3 (one cup)
Cola	10–15	0.75–1.5 (one cup)
Medication	(mg/tablet)	
Cafergot	100	3–6
NoDoz	100	3–6
Anacin	32	2–3
Midol	32	2–3

*Level dependent up on size of athlete and rate of metabolism. These figures represent general estimates based on average size and rate of metabolism.

tunate incident should underline the importance of careful evaluation of all medications—whether they be prescribed or provided over the counter—that are being used by athletes. Although earlier scientific studies demonstrated that the use of ephedrine or similar substances resulted in improved athletic performance, a recent double-blind study has shown that there was no significant improvement in performance in athletes using these drugs.[42] Because of concerns about the availability of approved substances to be used in asthmatics who demonstrate exercise-induced bronchospasm, the IOC has approved the use of the aerosolized selective β_2 agonists terbutaline, salbutamol (albuterol), bitolterol, orciprenaline, and rimiterol. These substances may be used only if the team physician notifies the IOC Medical Subcommission in writing concerning the use of these substances by individual athletes prior to their participation in Olympic competition.

NONSTEROIDAL ANTI-INFLAMMATORY DRUGS

The nonsteroidal anti-inflammatory drugs (NSAIDs) have become an important tool in the physician's treatment of common musculoskeletal disorders in athletes. They are frequently prescribed to assist in the management of tendinitis, sprains, strains, and other soft-tissue derangements. Although NSAIDs are extremely effective in the amelioration of soft-tissue inflammation, they do have known side effects, including dyspepsia, gastrointestinal bleeding, decreased platelet aggregation, and sedation. The antiprostaglandin activity of these drugs can result in reduced renal perfusion, and it is well known that the kidney can retain salt and water in response to the use of these medications. However, NSAIDs also uncouple oxidative phosphorylation in skeletal muscle, which can have an effect on oxygen consumption; they directly stimulate ventilation as well as promote sweating and dehydration.[19] Given this information, it is obvious that these drugs interfere with thermoregulatory mechanisms and may predispose athletes to heat illness. These facts should be considered by physicians prescribing these medications for common soft-tissue injuries. NSAIDs have analgesic properties and are frequently used in international competition for the management of pain, because they do not appear on the IOC's banned list.

RECREATIONAL DRUGS

Numerous recreational drugs are used on a regular basis by many athletes. These include alcohol, marijuana, and cocaine. As mentioned previously, cocaine does have a stimulatory effect on the central nervous system, and for this reason it appears on the IOC's banned list. This drug has previously been discussed in detail along with other psychomotor stimulants.

Alcohol

Alcohol is perhaps the drug most frequently used by inter-collegiate and elite athletes.[16,21] Social acceptance of this drug has been high, and it has not been until recently that abuse of this substance has been recognized as a significant problem. The physiologic effects of alcohol are well known and will not be reviewed here. What does deserve mention is the manner in which alcohol may affect performance. Much interest has been generated in this area because of the recent ingestion of alcoholic beverages by marathon runners as a carbohydrate source and a fluid and electrolyte replacement.

A position statement by the American College of Sports Medicine has addressed the use of alcohol by athletes and made several key statements that are substantiated by a thorough review of literature.[2]

1. The acute ingestion of alcohol has a deleterious effect on many psychomotor skills, including reaction time, hand-eye coordination, accuracy, balance, and complex coordination.

2. Alcohol consumption does not substantially influence physiologic functions crucial to physical performance ($\dot{V}O_2$ max, respiratory dynamics, cardiac function).

3. Alcohol ingestion will not improve muscular work capacity and may decrease performance levels.

4. Alcohol may impair temperature regulation during prolonged exercise in a cold environment.

Some have contended that alcohol may serve as a supplemental energy substrate. Animal studies, however, have demonstrated that ethanol ingestion results in depressed mitochondrial function in skeletal muscle.[22] Although mitochondrial respiration and cytochrome content were significantly depressed in sedentary animals given ethanol, these effects could be offset by exercise, as demonstrated by the normal levels present in trained animals given ethanol. Although there has been some interest in the possibility that alcohol dehydrogenase induction could supplement normal glucogenic pathways in the liver and boost endurance performance, no findings to date tend to support this conclusion.[43] It would appear that there are no advantages to using alcohol during or prior to athletic competition, and that the known effects of fine motor skill retardation and discoordination would speak against the use of this substance.

Marijuana

Marijuana is a recreational drug also used frequently by athletes. Its active ingredient, Δ-9 tetrahydrocannabinol (THC), results in the impairment of coordination, perception, and vigilance. It has been demonstrated that motor coordination is impaired by doses commonly taken in social settings by both naive and long-term users of this drug. Impairment of short-term memory and alteration of time sense also have been noted. An amotivational syndrome has been described that is characterized by apathy, difficulty in concentrating, loss of ambition, and decline in work performance.[8] Reduction in plasma testosterone levels, oligospermia, and gynecomastia are also well-recognized side effects in those individuals using marijuana chronically.

With regard to exercise performances, recent work by Renaud and Cormier has demonstrated a reduction of maximal exercise performance with premature achievement of maximal oxygen uptake after smoking marijuana.[40] No effect was noted on tidal volume, arterial blood pressure, or carboxyhemoglobin levels when compared with the control group.

While marijuana is not banned by the IOC, it has been banned by the National Collegiate Athletic Association (NCAA) and will result in disqualification if detected in athletes at NCAA Championships or post-season bowl games. Retention of this substance by adipose tissue results in the ability of sophisticated testing procedures to detect the drug as long as 2–4 weeks after it has been used. Depending upon the sensitivity of the testing procedures used, passive inhalation of secondary smoke theoretically could result in a positive test.

BLOOD DOPING

A discussion of doping could not be complete without a discussion of blood doping. This procedure, which also has been known as blood boosting or blood packing, results in the induction of erthyrocythemia. Blood is removed from an individual and stored in a frozen state while allowing the individual's red cell mass to re-equilibrate. At some later point in time after this equilibration, the red blood cells that have been donated previously are reinfused, resulting in a marked increase in red blood cell mass. The earliest report of this procedure appeared in the literature in 1947 and described the infusion of 2000 ml of freshly transfused blood from matched donors to armed forces personnel.[38] The infusion of fresh, matched blood resulted in a 26% increase in hematocrit over that of controls, as well as a 34% increase in endurance capacity. Subsequent studies using refrigerated blood failed to show increases as dramatic as those of this original study performed in 1947. However, in these instances the blood had been refrigerated, and one could expect that 30 to 40% of the red cells had been lost secondary to processing and normal cell aging during the storage period. Subsequent studies that have used blood frozen at minus 80°C have shown much more impressive results. Buick and colleagues studied the effect of blood doping on aerobic power in elite runners.[10] They demonstrated significant improvements in both maximal oxygen consumption and total exercise time, in addition to significant increases in hemoglobin concentration when compared with controls. Additional work has confirmed these results and demonstrated that the reinfused blood does not significantly compromise the cardiovascular system.[24,47,54] Although transfused blood does not represent a drug per se, it is a physiologic substance that is introduced into the body in a foreign manner with the explicit intent of improving performance, and therefore blood doping obviously is in violation of the definition of doping mentioned previously in this article.

The IOC, after reports of blood doping by American cyclists at the 1984 Summer Olympic Games, has officially banned the practice of blood doping. From a practical standpoint, however, techniques are not available for detecting the presence of transfused autologous or donor blood at the present time. Enforcement of this policy, therefore, will be extremely cumbersome, and effective deterrence of this practice by those athletes who wish to employ it will be difficult to accomplish.

Obviously there are considerable risks involved with the transfusion of blood or blood products. The use of improperly matched donor blood can result in transfusion reactions that can be fatal. The use of donor blood (as was done by some of the U.S. cyclists) also carries the potential risk of transmission of infectious disease. The use of blood products by athletes for purposes of enhancing performance contravenes the ethics of both sport and good medicine, and therefore this practice should be deplored by physicians and athletes alike.

BICARBONATE OR PHOSPHATE LOADING

The latest developments in doping have centered around ingestion of significant amounts of either bicarbonate or phosphate in an effort to favorably alter physiologic parameters that influence maximum performance. While neither of these substances is banned by the IOC, their ingestion solely for the purpose of artificially increasing performance violates the definition of doping presented earlier.

Bicarbonate Loading

During steady-state exercise, sufficient oxygen is supplied to and utilized by working muscle. Under these conditions lactic acid homeostasis is maintained. However, if exercise intensity increases and aerobic metabolism is insufficient to meet energy demands, anaerobic glycolysis contributes to energy requirements and lactic acid is formed. Almost all of the lactic acid generated during anaerobic metabolism is buffered by bicarbonate. However, regulation of pH becomes progressively more difficult during strenuous exercise secondary to an increase in hydrogen ion concentration from both carbon dioxide and lactic acid formation. Eventually intramuscular pH rises as a result of lactate accumulation, and this restricts not only glycolysis but also decreases lipolysis. This results in diminished energy production and decreased muscular work.

Since extracellular bicarbonate enhances diffusion of hydrogen and lactate ions from the intracellular to the extracellular space, it seems logical that increasing the concentration of bicarbonate available for these purposes would forestall fatigue and improve performance. In fact this has been demonstrated.[17,30] Pate and coworkers have studied the effect of orally administered bicarbonate on performance of high intensity exercise by highly trained endurance athletes.[39] They demonstrated that with a 0.3 g/kg oral dose blood pH was significantly increased immediately before, immediately after, and three minutes after exhaustive treadmill exercise as compared with placebo in a controlled, double-blind protocol. Additionally, run time to exhaustion was significantly increased (578 vs. 564 seconds) after athletes ingested bicarbonate rather than placebo.

Phosphate Loading

It is well known that increasing serum phosphate results in an increase in red blood cell 2,3 diphosphoglycerate (2,3 DPG) levels. Since increased 2,3 DPG levels shift the oxygen-hemoglobin dissociation curve to the right and thereby enhance oxygen delivery to tissues, it might seem logical that increasing serum phosphate would improve maximum oxygen consumption. Cade and colleagues at the University of Florida studied the effect of 1 gm of sodium phosphate taken four times daily for three consecutive days as compared with placebo in ten highly trained athletes who served as their own controls.[13] They found that after oral phosphate loading there was a significant increase in serum phosphate and red blood cell 2,3 DPG. Maximum oxygen consumption increased and correlated with the rise in 2,3 DPG (r = 0.81).

DRUG TESTING

Drug testing procedures have gained considerable notoriety recently as institution of the NCAA drug testing program resulted in the disqualification of 21 football players during the small school playoffs or prior to major postseason bowl games in 1986. Public awareness of the critical issues surrounding drug testing has heightened, including the cost of testing, its effectiveness in curtailing drug use, and, most importantly, the legality of testing and the reliability of results.

For the purist, doping of any type is antithetical to the nature of amateur or professional sport. Drug testing has been one means of attempting to enforce the presence of drug-free competition. Since the advent of drug testing at the Olympic Games in 1968, there has certainly been a greater awareness of the potential risks involved in the unethical use of drugs to enhance performance. This has not been without considerable expense. It cost approximately $3 million to equip the drug testing laboratory in Montreal in 1976; in 1984 the Olympic Organizing Committee spent approximately $1.8 million in funding the UCLA Olympic Analytic Laboratory in Los Angeles; and the NCAA estimates that it will spend $1 million this year testing its athletes. Nevertheless, drug testing remains the only effective way at the present time of attempting to enforce the definition of doping accepted by the International Olympic Committee, most international federations, and the NCAA. At the collegiate level, considerable interest has been expressed by universities with regard to drug testing. Many are developing their own drug testing programs to deal with the poten-

tial problems of drug abuse, and there is evidence that these programs are working. At Ohio State University, team physician Robert Murphy, M.D. has indicated that testing of athletes in 1984-85 revealed that 8% were using cocaine or marijuana, whereas in 1985-86 this dropped to 5%.[34]

Considerable attention has been drawn to the legal ramifications of drug testing. The courts have been asked to rule on the issue of constitutionality of mandatory, random drug testing, and to date they have ruled in favor of police officers, firefighters, prison guards, and teachers who have balked at providing urine samples. It is obvious that the issue of testing athletes would be contested, and indeed a New York court ruled favorably on the legality of testing jockeys and a Louisiana court upheld the disqualification of an intercollegiate player prior to the 1987 Sugar Bowl. However, it should be noted that the University of California at Berkeley recently declared a moratorium on testing athletes rather than contest a suit in court brought by the American Civil Liberties Union on behalf of an athlete who refused to be tested.

The reliability of testing procedures has also been raised and deserves mention. At present two screening procedures are commonly used by most laboratories, radioimmunoassay (RIA) and the enzyme-multiplied immunoassay technique (EMIT). The manufacturers of these tests claim that they are 97–99% accurate under ideal circumstances. In fact, such is usually not the case, and this underscores the need for a second, highly sensitive and specific test to confirm the presence of a banned substance to avoid false positive results. Gas chromatography/mass spectrometry (GC/MS) has served as the "gold standard" by which all other tests are measured, since it provides a precise "fingerprint" of the substance under question, thereby providing exact identification. All state-of-the-art laboratories, therefore, use GC/MS as a confirmatory procedure; however, the prohibitive cost of the equipment needed for this procedure, as well as the cost of conducting confirmatory tests on the equipment, frequently preclude the use of this technique by smaller laboratories.

Although drug testing procedures that utilize gas chromatography and mass spectrometry as a confirmation process are exquisitely sensitive and able to confirm with almost complete certainty the presence of a drug in an athlete's urine, the system is not 100% foolproof. Athletes are becoming more sophisticated in determining how to effectively "beat the system." In some instances this is being done by using drugs that currently cannot be detected by the system, such as growth hormone, or by carefully determining exactly how much time is required to excrete a given banned substance, such as anabolic steroid, so that it will not be detected in the urine during drug testing. The obvious solution to the latter problem would be the institution of random spot checking of athletes, and it is likely that this policy will be adopted and practiced by many in the near future.

SUMMARY

The use of drugs to enhance athletic performance poses tremendous potential risk to sport in general and athletes in particular. The incidence of drug usage by athletes is increasing, and many athletes are turning to new drugs or alternative doping methods in an effort to avoid detection by extremely sensitive and reliable drug testing procedures. Future success in eradicating drug usage by athletes will only result from increased efforts directed at enhancement of athlete education, development of strict policies dealing with those athletes who use banned substances, and refinement of drug testing procedures.

REFERENCES

1. Ad Hoc Committee on Growth Hormone Usage, the Lawson Wilkins Pediatric Endocrine Society, and the Committee on Drugs: Growth hormone in the treatment of children with short stature. Pediatrics 72:891–894, 1983.
2. American College of Sports Medicine: Position statement on the use of alcohol in sports. Med Sci Sports Exerc 14:ix–x, 1982.
3. American College of Sports Medicine: Stand on the use of anabolic-androgenic steroids in sports. American College of Sports Medicine, 1984.
4. Anderson WA, McKeag DB: The substance use and abuse habits of college student athletes. National Collegiate Athletic Association, June 1985.
5. Ariel G: The effect of anabolic steroid upon skeletal muscle contractile force. J Sports Med Phys Fitness 13:187–190, 1973.
6. Barnes L: Olympic drug testing: Improvements without progress. Phys Sportsmed 8:21–24, 1980.
7. Berg A, Keul J: Der Einfluss von anabolen Substanzen auf das Verhalten der freien Serumaminosauren von Normalperson und Scwerathleten in Rule and bei Korperarbeit. Oester Z Sportsmed 4:11–18, 1974.
8. Biron S, Wells J: Marijuana and its effect on the athlete. Athl Train 18:295–303, 1983.
9. Brown P, Gajdusek DC, Gibbs CJ, et al: Potential epidemic of Creutzfeldt-Jakob disease from human growth hormone therapy. N Engl J Med 313:728–731, 1985.
10. Buick FJ, Gledhill N, Froese AB, et al: Effect of induced erythrocythemia on aerobic work capacity. J Appl Physiol 48:636–642, 1980.
11. Burkett LN, Falduto MT: Steroid use by athletes in a metropolitan area. Phys Sportsmed 12:69–74, 1984.
12. Butts NK, Crowell D: Effect of caffeine ingestion on cardiorespiratory endurance in men and women. Res Q Exerc Sport 56(4):301–305, 1985.
13. Cade R, Conte M, Zauner C, et al: Effects of phosphate loading on 2,3 diphosphoglycerate and maximal oxygen uptake. Med Sci Sports Exerc 16:263–268, 1984.
14. Casal DC, Leon AS: Failure of caffeine to affect substrate utilization during prolonged running. Med Sci Sports Exerc 17:174–179, 1985.
15. Chandler JV, Blair SN: The effects of amphetamines on selected physiological components related to athletic success. Med Sci Sports Exerc 12:65–69, 1980.
16. Clement DB: Drug use survey: Results and conclusions. Phys Sportsmed 11:64–67, 1983.
17. Costill DL, Verstappen F, Kuipers H, et al: Acid-base balance during repeated bouts of exercise with HCO_3. Med Sci Sports Exerc 15:115, 1983.
18. Cregler LL, Mark H: Medical complications of cocaine abuse. N Engl J Med 315:1495–1500, 1986.
19. Day RO: Effects of exercise performance on drugs used in musculoskeletal disorders. Med Sci Sports Exerc 13:272–275, 1981.
20. Donike M: Personal communication, 1983.
21. Duda M: Drug testing challenges: College and pro athletes. Phys Sportsmed 11:64–67, 1983.
22. Farrar RP, Martin TP, Abraham LD, et al: The interaction of endurance running and ethanol on skeletal muscle mitochondria. Life Sci 30:67–75, 1982.
23. Frasier SD: Human pituitary growth hormone (hGH) therapy in growth hormone deficiency. Endocrinol Rev 4:155–170, 1983.
24. Goforth HW Jr, Campbell NL, Hodgdon JA, et al: Hematologic parameters of trained distance runners following induced erythrocythemia. Med Sci Sports Exerc 14:174, 1982.
25. Hervey GR: Are athletes wrong about anabolic steroids? Br J Sports Med 9:74–77, 1975.
26. Hervey GR, Knibbs AV, Burkinshaw L, et al: Effects

of methandienone on the performance and body composition of men undergoing athletic training. Clin Sci 60:457–461, 1981.

27. Ivy JL, Costill DL, Fink WJ et al: Role of caffeine and glucose ingestion on metabolism during exercise. Med Sports Exerc 10:66, 1978.

28. Isnek JM, Estes NAM, Thompson PD, et al: Acute cardiac events temporally related to cocaine abuse. N Engl J Med 315:1438–1443, 1986.

29. Johnson LD, Roundy ES, Allsen PE, et al: Effects of anabolic steroid treatment on endurance. Med Sci Sports 7:287–289, 1975.

30. Jones NL, Sutton JR, Taylor R, et al: Effect of pH on cardiorespiratory and metabolic responses to exercise. J Appl Physiol 43:959–964, 1977.

31. Koch TK, Berg BO, De Armand SJ, et al: Cruetzfeldt-Jakob Disease in a young adult with idiopathic hypopituitarism: Possible relation to the administration of cadveric human growth hormone. N Engl J Med 313:731–733, 1985.

32. Laurin CA, Letorneau G: Medical report on the Montreal olympic games. Am J Sports Med 6:54–61, 1978.

33. Loughton SV, Ruhline RO: Human strength and endurance responses to anabolic steroids and training. J Sports Med Phys Fitness 17:285–296, 1977.

34. Murphy RJ Personal communication, 1986.

35. MacDougall D: Anabolic steroids. Phys Sportsmed 11:95–99, 1983.

36. Mandell AJ, Stewart KD, Russo PV: The Sunday syndrome: From kinetics to altered consciousness. Fed Proc 40:2693–2698, 1981.

37. Overly WL, Dankoff JA, Wang BK, et al: Androgens and hepatocellular carcinoma in an athlete. Ann Intern Med 100:158, 1984.

38. Pace N, Lozner EL, Consolazio WV, et al: The increase in hypoxia tolerance of normal men accompanying the polycythemia induced by transfusion of erythrocytes. Am J Physiol 148:152–163, 1947.

39. Pate RR, Smith PE, Lambert MI et al: Effect of orally administered sodium bicarbonate on performance of high intensity exercise. Med Sci Sports Exerc 17:200–201, 1985.

40. Renaud AM, Cormier Y: Acute effects of marijuana smoking on maximal exercise performance. Med Sci Sports Exerc 18:685–689, 1986.

41. Ryan AJ: Anabolic steroids are fool's gold. Fed Proc

40:2682–2688, 1981.

42. Sidney KH, Lefcoe NM: The effects of Tedral upon athletic performance: A double blind cross-over study. Quebec City International Congress of Physical Activity Sciences, 1976.

43. Shepard RJ: 1982 Yearbook of Sports Medicine. Chicago, Year Book Medical Publishers, p. 140, 1982.

44. Smith GM, Beecher HK: Amphetamine sulphate and athletic performance. I. Objective effects. JAMA 170:542–547, 1959.

45. Smith GM, Beecher HK: Amphetamine, secobarbital and athletic performance. II. Subjective evaluation of performances, mood states, and physical states. JAMA 172:1502–1514, 1960.

46. Spiliotis BE, August GP, Hung W, et al: Growth hormone neurosecretory dysfunction: A treatable cause of short stature. JAMA 251:2223–2330, 1984.

47. Spriett LL, Gledhill N, Forese AB, et al: The effect of induced erythrocythemia on central circulation and oxygen transport during maximal exercise. Med Sci Sports Exerc 12:122, 1980.

48. Stamford BA, Moffatt R: Anabolic steroid: effectiveness as an ergogenic aid to experienced weight trainers. J Sports Med Phys Fitness, 14:191–197, 1974.

49. Stromme SB, Meen HD, Aakvaag A: Effects of an androgenicanabolic steroid on strength development and plasma testosterone levels in normal males. Med Sci Sports 6:203–208, 1974.

50. Underwood LE: Report of the conference on uses and possible abuses of biosynthetic human growth hormone. N Engl J Med, 311:606–608, 1984.

51. VanVliet G, Styne DM, Kaplan SL, et al: Growth hormone treatment for short stature. N Engl J Med 309:1016–1022, 1983.

52. Ward P: The effect of an anabolic steroid on strength and lean body mass. Med Sci Sports 5:227–282, 1973.

53. Welch JM, Aubier M, Jardin M, et al: Effect of caffeine on skeletal muscle function before and after fatigue. J Appl Physiol 54:1303–1305, 1983.

54. Williams MH, Wesseldine S, Somma T, et al: The effects of induced erythrocythemia upon 5-mile treadmill run time. Med Sci Sports Exerc 13:169–175, 1981.

5 Temperature Control, Heat Illness, and Safe Exercise in the Heat

Part I: Temperature Control and Heat Illness

MORRIS B. MELLION, M.D.
GUY L. SHELTON, R.P.T., A.T.C.

As people have increasingly modified their lifestyles to include regular aerobic exercise, especially in the warmer months, physicians have been expected to know more about how the body responds to the combined stresses of exercise and heat. This chapter will (1) explain the basic human mechanisms of temperature regulation; (2) discuss the common syndromes of heat injuries; (3) indicate special populations at high risk; (4) present general guidelines to prevent heat-related injuries; and (5) present relevant considerations for fluids and electrolytes. It is designed to meet the needs of a wide range of athletes, young and old, noncompetitive and high performance.

TEMPERATURE REGULATION

The human body is well adapted to exercise in the heat. Our muscles can generate 20 times as much energy during exercise as they do at rest. Conditioned endurance athletes can generate 1033 Kcal/hr of heat safely for up to three hours.[16] We have a highly efficient thermoregulatory system that allows us to dissipate this heat load into our environment. Otherwise, within 10–15 minutes of beginning intense exercise, our body temperature could rise to life-threatening levels.[10]

Heat Transfer and Heat Dissipation. Most of the heat generated by exercise is transported by the cardiovascular system from the working muscles back to the body core. Only a small amount is conducted passively from muscle through overlying tissue to skin for dissipation. Additionally, a small amount of heat is lost from superficial veins to the adjacent skin as the warmed blood is en route to the heart.

The blood from the working muscles mixes in the heart with the venous return from the rest of the body to form the cardiac output. Early in exercise heat production exceeds heat loss, producing an increase in body core temperature. The rise in core temperature is sensed by thermodetectors in the hypothalamus, spinal cord, and limb muscles, and provides a sympathetically mediated stimulus to increase the skin blood flow and initiate sweating.[16] Additional thermodetectors indicate skin temperature increases to the hypothalamus. High ambient temperature or severe radiant heat from the sun can trigger the heat-dissipating mechanisms even before exercise is begun.[10]

The warm blood from the body's core carries much of its heat load into the dilated vessels of the skin. When the ambient temperature is less than 68°F (20°C), most of the heat loss to the environment is by convection and radiation from the skin. When the environment itself is warm, these mechanisms are inefficient, and above 68°F most of the heat is lost through evaporative cooling.[16] Since the evaporative heat loss of a single liter of water at 30°C is 580 Kcal,[43] and the hypothetical 70-kg individual sweats 1–2 liters per hour during intense exercise in the heat, this is an extremely efficient way to dissipate heat.[10]

After the heat-dissipating mechanisms are brought into play, the core temperature reaches a plateau, where it remains until the exercise demand is past.[36] In elite endurance athletes this level may be as high as 104° F (40° C) without compromising performance. If the heat-dissipating mechanisms fail, or if there is an overwhelming heat stress, the core temperature may continue to rise, even to dangerous levels.

Distribution of Cardiac Output. There are competing demands for cardiac output and plasma volume in the exercising human. During the first 10–20 minutes of exercise, approximately 15% of the intramuscular fluid volume is shunted to the working muscles. Increases of skin blood-flow for cooling shunt additional blood from the central circulation and effectively lower central plasma volume. Additionally, sweating can easily cause losses of 1–2 liters/hour (more in larger athletes), thus causing further losses in plasma volume.

As central blood volume decreases, there is less blood returning to the heart to be pumped. Consequently, stroke volume decreases, and the body attempts to compensate by increasing heart rate in order to maintain cardiac output. Finally a point is reached at which a higher heart rate cannot be maintained. If adjustments are not made to this process, the system will collapse.[16,19,34]

The body does respond. Triggered by baroreceptor signals indicating hypovolemia and by osmolarity measures of hypertonic plasma, the vasomotor center transmits efferent messages that lower skin blood-flow and reduce sweat rate.[10] The obvious problem is that, if the cooling mechanisms are reduced significantly without a concurrent drop in the exercise level, and therefore in the heat load, core temperature may rise dangerously. The athlete can change this process favorably by reducing the exercise load (slowing down), or by building the plasma volume through hypotonic fluid (water) consumption, or preferably both.

Acclimatization and Training Effect. Both acclimatization to exercise in the heat and physical conditioning improve the individual's ability to tolerate heat stress, and the results are to some extent additive. Acclimatization consists of 4–7 episodes of exercise in

the heat for 1–4 hours each, with gradually increasing intensity over approximately 7–10 days for adults and slightly longer for children.[5] Table 1 demonstrates the physiological effects of acclimatization and physical conditioning that enable the athlete to tolerate a high level of exercise heat stress.

Fever, Exercise, and Antipyretics. Stimulated by endotoxin, microbes or immune system components, mononuclear phagocytes release the pyrogen interleukin-1, which, in turn, triggers the hypothalamus to raise the body's core temperature set point. The result is the form of temperature elevation known as fever. Core temperature rises caused by fever are additive to those caused by exercise. Temperature rises caused by fever may be reduced by antipyretics such as aspirin and acetaminophen, whereas those caused by exercising will not respond to these medications.[16,23,39]

EXERTIONAL HEAT ILLNESSES

There are four common syndromes of exercise-induced heat illness. Heat syncope is a transient hypovolemic syncopal episode. Heat cramps, heat exhaustion, and heat stroke form a spectrum of increasingly severe heat illnesses due to dehydration, electrolyte losses, and failure of the body's heat-dissipating mechanisms.

Heat Syncope. If an athlete who is maximally vasodilated and somewhat dehydrated after a workout or competition in the heat stops exercising abruptly and stands still, as some do at the end of a race, he or she may feel lightheaded and faint. Much of the athlete's central blood volume "pools" in the vessels of the lower extremities, and there is too little venous return for the heart to pump an adequate blood flow to the brain. This is a relatively trivial problem. Treatment consists of having the athlete lie down with legs slightly elevated in a cool or shaded place, drink cold water, and rest. Complications and sequelae are rare. This syndrome can be prevented by maintaining adequate hydration before and during exercise, acclimatizing properly to exercise in the heat, and ending exercise sessions with proper cool-down.

Heat Cramps. Heat cramps are a form of

TABLE 1. PHYSIOLOGIC EFFECTS OF ACCLIMATIZATION TO EXERCISE, HEAT STRESS, AND PHYSICAL CONDITIONING

Earlier initiation of sweating[5,10,16,27,34]
Increased rate of sweating[5,7,10,34]
Earlier skin vasodilatation[10,16]
Core and skin temperature lower at given work load and heat stress[5,10,27]
Increased basal plasma volume[19,34]
Heart rate lower at given work load and heat stress[5,27]
Sweat sodium concentration lower[5,27]
Perceived intensity of exercise reduced[5]
Thermal comfort increased[5]

muscle tightening and spasm occurring during or after intense, prolonged exercise in heat. They may be exquisitely painful, and they rarely respond to muscle kneading or massage. Typically, lower leg muscles are affected, but abdominal and intercostal muscles can be involved as well.

Hyponatremia has been implicated as the underlying cause of heat cramps. Typically, this syndrome occurs after prolonged sodium depletion with inadequate dietary replacement between exercise sessions. The already hyponatremic athlete exercises in the heat, loses more sodium in sweat, and then drinks large amounts of water during a break or after exercise. The further dilutional drop in serum sodium triggers the cramps. This problem is common in poorly acclimatized athletes, but it is also seen in well-acclimatized, highly conditioned athletes who lose large amounts of sodium relatively slowly over long bouts of exercise in the heat.[2] It also occurs in athletes on diuretics, particularly during the first few weeks of medication.

Treatment consists of rest and cooling down, gentle stretching, and oral hypotonic salt solutions (1 teaspoon salt/1 quart water). A liter of intravenous normal saline usually provides dramatic relief if these other measures fail.[6] If sodium replenishment fails to remedy heat cramps, evaluation of potassium, calcium, and magnesium levels may provide an answer.

The athlete should always be reminded that heat cramps may be a warning of impending heat exhaustion.

Heat Exhaustion. Heat exhaustion is a serious acute heat injury caused by dehydration, hyponatremia, or both. It is often seen in an unacclimatized athlete who has failed to replace adequately the water and salt lost in sweat for several days. The syndrome is characterized by severe fatigue, profound weakness, lightheadedness, profuse sweating, and nausea. Temperature elevations (103° F or less) and hypotension, if present, are moderate; and the patient usually exhibits a tachycardia.

A variety of "flu-like" symptoms may be present, including headache, myalgias, nausea, vomiting, or diarrhea. Mental status is generally normal or mildly impaired. Loss of consciousness is rare.

Treatment consists of rest, rapid cooling, and fluid electrolyte replacement. Hypotonic fluids may be given orally or intravenously. If cooling and oral fluids fail to induce a clinical improvement, it is generally safe to administer a liter of D5/½ normal saline intravenously over 30–60 minutes while obtaining serum electrolyte levels. When the serum sodium is markedly elevated, it is wise to continue hydration cautiously in order to avoid an iatrogenic cerebral edema.[2]

Heat Stroke. Exertional heat stroke is a medical emergency characterized by extreme hyperthermia, failure of the body's thermoregulatory mechanism, and profound central nervous system dysfunction. The key to the diagnosis is the level of temperature elevation. Rectal temperature is at least 105° F and often is as high as 107° F or 108° F. Frequently, the body's sweating mechanism has failed, and the patient is hot, flushed, and dry. Some patients retain the ability to sweat, but they still exhibit a form of thermoregulatory failure in that they cannot bring their elevated core temperature under control without external cooling. Heat stroke is not spontaneously reversible. Central nervous system impairment varies from confusion, disorientation, and agitation in milder cases to hysterical behavior, delirium, and coma in the more severe situations.

Heat stroke progresses inexorably to cardiovascular and central nervous system collapse unless there is prompt intervention. It involves a myriad of electrolyte and metabolic problems that require careful monitoring and therapy (Table 2) and cause severe complications to virtually every organ system (Table 3).

TABLE 2. COMMON ELECTROLYTE AND METABOLIC ABNORMALITIES IN EXERTIONAL HEAT STROKE

Hyperkalemia or hypokalemia
Hypernatremia or hyponatremia
Hypocalcemia
Hyperphosphatemia
Hypoglycemia
Lactic acidosis
Uremia

Heat Stroke Treatment. The cornerstone of heat stroke management is external cooling, because the patient's own thermal control system has failed. Treatment in the field or in an ambulance may involve removing the victim's clothing and packing him in ice. After transportation to a more controlled setting, such as a hospital emergency room, wetting the patient down with a tepid or cool spray and using a large fan to speed evaporation provide the most effective cooling.[4,15]

Heat stroke patients manifest incipient, if not actual, cardiac, respiratory, and metabolic collapse. Core temperature should be monitored rectally and external cooling may be stopped when the rectal temperature drops to 102° F. Vigorous management, preferably in a modern hospital emergency room or intensive care unit, is necessary. Heat stroke patients frequently require airway management, oxygenation, careful fluid and electrolyte administration, circulatory support, and cardiac, metabolic, and laboratory monitoring.

Similarities between some cases of heat stroke and the malignant hyperthermia syndrome seen in patients undergoing general anesthesia have been noted; and although some authors have suggested treating subsets of heat-stroke patients with dantrolene, the drug's efficacy has not been firmly established in this disease.[22,28,30] Its greatest promise appears to be in heat-stroke patients taking neuroleptic medications which predispose them to heat injury.[28,30,35]

POPULATIONS AT INCREASED RISK

Healthy Individuals. Certain populations are at increased risk for exertional heat injury. Those commonly encountered are listed in Table 4, and many deserve discussion. As already noted, inadequate acclimatization and conditioning create vulnerability. Athletes with lack of experience either in the sport or in exercising in the heat tend to have poorer judgment about heat risk. If the participant has become gradually water- or salt-depleted over several days, susceptibility is increased.

TABLE 3. SEVERE COMPLICATIONS OF HEAT STROKE

Cardiovascular:	Arrhythmias
	Myocardial infarction
	Pulmonary edema
	Shock
Central Nervous System:	Cerebral or spinal infarction
	Coma
	Seizures
Gastrointestinal:	Hepatocellular necrosis
	Upper gastrointestinal bleeding
Hematologic:	Disseminated intravascular coagulation
Musculoskeletal:	Rhabdomyolysis
	Myoglobinemia
Pulmonary:	Adult respiratory distress syndrome
	Pulmonary infarction
Renal:	Acute renal failure

TABLE 4. POPULATIONS AT INCREASED RISK FOR EXERTIONAL HEAT STROKE

HEALTHY INDIVIDUALS
Poorly acclimatized
Poorly conditioned
Inexperienced competitor
Salt or water depletion
Large and/or obese
Age extremes: children, elderly
Previous heat injury
Sleep-deprived
ACUTE ILLNESSES:
Febrile illnesses
Gastrointestinal illnesses
CHRONIC ILLNESSES:
Alcoholism and substance abuse
Cardiac disease
Cystic fibrosis
Diabetes, uncontrolled
Eating disorders
Hypertension, uncontrolled
MEDICATIONS:
Beta blockers, anticholinergics, antihistamines
Diuretics
Neuroleptics

Large athletes, even when well-conditioned, generate more heat to perform the same activity than smaller athletes; moreover, they dissipate the heat less efficiently due to a smaller body surface to mass ratio.[8,41] In addition to these factors, obese individuals have higher tissue temperature elevations for the same heat load because adipose tissue has a lower specific heat than lean tissue. They also have fewer heat-activated sweat glands in areas overlying adipose tissue.[25]

Children are less efficient in the heat than adults. They sweat less and they require a greater increase in core temperature to trigger perspiration. They acclimatize to heat more slowly. Since they have a lower cardiac output at a given metabolic rate, they are more likely to lack sufficient blood flow to maintain their activity level in the heat while providing adequate cooling flow to the skin. Children have a high surface area to body-mass ratio, which works well for them in a temperate environment; but when the sun is strong or temperature is high, they absorb relatively more heat from their environment than adults.[5]

At high levels of heat stress, the elderly are more prone to heat injury. This may be partly related to reduced fitness levels, but there also appears to be an age-related limitation on full heat acclimatization.[25]

Victims of previous heat injury have increased susceptibility to thermal heat stress.[38] This effect may be idiosyncratic, as with the malignant hyperthermia syndrome.[22] It may also be related to decreased work efficiency in the heat.[8] It is unclear whether the susceptibility is entirely premorbid or whether part is due to the effects of the first heat illness itself.

Sleep deprivation lowers both the sweat rate and skin blood-flow responses to exercise heat load.[37]

Acute Illnesses. Febrile illnesses reduce exercise heat tolerance by reducing the heart's ability to maintain cardiac output while, at the same time, increasing the metabolic demand for blood flow throughout the body. Gastrointestinal illnesses compromise heat tolerance by increasing blood flow to the gastrointestinal tract in competition with skin flow and by causing dehydration and electrolyte disturbances due to anorexia, vomiting, and diarrhea.

Chronic Illnesses. Alcohol and substance abuse predispose individuals to heat illness, but it is not clear whether the susceptibility is related to the substances themselves or to the related behaviors. Because many patients with cardiac diseases have reduced cardiac output, they manifest decreased heat-dissipating capacity. Cystic fibrosis patients are at increased risk due to marked sweat sodium losses. Uncontrolled diabetics are at increased risk due to their potassium and water balance problems, but well-controlled insulin-dependent diabetics without microangiopathy or neuropathy exhibit normal heat tolerance.[9] Anorexics and bulimics are prone to exercise-induced heat disorders, both because of their characteristic behaviors, which lead to dehydration and electrolytic disturbances, and because of the frequent obsessive patterns of over-exercise that they exhibit. Unmedicated or inadequately treated essential hypertensives exhibit reductions in heat transfer capacity and skin blood-flow when exercising in the heat.[24]

Medications. Many medications influence the body's capacity for exercise in the heat. This discussion is limited to those commonly demonstrating major effects. Anticholinergics, and, to a lesser extent, antihistamines, may reduce the body's sweating capacity. Beta blockers reduce the cardiac output necessary for heat dissipation. Additionally, noncardioselective beta blockers increase sweat production at a relatively low work load.[14] In a way, this is a protective effect, but it necessitates extra attention to adequate fluid replacement. Diuretics induce a contracted fluid volume that may reduce cardiac output and provide less plasma volume for sweating. They also induce frequent electrolyte abnormalities, which may be more significant in heat stress. Neuroleptic agents predispose to, and may trigger, malignant hyperthermia.

PREVENTION OF HEAT ILLNESS

Heat-related injuries in athletics are best treated through prevention. The adage that "an ounce of prevention is worth a pound of cure" is more than true in cases of heat illness. Several factors must be considered when advising athletes about how to prevent these injuries.

Medical History, Medical Evaluation, Level of Fitness, and Level of Acclimatization. Athletes who are susceptible to heat stress and those with conditions that would predispose them to heat stress should be identified and counselled. The preparticipation athletic evaluation should include screening for the heat stress risk factors listed in Table 4. Further work-up, correction of the risk factor, education of the athlete, and/or restriction of athletic activity should be instituted where appropriate.

Atmospheric Conditions. High levels of heat and humidity severely limit the exercising human body's ability to dissipate heat. Athletes, coaches, athletic trainers, and team physicians need an increased level of awareness of the prevailing atmospheric conditions during practice, competition, or workout. The exercising athlete cannot depend only on "how hot or humid it feels" to judge the situational heat stress from the environment. More objective measurements of temperature and humidity can be compared to published guidelines to give suggested adjustments in exercise intensity, duration, and precautions.

Weather reports from the United States Weather Service or local radio and television stations can provide approximate tempera-

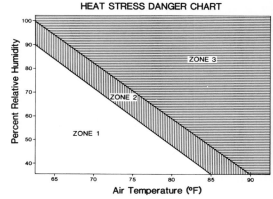

HEAT STRESS DANGER CHART

FIGURE 1. *Heat Stress Danger Chart.* Environmental conditions in **Zone 1** are fairly safe for participation. Normal heat stress precautions should be taken. In **Zone 2**, moderate heat stress precautions should be taken. Workouts should be less intense, shorter, and with more frequent fluid breaks, with more careful observation of individuals at increased risk. In **Zone 3**, heat stress danger is at its greatest. Workouts should be rescheduled to a cooler part of the day. Workouts should be relatively easy. Light clothing and a minimum of equipment should be worn. Extra fluids for everyone and close observation for early heat injury symptoms are essential. (Adapted from Fox EL, Mathews DK: The Physiological Basis of Physical Education and Athletics, 3rd Ed. Philadelphia, Saunders College Publishing, 1981.)

ture and humidity readings. Using Table 5 or Figure 1, relative degrees of heat stress can be determined. This is the most simple and convenient method for athletes involved in fitness, recreational, or individual sports ac-

TABLE 5.   HEAT STRESS*
(APPARENT TEMPERATURES IN ° F.)

		AIR TEMPERATURE (°F)									
		70	75	80	85	90	95	100	105	110	115	120
Relative Humidity (%)	0%	64	69	73	78	83	87	**91**	**95**	**99**	**103**	**107**
	10%	65	70	75	80	85	**90**	**95**	**100**	**105**	**111**	**116**
	20%	66	72	77	82	87	**93**	**99**	**105**	**112**	**120**	**130**
	30%	67	73	78	84	**90**	**96**	**104**	**113**	**123**	**135**	**148**
	40%	68	74	79	86	**93**	**101**	**110**	**123**	**137**	**151**	
	50%	69	75	81	88	**96**	**107**	**120**	**135**	**150**		
	60%	70	76	82	**90**	**100**	**114**	**132**	**144**			
	70%	70	77	85	**93**	**106**	**124**	**144**				
	80%	71	78	86	**97**	**113**	**136**					
	90%	71	79	88	**102**	**122**						
	100%	72	80	**91**	**108**							

DANGER ZONE = +90° F. (temperatures in bold-faced type, above)
*Source: National Weather Service

tivities. However, these remote temperature and humidity readings do not allow for variances due to local geography or distance between the weather reporting site and the workout area.

A *sling psychrometer* (Fig. 2) is used to measure dry bulb (DB) and wet bulb (WB) temperature at the activity site. The relative humidity can then be determined from a chart supplied with the instrument. Table 5 or Figure 1 can be consulted to determine the degree of environmental heat stress for the given workout time. The sling psychrometer is readily available (School Health Supply, Addison, Illinois), reasonably inexpensive, accurate, portable, and easy to learn to use.

The *heat index thermometer* is a more complex and expensive system used to measure DB, WB, and black bulb (BB) temperatures. The BB thermometer is enclosed in a black globe. First used in the military,[31] it provides for a measure of the radiant heat gained in the heat stress index. Figure 3 shows a home-made heat index thermometer system. The Wet Bulb Global Temperature (WBGT) index is then calculated, using the following formula:

$$WBGT = 0.7 \, (WB) + 0.1 \, (DB) + 0.2 \, (BB)$$

The WBGT index can also be determined using a commercially available heat index thermometer (Reuter-Strokes, Cambridge, Ontario).

The WBGT index is compared to published guidelines that indicate relative levels of heat-stress risk and provide suggestions for activity modifications. Such guidelines have been outlined for football[3,7,12,18] and distance running[1,21] and can be adapted for other activities.

Workout Schedule. Identifying stressful environmental conditions has absolutely no benefit unless appropriate steps are taken to adjust the practice or competition schedule. Several authors have suggested various levels of modification in the football practice schedule in the presence of different levels of heat stress.[3,7,12,18] The American College of Sports Medicine[1] has proposed a system of flags to advise race participants of heat stress conditions during races. Each flag color suggests certain adjustments in running intensity.

During times of the year when environmental stress is likely to be the greatest, competition and workouts should be scheduled away from the middle of the day. Other extra precautions should also be taken (Fig. 1). These general suggestions should also be applied to athletes who participate in sports and activities other than football or running.

Clothing. As ambient temperatures increase, evaporation becomes the primary means for the body to dissipate heat. Restrictive clothing can severely limit evaporative cooling. Core temperature, heart rate, and weight loss are significantly increased during exercise in football gear compared to exer-

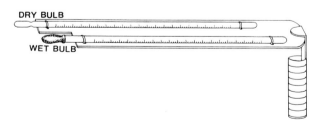

FIGURE 2. *Sling Psychrometer.* Wick on wet bulb is moistened with distilled water and the unit is rotated overhead. Evaporative cooling causes the wet bulb temperature to decrease. The dry bulb and wet bulb readings are used to determine percent of relative humidity.

HEAT INDEX THERMOMETERS

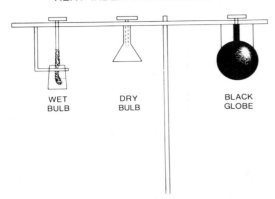

WET BULB   DRY BULB   BLACK GLOBE

FIGURE 3. *Heat Index Thermometers.* Homemade unit consists of three thermometers mounted on a board. The bulb of the wet thermometer is enclosed in a moistened wick. The bulb of the dry thermometer is in an inverted funnel to shield it from direct sunlight. The bulb of the black globe thermometer is enclosed in a black copper globe to absorb radiant energy.

cise in shorts, even in mild environmental conditions.[29] Excessive protective equipment limits the skin-surface area available for evaporative cooling.[3]

Air trapped next to the skin and in the clothing itself creates an insulating layer, limiting convective air currents from assisting evaporation.[17] Rectal temperatures in exercising subjects wearing vapor-impermeable garments are increased significantly compared to those in exercising subjects dressed in vapor-permeable garments.[13] The use of rubberized workout suits creates a super-saturated environment around the skin and limits evaporative cooling. It has been suggested that certain sunscreens containing an oil or gel base allow sweat to run off before evaporative cooling takes place.[42]

Several authors have suggested the use of short-sleeved, short-midriff shirts under football shoulder pads and loose-fitting, open-weave "fishnet" jerseys to facilitate evaporative cooling.[3,12,33,40] Light-colored uniforms[3,12] help reflect radiant energy. Murphy[32] advocates changing sweat-soaked clothing to decrease the humidity directly adjacent to the skin. In males, wearing no shirt further facilitates evaporative cooling but may allow some radiant heat gain.[1]

Body Weight. Hecker and Wheeler[20] showed that acute weight loss of as little as 2% can impair thermoregulatory ability. Greater than 3% weight loss causes deterioration of performance parameters. Dehydration is evidenced by acute weight loss. Therefore, ongoing monitoring of the athletes' weight is a reasonably accurate method of assessing their state of hydration. Several authors have suggested having the athlete weigh before and after workouts.[3,12,32] These recorded weights should be checked daily by the athletic trainer, coach, or other responsible person. Caution should be exercised with individuals showing a practice weight loss of 3%–5%. Particular caution should be conveyed to athletes who have not regained the previous day's weight loss by practice time the next day. This residual weight loss is due to dehydration. Athletes with large or persistent acute weight loss should be restricted from activity until rehydrated.

Observation. Careful observation of athletes identified as being at risk is essential to preventing heat illness. Particular attention should be paid to those athletes who are out of shape or overweight. Athletes who give 100% may not recognize the early signs of heat illness.[40] In extreme environmental heat stress and before acclimatization, all athletes should be watched more carefully for signs of heat illness. Those with excessive practice weight loss and/or failure to rehydrate should be closely monitored, even once their weight is regained.

Education. All people involved with athletics and fitness should have a basic understanding of heat illness, its causes, treatment, and prevention. Medical personnel should be able to provide sound advice on the prevention, recognition, and treatment of various types of heat illness. Good communication with the coaches and athletes is essential.

Coaches must set aside all of the myths that can contribute to additional heat stress.[26] They must be trained to recognize early signs of heat illness and apply appropriate first aid measures. The coach also serves as the coordinator of the prevention program in the absence of an athletic trainer.

The athlete must be taught to recognize the early signs and symptoms of heat illness and the appropriate initial steps to take in treating it. The athlete should have a working knowledge of heat illness prevention principles. Emphasis should be placed on environmental factors, fluid replacement, acclimatization, and clothing. Further, the athlete should be versed in how to adjust his or her training program to accommodate to the heat.

REFERENCES

1. American College of Sports Medicine: Position stand on prevention of thermal injuries during distance running. Sports Medicine Bulletin 19(3):8, 1984.
2. Anderson RJ, Reed G, Knochel J: Heatstroke. Adv Intern Med 28:115–140, 1983.
3. Andrews JR, Massey M, Mullins L, et al: Heat illness in athletes. Journal of the Medical Association of the State of Alabama 45(2):29, 1975.
4. Barner HB, Masar M, Wettach GE, Wright DW: Field evaluation of a new simplified method for cooling heat casualties in desert. Milit Med 149:95–97, 1984.
5. Bar Or O: Climate and the exercising child. In Bar Or O: Pediatric Sports Medicine for the Practitioner: From Physiologic Principles to Clinical Applications. New York, Springer-Verlag, 1983, pp 260–299.
6. Crawshaw JP, Bar Or O, Burch GE, Knochel JP: Hot weather ills: Beating the summer heat syndromes. Patient Care 20(9):66–78, May 15, 1986.
7. Davidson M: Heat illness in athletics. Athletic Training 20(2):96, 1985.
8. Epstein Y, Shapiro Y, Brill S: Role of surface area-to-mass ratio and work efficiency in heat intolerance. J Appl Physiol 54:831–836, 1983.
9. Fortney SM, Koivisto VA, Felig F, Nadel ER: Circulatory and temperature regulatory responses to exercise in a warm environment in insulin-dependent diabetics. Yale J Biol Med 54:101–109, 1981.
10. Fortney SM, Vroman NB: Exercise, performance and temperature control: Temperature regulation during exercise and implications for sports performance and training. Sports Med 2:8–20, 1985.
11. Fox EL, Mathews DK: The Physiological Basis of Physical Education and Athletics (3rd ed). Philadelphia, Saunders College Publishing, 1981.
12. Gieck J: Heat and activity. Athletic Training 9(2):78, 1974.
13. Gonzalez RR, Cena K: Evaluation of vapor permeation through garments during exercise. J Appl Physiol 58(3):928, 1985.
14. Gordon NF: Effect of selective and nonselective beta-adrenergic blockade on thermoregulation during prolonged exercise in the heat. Am J Cardiol 55:74D–78D, 1985.
15. Graham BS, Lichtenstein MJ, Hinson JM, Theil GB: Nonexertional heatstroke: Physiologic management and cooling in 14 patients. Arch Intern Med 146:87–90, 1986.
16. Grisolfi CV, Wenger CB: Temperature regulation during exercise: Old concepts, new ideas. In Terjung, RL (ed): Exercise and Sports Science Review, Vol 12. Lexington, MA, D.C. Heath, 1984, pp 339–372.
17. Guyton AC: Textbook of Medical Physiology (7th ed). Philadelphia, W.B. Saunders Company, 1986.
18. Harrelson GL: The WBGT index. The First Aider (Cramer Products Company), Sept 1983, p 4.
19. Harrison MH: Heat and exercise: Effects on blood volume. Sports Med 3:214–223, 1986.
20. Hecker AL, Wheeler KB: Impact of hydration and energy intake on performance. Athletic Training 19(4):260, 1984.
21. Hughson RL, Staudt LA, Mackie JM: Monitoring road racing in the heat. Phys Sportsmed 11(5): 94, 1983.
22. Jardon OM: Heat stroke, stress, and malignant hyperthermia. Neb Med J 195–199, 1985.
23. Johnson SC, Ruhling RO: Aspirin in exercise-induced hyperthermia: Evidence for and against its role. Sports Med 2:1–7, 1985.
24. Kenney WL: Decreased core-to-skin heat transfer in mild essential hypertensives exercising in the heat. Clin Exp Hypertens A7:1165–1172, 1985.
25. Kenney WL: Physiologic correlates of heat intolerance. Sports Med 2:279–286, 1985.
26. Knochel JP: Dog days and siriasis: How to kill a football player. JAMA 233(6):514, 1975.
27. Kobayashi Y, Ando Y, Takeuchi S, et al: Effects of heat acclimatization of distance runners in a moderately hot environment. Eur J Appl Physiol 45:189–198, 1980.
28. Lydiatt JS, Hill GE: Treatment of heat stroke with dantrolene. JAMA 246:41–42, 1981.
29. Mathews DK, Fox EL, Tanzi D: Physiological responses during exercise and recovery in a football uniform. J Appl Physiol 26(5):611, 1969.
30. Meyers EF, Meyers RW: Thermic stress syndrome. JAMA 247:2098–2099, 1982.
31. Minard D, O'Brien RL: Heat casualties in the Navy and Marine Corps, 1959–1962, with appendices on the field use of the wet globe thermometer index. U.S. Navy Medical Research Institute Report 7:1,1964.
32. Murphy RJ: Heat illness. J Sports Med 1(4):26, 1973.
33. Murphy RJ: Heat illness in the athlete. Am J Sports Med 12(4):258, 1984.
34. Nadel ER: Recent advances in temperature regulation during exercise in humans. Fed Proc 44:2286–92, 1985.
35. Paasuke RT: Drugs, heat stroke, and dantrolene. Can Med Assoc J 130:341–343, 1984.
36. Pugh LGE, Corbett JL, Johnson RH: Rectal temperatures, weight losses, and sweat rates in marathon running. J Appl Physiol 23:347–352, 1967.
37. Sawka MN, Gonzalez RR, Pandolf KB: Effects of sleep deprivation on thermoregulation during exercise. Am J Physiol 23:347–352, 1967.
38. Shapiro Y, Magazanik A, Udassin R, et al: Heat intolerance in former heatstroke patients. Ann Intern Med 90:913–916, 1979.

39. Simon HB: Extreme hyperpyrexia. Hosp Pract 21(5A):123–129, 1986.
40. Spickard A: Heat stroke in college football and suggestions for prevention. South Med J 61:791, 1968.
41. Wailgum TD, Paolone AM: Heat tolerance of college football linemen and backs. Phys Sportsmed 12:81–86, 1984.
42. Wells, TD, Jessup GT, Langlotz KS: Effects of sunscreen use during exercise in the heat. Phys Sportsmed 12(6):132, 1984.
43. Wenger CB: Heat of evaporation of sweat: Thermodynamic considerations. J Appl Physiol 32:456–9, 1972.

Part II: Fluids and Electrolytes

ANN C. GRANDJEAN, M.S., R.D.

The subject of fluids and electrolytes is important in all of medicine, and sports medicine is certainly no exception. Water, more than electrolytes, has a crucial role in athletic endeavors, especially in thermoregulation. Hypohydration can not only affect performance but also cause serious physical disorders, even death, if not managed properly.

WATER

Water has many functions in the body. One extremely important function of water in the athlete is thermal regulation. Normally, body heat is dissipated by convection and radiation, but when large amounts of metabolic heat are produced, such as by muscular exercise, these systems are not sufficient and sweating becomes the primary cooling system.

It is important that the athlete understand the role of sweating in maintaining body temperature and the importance of replacing the lost water. A survey of 171 college athletes revealed that 86% knew that drinking ample amounts of water during events and practices helps to prevent heat exhaustion.[12] However, the athletes were not as knowledgeable about questions pertaining to the amount of water they should drink; 53% of athletes did not know *how much* water was adequate and erred on the side of under-consumption. This study indicated that educators of athletes have been fairly successful in stressing the importance of water; however, they have not adequately provided usable measures of optimal intake.

It has long been known that dehydration can affect both body temperature and performance. Pitts et al.[33] demonstrated that without water, rectal temperature rose steadily to high levels with no sign of reaching a steady state, and that without water for the first hour, even though water was available ad libitum after that time, rectal temperature continued to increase. Their study also revealed that thirst is not a sensitive indicator of water need, that consumption of water combats all undesirable changes seen in dehydration, and that, in general, the more nearly water intake approximates sweat loss the better off the subject. Unfortunately, more than 40 years later, this information has still not been received and/or accepted by some coaches and athletes, and deaths continue to be caused by heat stroke.[2,30]

Hypohydration can cause decrements in performance and the impact can be immediate.[1] Olsson and Saltin[32] noted that several studies have shown that a reduction in body water causes pronounced impairment of work ability and that increases in body temperature and pulse rate occur when there is fluid loss corresponding to 1% of body weight.

A sweat loss equal to as little as 2–3% of body weight can cause measurable impairments of cardiovascular performance and thermal regulation.[31] Additionally, unreplaced water loss may cause reductions in strength, power, endurance, and aerobic work capacity in some athletes.[35,38]

Several athletic events require nonstop strenuous performance for an hour or more. Such athletic events are collectively referred to as endurance events and include such sports as long-distance running, road cycling, and cross-country skiing. It is well established that prolonged exercise may lead to a state of hypohydration and that success in endurance events is closely related to the cardiovascular capacity for oxygen transport.[10] During endurance events, the amount of oxygen that can be delivered to the exercising muscles depends on the volume of blood available for distribution and the ability to divert large amounts to the working muscles. Any factor that compromises the blood flow to the muscle will impair performance. Marathon runners can incur sweat losses in excess of 6 liters during a race, and, despite efforts to ingest fluids, body weight may be reduced by 8%[8]

The obvious goal for the athlete is to replace water that is lost and to prevent hypohydration. There are well-documented benefits to ingesting fluids during endurance events, especially during hot weather. Hypohydration can be acute or chronic. For example, chronic fluid loss can result from cumulative water loss on consecutive days of football practice.[9]

Thirst is not an adequate indicator of water need for the exercising athlete. When Pitts et al.[33] offered subjects water as desired, the subjects were not able to maintain normal body temperature. The authors observed "It should be emphasized that during work men never voluntarily drink as much water as they sweat, even though this is advantageous for maintaining heat balance, but usually drink at a rate approximating about two-thirds of the water loss in sweat."

Mechanisms of drinking have been studied extensively in laboratory animals but comparatively little information is available on human consumption of fluid.[13] Unlike some mammals, humans have a delay in rehydration (involuntary dehydration) after fluid loss. According to Greenleaf, two factors unique to humans that probably contribute to involuntary dehydration are upright posture and extracellular fluid and electrolyte loss by sweating from exercise and heat exposure.

The most accurate method of monitoring hydration is for athletes to weigh themselves, nude, before and after practice sessions or competitions. Monitoring daily weights over a period of time will not only help to identify athletes who sweat heavily, but will also help coaches and trainers identify athletes who may be suffering from cumulative hypohydration.

A major consideration in fluid replacement is how rapidly the fluid empties from the stomach. A number of factors affect the rate of gastric emptying, including the type of drink, volume, temperature, and osmolality.[11] Larger volumes (500 to 600 ml) empty more rapidly from the stomach; however, smaller amounts, 150 to 250 ml, every 10 to 15 minutes, may be easier for an athlete to handle.[6] Cold fluids are reported to empty from the stomach faster than warmer fluids.[36] Drinks containing large amounts of carbohydrate

(sucrose, fructose, and galactose) or electrolytes can delay gastric emptying and result in dehydration.[4] Water is the fluid of choice for replacing sweat losses.

Please note the handout titled "The Athlete's Most Important Nutrient—Water," which appears at the end of this chapter.

ELECTROLYTES

Although sweat is composed primarily of water, it does contain a number of nutrients. Three of these nutrients—sodium, chloride, and potassium—function as electrolytes and are often added to sport drinks that are designed and promoted to replace sweat losses incurred during exercise.

Electrolytes play a fundamental role in regulation of body water distribution in various fluid compartments. Sodium, in particular, has a major influence on fluid regulation. Changes in the extracellular concentration of sodium will stimulate adjustments in thermal regulation, water and ion excretion, and drinking behavior. Electrolytes are essential to muscle and nerve excitation, electromechanical coupling in muscle contraction, and enzymatic control of cellular reactions.

Theoretically, any great disturbance in the balance of electrolytes in body fluids could interfere with performance. Electrolyte supplementation during heavy physical work with profuse sweating is based on the concept that large quantities of electrolytes are lost in sweat and need to be replaced. The electrolytes that have been the subject of the most research are sodium, chloride, and potassium.

Table 1 compares the concentrations of sodium and chloride in sweat to those in other body fluids. Compared with other body fluids, sweat is hypotonic. The ionic concentration of sweat varies among individuals, however, and is influenced by the rate of sweat, the athlete's state of heat acclimatization, and the dietary intake of electrolytes.[7,9] Excessive sweating during heavy physical activity can produce large losses that can potentially disturb fluid and electrolyte balances.

Costill et al.[6] dehydrated subjects by 3% of

TABLE 1. ELECTROLYTE CONCENTRATIONS AND OSMOLALITY IN SWEAT, MUSCLE, AND PLASMA*

	ELECTROLYTES (mmol/L)				OSMOLARITY (mOsmol/L)
	Na	*Cl*	*K*	*MG*	
Sweat	40-60	30-50	4-5	1.5-5	80-185
Plasma	140	101	4	1.5	302
Muscle	9	9	162	31	302

*From Costill DL, Miller JM, with permission.[9]

of body weight on five successive days. During the first five-day sequence, the subjects replaced fluid losses with a glucose-electrolyte solution, whereas water was the only fluid ingested during a second five-day series. Water and electrolyte losses in sweat and urine revealed a positive balance for body sodium, potassium, and chloride during both the water and glucose-electrolyte solution treatments. If the supplemental electrolytes provided in the electrolyte drink were needed to offset excessive water and electrolyte losses incurred during the dehydration, it would be expected that the subjects would retain a portion of the electrolytes provided. Apparently, the needs for sodium, potassium, and chloride were adequately met by food intake with no need for electrolyte supplementation. This was evidenced by a larger loss of electrolytes in urine during the electrolyte solution experiment. The additional urine excretion of these electrolytes during the electrolyte solution treatment were nearly identical to the daily quantities of the electrolytes consumed in the electrolyte solution. The researchers thus concluded that the addition of electrolytes to drinking water is of minimal value for subjects who dehydrate 3% of body weight on repeated days if they are permitted to ingest food and drink ad libitum. Although the investigators limited the food items the subjects could consume during the study, they did not report the levels of electrolytes ingested in the diet. Food intake was ad libitum but discretionary use of salt was not allowed. Most subjects indicated that they would have added salt to some food items if permitted. Therefore, an additional variable in this study may have been reduced sodium intake.

Sodium

Sodium is the mineral most affected by physical exercise, and studies have shown that sodium deficiency can impair performance. For this reason, salt tablets and electrolyte beverages have become popular among many athletes; however, they are unnecessary.

It is widely believed by athletes and coaches that heat cramps are caused by an inadequate sodium intake. While this may be true on a cumulative basis, sodium deficiency will not produce heat cramps in a single day even under the most severe environment conditions.[3] Replacement of salt is not an immediate problem in that salt need not be replaced on an hourly basis. It can be replaced at the end of the day. However, replacement day by day, especially during acclimatization, is important and must be made prior to another day of heat exposure and heavy physical activity. The best method of maintaining salt balance is by salting food during meals.[3]

Exercise-induced sweating initiates renal conservation of sodium. Under extreme conditions, athletes who sweat profusely, who are not acclimated to working in the heat, or who have low sodium intakes may experience heat cramps or exhaustion due to sodium depletion. This can be easily prevented or treated by consuming foods high in sodium (salted snack foods, ham, pizza) or by adding salt to food at meals. For those who prefer to use salt water during practice, the concentration should be no more than 1 tablespoon of salt per gallon of water.

Salt tablets are irritating to the stomach and can increase the danger of dehydration. Electrolyte beverages generally have a high osmolality and can cause fluid retention in the stomach and intestines.[19] The greater the sugar content of the drink, the slower the rate of emptying. A gastric emptying time is increased for beverages with a glucose or sucrose concentration of more than 2.5% (2.5 gm/100 ml). If an athlete uses any of the "sport beverages" or commercial preparations, they should be diluted with water to decrease the concentration of sugar and therefore decrease the time the fluid stays in the stomach. Recommended dilutions are given in Table 2.

TABLE 2. DILUTION FACTOR

The following replacement fluids should be diluted:

Fruit Juices	1 part juice: 3 parts water
Soft Drinks	1 part pop: 3 parts water
Vegetable Juices	1 part juice: 1 part water
Gatorade	1 part drink: 1 part water
Pripps Pluss	1 part drink: 3 parts water
Quickick (orange flavor)	1 part drink: 3 parts water

Sport drinks that use glucose polymers as the carbohydrate source are beginning to appear on the market. The use of polymers increases the amount of carbohydrate contained in the beverage per 100 ml without changing the osmotic concentration. A 5-7% polymer solution is equivalent to water in terms of gastric emptying time.

Pitts and colleagues[33] and Rose[34] conducted several studies evaluating the effect on performance of water, saline solutions (0.1%, 0.2%, and 10%), and salt tablets. Ingestion of water, 0.1% saline, and 0.2% saline resulted in good performance. Salt tablets and 10% saline resulted in "a distressing situation" (gastrointestinal disturbances) for the subjects.

Overloading with salt has also been associated with body potassium depletion. It has been suggested that there is a direct relationship between potassium depletion and the high incidence of heat stroke among troops in training or in athletes during preseason conditioning.[3]

Potassium

Potassium plays an essential role in muscular contraction and nerve conduction. It helps in the transport of glucose across cell membranes and in the storage of glycogen, thus playing an important role in the energy schema. Potassium is lost in sweat, although levels are not exceptionally high and losses can be replaced with a balanced diet. If potassium losses are not replaced, however, hypokalemia could adversely affect physical performance.[18] Sodium supplementation has been the traditional procedure for preventing heat stress. Knochel and Vertel[16] cautioned that the indiscriminate use of salt by a heat-acclimatized person could lead to serious potassium depletion and resultant abnormalities in carbohydrate and protein metabolism, electrochemical effects, renal function, and specific enzymatic function. Additionally, potassium depletion may play a role in the type of heat illness seen after a week or two of training.[15]

The effect of potassium supplementation on potassium balance in athletes performing vigorous exercise in a hot, humid environment was investigated by Lane et al.[17] Seven healthy males who ran 9 to 10 miles twice daily served as subjects. During two different tests the subjects were given either a "high" or "low" potassium beverage. They drank 9.60 ml/kg of body weight of a supplement 1 to 2 hours before their afternoon run. The "low potassium" and "high potassium" beverages contained 4.3 and 98.25 mEq potassium/liter respectively. Both also contained sodium and glucose. The control beverage was "zero potassium" and consisted of sodium chloride and water. Fecal, urinary, and sweat losses of potassium and sodium were measured and total body potassium was determined using a whole body counter. The results indicated that the potassium requirements of subjects doing hard physical work in hot climates are much higher than those recommended by the National Academy of Sciences. The investigators concluded that the potassium requirement of athletes running 9 to 10 miles in an hour is greater than 3.0 gm/day.

Costill and Miller[9] reviewed the nutritional needs of endurance athletes. They noted that during acute bouts of prolonged exercise in the heat, endurance athletes must ingest fluids to minimize dehydration and the threat of hyperthermia. Electrolyte concentration of sweat varies markedly among individuals and is strongly influenced by the rate of sweating (which varies greatly) and the athlete's state of heat acclimatization. Despite the electrolyte losses incurred, the endurance athlete probably maintains a positive sodium, potassium, and chloride balance by dietary intake and renal conservation, provided that food and drink are provided ad libitum.

In an attempt to study the changes in potassium content of muscle and blood during repeated days of heavy exercise and sweating, Costill et al.[5] tested subjects during two exercise regimens. In one sequence, the diets contained 80 mEq of potassium, while 25 mEq was provided in the other. Sodium intake in both regimens was 190 mEq. Electrolyte analysis of muscle biopsies, blood, sweat, and urine was performed. The researchers found that despite their efforts to induce a body potassium deficit by combining heavy exercise/sweating with repeated days of a low potassium diet, there was no indication that muscle tissue potassium was significantly reduced. The investigators did qualify the results by stating that their results do not preclude the possibility that potassium deficits could occur when dietary sodium intake is large and sodium potassium excretion is substantially greater than those seen in their study. It must also be considered that four days is not a long enough period for a cumulative potassium deficiency to occur.

In a discussion of the prevention of heat disorders in sports, Smith[37] observed:

Recent balance studies have demonstrated that the athletes who are training most actively will replace all electrolytes and nutrient losses in sweat with the electrolytes and nutrients contained in a mixed diet that is sufficient in amount to satisfy their energy needs. Electrolyte-containing beverages and salt tablets in particular serve no purpose, are needlessly expensive, and are potentially dangerous.

Athletes and coaches should be advised about the adverse effects of using the so-called athlete drinks and sport beverages for replacing sweat losses.... As a result of their hypertonicity, they leave the stomach very slowly, which produces a sensation of satiety that discourages the athlete from ingesting much needed water.

There is currently no substantial evidence to support the use of supplements or potassium-rich beverages or electrolyte beverages containing potassium, even for individuals who perform prolonged exercise in the heat on repeated days.[14] Under such conditions daily potassium losses remain low and can easily be offset by increasing the natural potassium-containing foods in the diet. Ingestion of potassium in chemical forms should be discouraged because of the possibility of sharp elevation of plasma potassium and risk of cardiac toxicity.

A typical mixed diet should provide ap- proximately 1950 to 5850 mg/day potassium.[19] Potassium needs can be met by including potassium-rich foods in the daily diet (Table 3).

SUMMARY

Plain cold water is the most effective replacement fluid for athletes before, during, and after exercise. The need to replace body water is far greater than any immediate need for electrolytes. A typical diet should provide adequate amounts of sodium, chloride, and potassium, and other nutrients to replace sweat losses.

TABLE 3. FOODS THAT PROVIDE 5.0 mEq (200 mg) OR MORE OF POTASSIUM PER AVERAGE SERVING

CEREALS		
	All Bran	Bran Buds
	100% Bran	Bran Chex
FISH		
	Bass	Perch
	Carp	Pike
	Catfish	Pollack
	Cod	Red snapper
	Flounder	Salmon
	Haddock	Sole
	Halibut	Tuna
	Herring	
FRUITS		
	Apricots	Orange Juice
	Banana	Pear-fresh
	Blackberries	Prune juice
	Cantaloupe	Prunes
	Grapefruit juice	Rhubarb
	Honeydew melon	Strawberries
	Orange	Tangelos
MEAT		
	Beef	Pork (except
	Lamb	bacon)
		Veal
MILK		
	Buttermilk	Skim
	Lowfat	Whole
VEGETABLES		
	Asparagus	Kidney beans
	Avocado	Mustard greens
	Black-eyed peas	Parsnips
	Broccoli	Potato
	Brussels sprouts	Pumpkin
	Cabbage—raw	Radishes
	Green pepper	Spinach
	Lentils	Squash—winter
	Lima beans	Tomato
	Kale	Zucchini

REFERENCES

1. Armstrong LE, Costill DL, Fink WJ: Influence of diuretic-induced dehydration on competitive running performance. Med Sci Sports Exercise 17: 456–461, 1985.
2. Committee on Nutritional Misinformation: Water Deprivation and Performance of Athletes, A Statement of the Food and Nutrition Board. Washington, DC, National Academy of Sciences, May 1974.
3. Consolazio CF: Nutrition and performance. In Johnson RE (ed): Progress in Food and Nutrition, Vol. 7. Oxford, Pergamon Press, 1983.
4. Costill DL: Water and electrolyte requirements during exercise. Clin Sports Med 3:639, 1984.
5. Costill DL, Cote R, Fink W: Dietary potassium and heavy exercise: effects on muscle water and electrolyte. Am J Clin Nutr 36:266–275, 1982.
6. Costill DL, Cote R, Miller E, et al: Water and electrolyte replacement during repeated days of work in the heat. Aviation Space Environ Med 46:795–800, 1975.
7. Costill DL, Gisolfi C, Murphy RJ, Westerman RL: Balancing heat stress, fluids, and electrolytes. 43:52, 1975.
8. Costill DL, Kammer WF, Fisher A: Fluid ingestion during distance running. Arch Environ Health 21:520–525, 1970.
9. Costill DL, Miller JM: Nutrition for endurance sport: carbohydrate and fluid balance. Internat J Sports Med 1:2–14, 1980.
10. Costill DL, Sparks K: Rapid fluid replacement following thermal dehydration. J Appl Physiol 34:299–303, 1973.
11. Costill DL, Saltin B: Factors limiting gastric emptying during rest and exercise. J Appl Physiol 37:679, 1974.
12. Grandjean AC, Hursh, LM, Majure WC, Hanley DF: Nutrition knowledge and practices of college athletes. Med Sci Sports Exercise 13:82, 1981.
13. Greenleaf JE: The body's need for fluids. In Haskel W, Scala J, Whittam J (eds): Nutrition and Athletic Performance. Palo Alto, CA, Bull Publishing, 1982.
14. Herbert WG: Water and electrolytes. In Williams MH (ed): Ergogenic Aids in Sports. Champaign, IL, Human Kinetics Publishers, 1983.
15. Knochel JP: Potassium deficiency during training in the heat. Ann Acad Sci 301:175–189, 1977.
16. Knochel JP, Vertel RM: Salt loading as a possible factor in the production of potassium depletion, rhabdomyolysis, and heat injury. Lancet 9:659–661, 1967.
17. Lane HW, Roessler GS, Nelson EW, Cerda JJ: Effect of physical activity on human potassium metabolism in a hot and humid environment. Am J Clin Nutr 31:838–843, 1978.
18. Macaraeg PVJ: The importance of fluid and electrolytes in athletics. J Sports Med Phys Fitness, 14:213–217, 1974.
19. Manjarrez C, Birrer R: Nutrition and athletic performance. Fam Phys 28:105, 1983.
30. Mueller FO, Schnidler RD: Annual Survey of Football Injury Research 1931–1985. Orlando, FL, The American Football Coaches Association, 1986.
31. Nadel ER, Fortney SM, Wenger CB: Effect of hydration state on circulatory and thermal regulations. J Appl Physiol: Respirat Environ Exercise Physiol 49:715–721, 1980.
32. Olsson KE, Saltin B: Diet and fluids in training and competition. Scand Rehabil 3:31–38, 1971.
33. Pitts GC, Johnson RE, Consolazio CF: Work in the heat as affected by intake of water, salt, and glucose. Am J Physiol 142:253, 1944.
34. Rose KD, Schneider PJ, Sullivan GF: A liquid pregame meal for athletes, report on a field trial. JAMA 178:30–33, 1961.
35. Sawka MN, Francesconi RP, Young AJ, Pandolf KB: Influence of hydration level and body fluids on exercise performance in the heat. JAMA 252:1165–1169, 1984.
36. Shephard RJ: Physiology and biochemistry of exercise. New York, Praeger, 1982.
37. Smith NJ: The prevention of heat disorders in sports. Am J Dis Child 138:786–790, 1984.
38. Williams MH: Nutritional Aspects of Human Physical and Athletic Performance, 2nd ed. Springfield, IL, Charles C Thomas, 1985.

The Athlete's Most Important Nutrient—Water

Water loss for an athlete can be critical and, in severe cases, can lead to death. Maintaining an adequate level of water in the body can be easy if you understand the importance of water and you remember to weigh.

The body cools itself much like the cooling system of an automobile. As muscles produce the energy needed for training and competition, they generate heat. This heat, in turn, causes your body temperature to rise. Blood picks up heat from the muscles and carries it to the skin's surface, where it is lost as sweat evaporates. Sweat is your body's main method for cooling itself.

As you sweat, you lose water—water which must be replaced if you want to perform your best. Losing as little as 2 to 3 percent of your weight via sweat can cause a decrease in concentration, coordination, strength and stamina. More importantly, if lost water is not replaced, your body begins to conserve water by slowing the sweating and, thus, the cooling process.

YOU MUST REPLACE LOST WATER.

This is especially important when rising temperatures combine with high humidity. As temperatures rise, sweating is the main means of keeping the body cool. However, as humidity worsens, evaporation of sweat is slowed.

If you think of the air as a paper towel, a dry towel (low humidity) will easily absorb sweat. A wet paper towel (high humidity) absorbs little. You may appear to sweat more in high humidity, but the moisture that appears is not evaporating, which greatly lessens the cooling effect—and further reinforces the need to replenish lost water.

Normally you need an average of two liters (eight glasses) of water a day. During competition or training, some athletes lose as much as three to five liters of water, and even more in hot, humid weather.

Thirst is not always the best indicator that the body needs water. In addition to drinking water before, during and after practice or competition, you should keep a close watch on weight changes that occur. Weighing before and after competition or practice will help determine how much water you have lost. One-half liter (16 ozs.) of water equals one pound. If drinking water doesn't achieve water recovery, the team physician should be consulted.

The most common form of heat illness results from a large loss of body water. Aiding in its development is the wearing of sweatsuits and other clothing that prevent evaporation. This slows the cooling process and causes body temperature to rise. To prevent heat illness such as cramps, exhaustion and heat stroke, you should wear light, loose clothing that allows free circulation of air; move to the shade for rest and water breaks; and drink water before, during and after practice sessions or competition.

Finally, do not take salt tablets. Water will be pulled from the body to dilute the salt. If the team physician or trainer feels that additional salt is needed, it should be added to food at meals or you should eat salty foods such as ham, nuts, chips or other snack foods.

Prepared by the Swanson Center for Nutrition and the United States Olympic Committee. The reader is invited to photocopy this page for distribution to individual athletes and teams.

6 Special Issues in Youth Sports

MORRIS B. MELLION, M.D.

One of the most difficult tasks facing the physician who treats children is to counsel them and their parents about a broad range of perplexing, often controversial, issues involving youth sports. Questions about organized sports programs, weight lifting, safety, motivation, and injuries often indicate both a desire for information and a need for family guidance in dealing with important matters. This chapter examines some of the more commonly encountered issues that transcend the boundaries of sports, medicine, psychology, and physiology.

ORGANIZED COMPETITIVE YOUTH SPORTS

"Should my child play competitive sports?" How many times does the practicing physician encounter this simple question to which there is no simple answer? The increasing popularity of organized competitive youth sports has paralleled the growing recognition that physical fitness is a basic component of a healthy lifestyle for all ages. It is important to understand that children are not merely small adults, and their needs are not the same as those of their parents. Youth sports programs, properly organized and run, offer an excellent opportunity for a positive growth experience for children. Unfortunately, not all youths sports programs live up to this potential.

Effective Coaching

The key to a successful youth sports program is the coach, particularly at the entry level. There are approximately 20 million children coached by 2.5 million adult volunteers participating in nonschool youth sports programs.[23] Many of these volunteer coaches have little or no formal training and tend to fall back on their past sports experience, usually at the high school or college level, for coaching young children. On the other hand, there are training programs that teach the educational and motivational skills essential to good coaching.

In order to meet the training needs of prospective youth coaches Rainer Martens, Ph.D., a leading sports psychologist, founded the American Coaches Effectiveness Program (ACEP). ACEP sponsors coaching effectiveness clinics to prepare entry level coaches and leadership clinics to train coaching effectiveness instructors around the country. The YMCA, the Boys Clubs of America, 19 of the 37 National Governing Bodies of Olympic Sports, a long list of other national and state sports organizations, as well as many colleges and universities use the ACEP. Table 1 provides the addresses of ACEP and two other major organizations concerned with the training and competency of youth coaches.

Coaching Young Athletes, the text for ACEP level 1 Courses, is available to the public.[24] The authors start from the premise "Athletes First—Winning Second." By doing so, they confront the central issue. Youth sports have value only in as much as they contribute to the child's *growth* as a person and as an athlete while simultaneously providing an opportunity for the child to have *fun.* We live in an extremely competitive society, in which the notion of "winning" in sports is carried to almost every home virtually every day by electromagnetic waves. Television sports are an entertainment medium in which the focus on winning and the hype of stardom tend to

TABLE 1. ORGANIZATIONS CONCERNED WITH THE TRAINING AND COMPETENCY OF YOUTH COACHES

American Coaching Effectiveness Program
P. O. Box 5076
Champaign, IL 61820

Canadian National Certification Program
Coaching Association of Canada
333 River Road
Ottawa K1L 8H9
Canada

National Youth Sports Coaches Association
2611 Okeechobee Road
West Palm Beach, FL 33409

be overemphasized. It is important that these exaggerations not be carried over to the sports experience of youngsters.

Although we are rightly concerned with the threat to our children of an unbridled concentration on winning, there is a legitimate merit to competition, which Martens defines as "a process of striving for a valued goal." Indeed, youth sports may provide an excellent setting in which to teach children about achieving a balance between competition and cooperation in their lives.[22] "The intensity of competition should be low, increasing only as the children's skill level and interest increase."[25]

A high level of self-esteem is essential for emotional health, and research has shown that children led by coaches with effectiveness training made significant gains in self-esteem when compared to a control group supervised by untrained coaches. Moreover, "it is the low self-esteem child who probably is in the greatest need of a positive athletic experience and who appears to respond most favorably to the desirable coaching practices and most unfavorably to negative practices."[37] The coach makes the biggest impact on the most vulnerable children. The well trained coach can provide the most positive experience for the child who needs it the most.

Parents of Athletes

The other major influence determining the quality of a child's experience in organized sports is the role the parents play. The interactions among athlete, parents, and coach are so important that the relationship is often called the "athletic triangle." With skillful parenting and coaching the triangle is filled with fun and growth (Fig. 1); but when the skill is lacking, the triangle may be hollow.

Parental involvement can produce a wide variety of responses ranging from pleasure and elation to anger and sadness in the young athlete. Parents who know how to encourage their children's efforts and praise their successes, no matter how small, enhance the sports experience greatly. Those who are overly critical about their children's performance may trigger an undesired response that endures long after the time spent on the playing field.

Here again, self-esteem is the issue. Children tend to view their worlds globally. Frequent criticism of their performance on the athletic field may lead children to think that they are a general disappointment to their parents. This reaction may diminish their self-esteem and reduce their motivation to perform well, not only in athletics but also in other aspects of their lives as well.

There is a particularly difficult type of parent who may be appropriately called "The Vicarious Athlete." This parent pressures the child to excel in athletics so that the parent can experience the child's successes vicariously. The Vicarious Athlete generally recruits the spouse into an alliance in which they both provide an extremely confining bizarre form of support and encouragement for the child. They may become overly in-

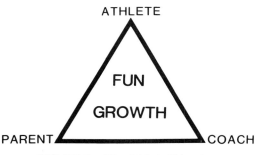

FIGURE 1. The Athletic Triangle.

volved in the administration and logistics of the youth sports program often to the point of manipulating the coach or other parents. They place ever increasing expectations on their child-athlete. In response, the child must narrow his or her athletic participation to a single sport, which then becomes a year-round endeavor. The parents reward improving performance with a seemingly never-ending round of athletic camps and sports clinics in order to ensure their child's path to championship. The normal activities of childhood are set aside to allow more time for practice. If the child has the natural potential to become a truly elite athlete, this process may go on for many years.

Most children of Vicarious Athletes reach a point at which they can no longer achieve the ever increasing expectations of their parents. The children have been trapped in this aberrant parent-child relationship for so many years that it is unthinkable to tell the parents that it is time to stop. Instead, they develop an injury that is typical of their sport. Gymnasts get back pain, skiers get knee pain, and swimmers get shoulder pain. When these children present in the physician's office, they present a major diagnostic challenge. Are they elite athletes with overuse injuries, as their parents contend; or are they burned out child athletes in whom the pain is a psychosomatic attempt to get out of what they subconsciously, or perhaps consciously, perceive is a trap their parents have set? The answer to the physician's dilemma is rarely obtained in one or two visits but over time as the patient has the opportunity either to heal or reveal the underlying problem. In the latter case, the physician's task at hand is to help the family establish a new basis for communications to replace the child's athletic career so that the child may branch out to perform many of the other activities of normal childhood which had been previously set aside.

Fortunately, most parents do not fall into this pattern. They are able to let their children know that they are loved for what they are, not for how they perform, either on the playing field or in the classroom. The important issue is that the child learns that his or her worth is as a person, not as a performer.

Parents as Coaches

"Should I coach my own child?" This question is asked so often in youth sports. The answer usually is found in practical necessity. Since one coach is needed for roughly every eight children, and there are 20 million children participating in organized youth sports in the United States, many parents will find that they have to coach in order to provide an opportunity for their children to play.

It is a major challenge for parents to coach their own children, but one that can be met with proper training and preparation. The first step in meeting this challenge is to undergo ACEP or other coaching effectiveness training. If this training is not available through the community league or the local YMCA, assistance in finding or even establishing a coaching effectiveness program can usually be obtained by contacting the physical education department of a nearby college or state university.

The trained parent-coach will still have to walk the fine line between appearing too critical or too approving of his or her own child at practice or during a competition. It is helpful to learn to focus approval or criticism to the specific effort made or skill demonstrated. Global criticism is never appropriate with children. Parent-coaches are generally well advised to praise their own children's efforts moderately on the field and more generously in the car on the way home.

ISSUES OF PARTICIPATION

Age Guidelines. Children vary in their rates of emotional and physical maturity; consequently, there is no specific age at which all children should begin to participate in organized or competitive sports. Generally, children will cue their parents in many subtle and not-so-subtle ways that they are ready to play. Guidelines currently accepted by physical educators based on average rates of maturity are provided in Table 2.

Maturity and Matching. One of the most difficult problems in organized youth sports is how to organize the programs into dif-

AGE	TYPE OF SPORT	EXAMPLES
6	Noncontact	Swimming Tennis Track and field
8	Contact	Basketball Soccer Wrestling
10	Collision	Tackle football Ice Hockey

*Adapted from Martens R: The uniqueness of the young athlete: Psychological considerations. Am J.Sports Med 8:382–385, 1980.

ferent levels of participation. The problem is most acute in the peripubertal years because the hormonal changes of puberty accelerate growth in size, strength, coordination, and endurance, as well as epiphyseal closure. The onset of puberty varies normally from 8.5 to 13.0 years in girls and 9.5 to 13.5 years in boys. Even more significantly, the period of most rapid growth, known as peak height velocity, varies greatly as well, averaging 12.1 years in girls and 14.1 years in boys.[20,21]

Traditionally, children have been matched by age or grade in school. This method results in frequent mismatches in size, strength, speed, and agility and weakens the quality of the sports program. A much preferred method is to match participants, especially in contact and collision sports, by level of sexual maturation using the generally accepted Tanner scales.[20,21] In pubertal girls age at menarche is also extremely useful. Matching by sexual maturation requires a very tactful sensitive approach. The greatest problem for this method is that it often cuts across school grades and other social patterns.

Boys and Girls Together? "Should boys and girls play organized sports together on the same teams?" This question was rarely, if ever, seriously asked until the 1970s. As social assumptions have changed, however, physicians and physical educators have addressed the issue. There is now a general consensus that prepubertal boys and girls can

play together without concern for increased physical or emotional risk.[4]

After puberty, the situation is much more complicated. The differences in strength and size between pubertal and postpubertal boys and girls is often great enough to pose an increased risk for coeducational participation in contact or collision sports. This risk is only one factor, however, because in most situations where schools or sports leagues have resisted participation by girls in boys' sports programs, court rulings have allowed the girls to play.

Every Child Plays. If the main reason for developing youth sports programs is to provide a safe setting for children to develop athletically while also having fun, then all children have the right to play. It is grossly unfair to allow youngsters to commit large amounts of time and energy to learning and practicing a sport without the benefit of actually playing. Children agree. When surveyed, " . . . more than 90% of the boys questioned would rather play on a losing team than sit on the bench of a winning team. In short, playing is more valued than winning."[23]

Dangerous Sports. Although there is inherent risk involved in most sports, there are two sports that present extreme risks—boxing and trampoline.

Because of the high risk of head injury and chronic brain damage the American Medical Association, the American Academy of Family Physicians, and the American Academy of Pediatrics have all opposed boxing. It is difficult to find any benefits from boxing that cannot be obtained from other safer, more appropriate sports.

Because of growing public awareness that trampoline accidents produce frequent severe head and neck injuries and because of ensuing liability insurance problems, trampoline availability and use have dropped way off. There is a valid limited role for the trampoline in youth sports but it should be used only under the immediate supervision of highly trained instructors. It has no place in the home or recreational settings, and it should not be left unsecured in an open space when a qualified instructor is not present.[1] When used properly, it may be a valuable tool for teaching athletic skills, especially in gymnastics and diving.

Safety in Youth Sports. There are several aspects of youth sports programs that can reduce the risk of injury inherent in athletics. Preparticipation physical examination can identify children with limiting conditions and those with problems warranting treatment and rehabilitation. Proper supervision by well-trained coaches and officials is the cornerstone of a safe program. The rules of play should be designed to protect the young athlete. Adequate physical conditioning reduces the frequency and severity of injuries, as does matching for maturity already discussed. Properly fitting protective equipment, adequate footwear, and well-maintained practice and competition facilities are essential. The importance of all of these factors is demonstrated by the existence of the Bill of Rights for Young Athletes (Fig. 2).

THE BILL OF RIGHTS
FOR YOUNG ATHLETES

Right to participate in sports

Right to participate at a level commensurate with each child's maturity and ability

Right to have qualified adult leadership

Right to play as a child and not as an adult

Right of children to share in the leadership and decision-making of their sport participation

Right to participate in safe and healthy environments

Right to proper preparation for participation in sports

Right to an equal opportunity to strive for success

Right to be treated with dignity

Right to have fun in sports

FIGURE 2. The Bill of Rights for Young Athletes. (Reprinted with permission of the American Alliance, for Health, Physical Education, Recreation and Dance, 1900 Association Drive, Reston, Virginia 22091.)

STRENGTH TRAINING AND
WEIGHT LIFTING

Athletes are constantly searching for ways to enhance performance, and strength training is a well-documented technique for doing so in the physically mature athlete. There is a trend for training methods successfully employed by high level competitors to spread to lower echelons of competition and younger athletes. After all, youngsters may share the desire to become stronger and faster. Consequently, there has been increasing interest in strength training in prepubertal and pubertal athletes. At the same time, there has been concern over the value and safety of strength training at these levels of maturity.

Recently, three major national organizations with interests in sports medicine and athletics published position papers on strength training and weight lifting in young athletes.[3,11,27] One, the National Strength and Conditioning Association, presented the following definitions, which have already received widespread acceptance:

Resistance training is any method or form used to resist, overcome, or bear force.

Weight training is the use of barbells, dumbbells, or machine type apparatuses as resistance.

Weight lifting and *power lifting* are the competitive sports that contest maximum lifting ability in the Olympic snatch and clean and jerk, or squat, bench press and dead lift, respectively.

Strength training is the use of resistance methods to increase one's ability to exert or resist force. The training may utilize free weights, the individual's own body weight, machines and/or other devices to attain this goal. In order to be measurably effective, the training sessions must include timely progressions in intensity which impose sufficient demand to stimulate strength gains that are greater than those associated with normal growth and development.[27]

With these definitions in mind, this discussion will address the following questions: (1) Can prepubertal and pubertal athletes gain significant strength through strength training? (2) Does strength training cause injuries to children at these levels of maturity? (3) Does strength training reduce the incidence of sports-related injuries at these levels of maturity? (4) If strength training is safe and useful, are there guidelines available for the young athlete's benefit? (5) Is there a role for weight lifting and power lifting before puberty is completed?

Strength Gains

The traditional view in sports science has been that before the hormonal changes of puberty children are unable to produce significant muscle response to strength training. It was thought that apparent gains in strength were really the result of attaining new skills and and improving coordination by repetition. Several recent studies in prepubertal and pubertal athletes challenge this conception by demonstrating significant strength gains.[29,31,34,35]

Safety of Strength Training

There are many concerns frequently expressed about the safety of strength training, with only a paucity of data to substantiate or refute them. A large controlled prospective study focusing on the safety of strength training is lacking in the sports medicine literature at this time. In the well-controlled studies demonstrating the efficacy of strength training in prepubertal and pubertal athletes, there was no evidence of an increased incidence of injuries, but these studies were small, relatively short-term, and well supervised.

There are, however, both documented reports and an extensive mythology about injuries related to strength training, weight lifting, and power lifting. Since resistance training for sports conditioning has become common practice for so many junior high school and high school athletes, it is important that the practicing physician be able to provide credible advice to young athletes and their parents.

First, at least two types of injuries appear to be common in this population when performing unsupervised or poorly supervised overhead weight lifting: epiphyseal fractures of the wrists and damage to the pars interarticularis. Proponents of strength training maintain that the epiphyseal wrist injuries

are the product of competitive style lifting, and the reports in the literature tend to support their analysis as far as they go.[6,14,30]

The pars interarticularis injuries are much more problematic. There is little question that spondylolysis and spondylolisthesis are encountered in young athletes performing strength training and Olympic-style weight-lifting more frequently than previously observed.[6,17,18] It is also clear that certain types of resistance training equipment are more likely to cause low back injury and require competent supervision when and if they are used.[5] Many of the young athletes using various forms of resistance training to develop strength are also stressing their backs by playing football or performing gymnastics at the same time.[16,41] It is not clear whether strength training with proper equipment and competent on-site supervision increases the risk of pars damage in young athletes. Good prospective controlled studies are needed.

Second, a group of overuse syndromes is seen in athletes performing resistance training. Most common among these are musculotendinous strains and patellofemoral syndrome. They are often related to attempting too much too fast and/or using improper technique. Generally speaking, these problems respond well to rehabilitation and, thus, are not as worrisome. They do, however, teach the importance of having a knowledgeable coach or teacher individualize and supervise strength training for young athletes.

Third is the accusation that strength training will reduce flexibility and make the young athlete "muscle bound." In fact, there is evidence that just the opposite is true. Well-designed strength programs in which the exercises are performed throughout the full range of joint motion tend to increase flexibility.[7,35] The athlete who is extremely inflexible initially may be well advised to perform an intensive stretching program prior to or along with strength training.

Protective Aspect of Strength Training

One benefit of strength training appears to be that it seems to confer on the athlete an element of protection against injury. Preseason conditioning has been shown to reduce the incidence and severity of knee injuries in high school football players.[7] It has also been associated with a dramatic reduction in the incidence of injuries in a cohort of strength-trained high school boys and girls participating in a variety of sports compared with an untrained control group. Additionally, when injuries did occur, those in the strength-trained group had a greatly reduced average recovery and rehabilitation time.[15] Certainly, more research about the potential protective role of strength training is needed.

Guidelines for Safe Strength Training

Whether physicians agree with the notion that strength training is valuable or not, they often find themselves faced with the reality that there are such programs already in place in their communities and wonder if there are some guidelines available that are designed to make strength training as safe as possible. In 1985 the American Orthopedic Society for Sports Medicine (AOSSM) convened a workshop including representatives of eight organizations involved in sports medicine to establish such a set of guidelines. Their recommendations were published the following year.[11] Also in 1985, the National Strength Coaches Association published its Position Paper on Prepubescent Strength Training.[27]

Most major issues are treated with similar recommendations by the two documents. Common guidelines suggested by both groups include: (1) the need for a preparticipation physical examination; (2) the requirement that the child have adequate emotional maturity to accept coaching; (3) supervision by competent coaches trained in strength training specifically for this age group; (4) strength training only as part of a broader program designed to increase other motor skills and fitness level; (5) adequate warm-up and cool-down; (6) all exercises performed through full joint range of motion; (7) no lifting to attain the individual's maximum single repetition capacity; (8) initial training without resistance to learn proper techniques; (9) six to fifteen repetitions per set; (10) small load increments (maximum 3 pounds) when building up resistance level; and (11) 20- to 30-minute strength training sessions up to 3 times per week.[11,27] The AOSSM recommendations also prohibit competition and call for em-

phasis on dynamic concentric contractions (exercises in which the major resistance occurs while the muscles are shortening and tightening rather than while lengthening and releasing).[11]

Weight Lifting and Power Lifting

As defined earlier, weight lifting and power lifting are competitive sports, whereas strength training is a type of physical conditioning. Because of concerns about the higher injury potential of these sports the AOSSM and the AAP guidelines consider them inappropriate for prepubertal children.[3,11] Extreme caution and close supervision are warranted for participation of pubertal and postpubertal athletes in any form of overhead or competitive lifting.

Some Reservations

The evidence about the safety of strength training is thin, and more research is necessary. The present guidelines are valuable interim measures because they provide the practicing physician a basis for counselling patients and parents, but they will require a great deal of refinement over the next few years as more data become available. Other concerns that must be addressed include the relationship between resistance training and the development of hypertension, the relationship between increased upper body mass and the incidence of knee injuries, and the clinical syndrome of syncope during heavy lifting.

INJURIES

The risk of injury to children in sports is an important concern for athletes, parents, coaches, and administrators. Not many years ago, organized medicine openly opposed contact sports for young children because it was feared that youngsters would be more susceptible to injury than high school or college athletes.[2] In fact, research has shown that their fears were unfounded; contact and even collision sports are now regularly played in some elementary and most middle level schools as well as in a myriad of community leagues.

A community-wide study in a midwestern city of 100,000 demonstrated that younger children had fewer injuries and that the rate of injury increased with age until high school age was attained: 3% of elementary school students, 7% of junior high school students, and 11% of high school students sustained injuries severe enough to be treated by a physician, noted in official sports records or reported to the school insurance carrier over the course of a year. There were approximately twice as many injuries in nonorganized sports and in physical education classes as there were in organized sports, but it is possible that these data merely reflect the numbers of children participating in these activities. Twenty percent of the injuries were considered serious but only 1.2% caused permanent damage. The authors felt that 27% of the injuries "could have been avoided had nominal safety precautions been observed."[42] Other authors have suggested that 63% of youth sports injuries evaluated in a different setting could have been avoided.[13]

Boys and girls have similar injury rates in sports played by both sexes.[12,39] However, the overall injury rate for boys is much higher due to greater participation in contact and collision sports.[12,36,42]

At the high school level, most athletes are postpubertal and therefore stronger, larger, and faster. Here, the injury rate rises precipitously in proportion to the intensity of contact involved in the sport. Additionally, overuse injuries in the running sports begin to be frequent problems in this age group. Table 3 provides data on injuries sustained by athletes in four large metropolitan high schools.

Epiphyseal Injuries

Injuries involving the bony growth plate deserve special attention in any discussion of youth sports medicine. Although a thorough analysis of the diagnosis and management of these problems is more appropriate for an orthopedic text, a general understanding of some basic issues is essential for any physician treating young athletes.

In growing children the physis, or bony growth plate, is considerably weaker than the surrounding ligamentous tissue. This difference in strength between the two types of tissue appears to be greatest at puberty, the

TABLE 3. INJURY RATE PER SEASON IN FOUR METROPOLITAN HIGH SCHOOLS*

SPORT	BOYS (%)	GIRLS (%)
Badminton	—	6
Baseball	—	18
Basketball	31	25
Cross-country	29	35
Football	81	—
Gymnastics	28	40
Soccer	30	—
Softball	—	44
Swimming	9	1
Tennis	3	7
Track and field	35	33
Volleyball	—	10

*Adapted from Garrick JG, Requa RK: Injuries in high school sports. Pediatrics 61(3):465–469, 1978.

time of peak bone growth.[28,40] Consequently, an injury that would likely result in a torn ligament in a postpubertal athlete is more likely to cause a disruption of the growth plate in the prepubertal or pubertal competitor. The physician, aware of this phenomenon, will often wisely obtain stress x-rays of joints that appear to be "sprained" but that actually have sustained growth plate fractures.

Growth cartilage also occurs in bony prominences where major muscle tendons insert. These sites, called apophyses, are prone to two types of injury: avulsion and traction. Where the older athlete might sustain a muscle "pull," the peripubertal athlete is vulnerable to the avulsion of the tendinous insertion.[40] When a physician is suspicious of a muscle strain at either end of the muscle in this age athlete, it is worthwhile to obtain x-rays in order to rule out epiphyseal avulsion at the origin or apophyseal avulsion at the insertion.

Repetitive forceful contractions of large muscles may cause traction injuries of the apophysis, known variably as apophysitis and epiphysitis. The process appears to start as an inflammatory reaction to repeated stress at the tendinous insertion and is followed by reactive bone formation. There is growing acceptance of the theory that these lesions are "the result of tiny avulsion fractures and the body's resultant healing processes."[26] The most common traction apophysitis is Osgood-Schlatter's disease, which occurs at the insertion of the patella tendon and often produces painful bony hypertrophy of the tibial tubercle. It is discussed in greater detail in Chapter 18.

The popularity of endurance running and even marathon competition in recent years has spread to children, and many are undergoing intensive training programs with extremely high mileage. The research literature does not provide a clear understanding about whether this rigorous activity can be tolerated safely by the growth plates of the weight-bearing bones in the young athlete. Until better information is available, most authorities are recommending a cautious approach to extreme distance running until puberty is complete.[8]

For many years physicians were concerned that the epiphyses were so prone to injury that children should avoid contact sports until completing puberty. Larson dispelled these concerns by demonstrating that only 933 (19%) of 4854 athletic injuries evaluated in a group orthopedic practice occurred in children 15 years old or younger. Of this number, 933 84 (9%) involved disruptive injuries and 54 (6%) were other epiphyseal problems, mostly apophysitis.[19]

Concussion

Concussion is defined as "a clinical syndrome characterized by immediate and transient posttraumatic impairment of neural function, such as the alteration of consciousness, disturbance of vision, equilibrium, etc, due to brainstem involvement."[10] Although on-the-field management of head injury is beyond the context of this book, the issue of when and if it is safe for the athlete who has sustained one or more concussions to return to collision sports is extremely germane.

The physician reading the current sports medicine literature regarding concussion is likely to be confused and frustrated. There are well over a half dozen classification and grading systems for concussion, each with a different set of guidelines for return to play. There is a well-justified general trend, however, to be much more conservative in decision making.

In 1984 Saunders and Harbaugh defined what has since become known as the second impact syndrome. They noted that "sequential minor impacts may occasionally lead to major cerebral pathological conditions." The initial minor head injury reduces the compliance of the brain and, thereby, its ability to withstand the shock of a second relatively minor blow. The result may be severe intracranial injury and death.[32] Two cases of athletes developing almost immediate cerebral edema and dying after having sustained prior concussions had been reported previously.[33] Similarly, athletes recovering from infectious mononucleosis with encephalitis have sustained major head injury from minor trauma.[38]

Our current understanding of the second impact syndrome makes it clear that there is no justification for an athlete with *any* persisting signs or symptoms related to a concussion or postconcussion state to return to play in a contact sport until long after the sequelae have resolved. The athlete with even brief loss of consciousness or posttraumatic amnesia should be kept out of contact play until symptom free for a week, or longer if it is a recurrent concussion in the same season.[9] The athlete with symptoms that persist several days after even mild concussion or with symptoms that progress at any time warrants CT scan evaluation. Three mild concussions should lead to termination of the athlete's season.[9] At the high school level or below, three concussions with flaccid unconsciousness should end participation in collision sports.[4]

CONCLUSION

The issues discussed in this chapter are of vital concern to all who are involved in youth sports. The responsibility for counseling athletes, their parents and their coaches often falls on the shoulders of the physician. In view of the complexity of the matter, this is a responsibility that should always be treated with extreme care.

REFERENCES

1. American Academy of Pediatrics: Committee on Accident and Poison Prevention and Committee on Pediatric Aspects of Physical Fitness, Recreation, and Sports. Trampolines II. Pediatrics 67:438, 1981.
2. American Academy of Pediatrics: Committee on School Health. Competitive athletics: A statement of policy. Pediatrics 18:672–676, 1956.

3. American Academy of Pediatrics: Committee on Sports Medicine. Weight training and weight lifting: Information for the pediatrician. Phys Sportsmed 11:157–161, 1983.
4. American Academy of Pediatrics: Committee on Sports Medicine. Smith NJ (ED.) Sports medicine: health care for young athletes. Evanston, IL, American Academy of Pediatrics, 1982.
5. Brady TA, Cahil BR, Bodnar LM: Weight training-related injuries in the high school athlete. Am J Sports Med 10:1–4, 1982.
6. Brown EW, Kimball RG: Medical history associated with adolescent powerlifting. Pediatrics 72:636–644, 1983.
7. Cahill BR, Griffith EH: Effect of preseason conditioning on the incidence and severity of high school football knee injuries. Am J Sports Med 6:180–184, 1978.
8. Caine DJ, Lindner KJ: Growth plate injury: A threat to young distance runners? Phys Sportsmed 12:118–124, 1984.
9. Cantu RC: Guidelines for return to contact sports after a cerebral concussion. Phys Sportsmed 14:75–83, 1986.
10. Congress of Neurologic Surgeons: Ad hoc Committee to Study Head Injury Nomenclature. Glossary of head injury including some definitions of injury to the cervical spine. Clin Neurosurg 12:386–394, 1966.
11. Duda M: Prepupescent strength training gains support. Phys Sportsmed 14:157–161, 1986.
12. Garrick JG, Requa RK: Injuries in high school sports. Pediatrics 61:465–469, 1978.
13. Goldberg B, Witman PA, Gleim GW, Nicholas JA: Children's sports injuries: Are they avoidable? Phys Sportsmed 7:93–101, 1979.
14. Gumbs VL, Segal D, Halligan JB, Lower G: Bilateral distal radius and ulnar fractures in adolescent weight lifters. Am J Sports Med 6:375–379, 1982.
15. Hejna WF, Rosenberg A, Buturusis DJ, Krieger A: The prevention of sports injuries in high school students through strength training. Nat Strength Condit Assoc J 4:28–31, 1982.
16. Jackson DW, Wiltse LL, Cirincione RJ: Spondylolysis in the female gymnast. Clin Orthop 117:68–73, 1976.
17. Jackson DW, Wiltse LL, Dingeman RD, Hayes M: Stress reactions involving the pars interarticularis in young athletes. Am J Sports Med 9:304–312, 1981.
18. Jesse JP: Olympic lifting movements endanger adolescents. Phys Sportsmed 5:61–67, 1977.
19. Larson RL: Epiphyseal injuries in the adolescent athlete. Orthop Clin North Am 4:839–851, 1973.
20. Marshall WA, Tanner JM: Variations in the pattern of pubertal changes in boys. Arch Dis Child 45:13–23, 1970.
21. Marshall WA, Tanner JM: Variations in the pattern of pubertal changes in girls. Arch Dis Child 44:291–303, 1969.
22. Martens R: Kids sports: a den of iniquity or a land of promise. In Magill RA, Ash MJ, Smoll FL (eds): Children in Sport: A contemporary Anthology. Champaign, IL, Human Kinetics, 1978, 201–216.
23. Martens R: The uniqueness of the young athlete: psychological considerations. Am J Sports Med 8:382–385, 1980.
24. Martens R, Christina RW, Harvey JS, Sharkey BJ: Coaching Young Athletes. Champaign, IL. Human Kinetics Publishers, Inc., 1981.
25. Martens R, Seefeldt V (eds): Guidelines for children's sports. Reston, VA, American Alliance for Health, Physical Education, Recreation and Dance, 1979.
26. Micheli LJ: Overuse injuries in children's sports: The growth factor. Orthop Clin North Am 14:337–360, 1983.
27. National Strength and Conditioning Association: Position paper on prepubescent strength training. Nat Strength Condit Assoc J 7:27–31, 1985.
28. Pappas AM: Epiphyseal injuries in sports. Phys Sportsmed 11:140–148, 1983.
29. Pfeiffer RD, Francis RS: Effects of strength training on muscle development in prepubescent, pubescent, and postpubescent males. Phys Sportsmed 9:134–143, 1986.
30. Ryan JR, Salciccioli GG: Fractures of the distal radial epiphysis in adolescent weight lifters. Am J Sports Med 4:26–27, 1976.
31. Sailors M, Berg K: Comparison of responses to weight training in pubescent boys and men. J Sports Med Phys Fit in press, 1987.
32. Saunders RL, Harbaugh RE: The second impact in catastrophic contact-sports head trauma. JAMA 252:538–539, 1984.
33. Schneider RC: Head and Neck Injuries in Football; Mechanisms, Treatment, and Prevention. Baltimore, Williams & Wilkins Co., 1973.
34. Servedio FJ, Bartels RL, Hamlin RL, et al: The effects of weight training, using olympic style lifts, on various physiological variables in prepubescent boys. Med Sci Sports Exerc 17:238; 1985.
35. Sewell L, Micheli LJ: Strength training for children. J Pediat Orthop 6:143–146, 1986.
36. Shively RA, Grana WA, Ellis D: High school sports injuries. Phys Sportsmed 9:46–50, Aug 1981.
37. Smith RE, Smoll FL, Curtis B: Coach effectiveness training: a cognitive-behavioral approach to enhancing relationship skills in youth sport coaches. J Sports Psychol 1:59–75, 1979.
38. Torg JS, Beer C, Bruno LA, Vegso J: Head trauma in football players with infectious mononucleosis. Phys Sportsmed 8:107–110, Jan 1980.
39. Tursz A, Crost M: Sport-related injuries in children: A study of their characteristics, frequency, and severity, with comparison to other types of accidental injuries. Am J Sports Med 14:294–299, 1986.
40. Wilkins KE: The uniqueness of the young athlete: Musculoskeletal injuries. Am J Sports Med 8:377–382, 1980.
41. Wiltse LL, Widell EH, Jackson DW: Fatigue fracture: The basic lesion in isthmic spondylolisthesis. J Bone Joint Surg 57A:17–22, 1975.
42. Zaricznyj B, Shattuck LJM, Mast TA, et al: Sports-related injuries in school-aged children. Am J Sports Med 8:318–324, 1980.

7 The Athletic Woman

ROSEMARY AGOSTINI, M.D.

This chapter, intended to be a resource for physicians caring for active and athletic women, focuses on the specific problems encountered by women in sports. In giving health care to active women the physician needs to be empathetic, to demonstrate respect for the patient's athleticism, and to be willing to research or refer problems that may be special to the athletic woman. The last thing a woman who participates in sports and athletic activities wants to be told is to curtail her active lifestyle. The patient will rarely do so; instead, the doctor will lose the patient, and the patient will lose the opportunity to receive the information and medical care she needs.

To evaluate the myth that women are weak and unathletic the Armed Forces conducted two major studies. The investigators concluded that the gross differences between men and women are primarily the results of traditional sex bias, which, rather than actual physiologic differences, has resulted in women rarely exercising to their potential fitness levels. Furthermore, they noted that the present national fitness standards for women are far below women's true physiologic potential.[2,27,31]

Topics addressed in this chapter include gynecologic concerns, pregnancy and women athletes, eating disorders and women athletes, musculoskeletal problems, osteoporosis, and psychological issues.

GYNECOLOGIC CONCERNS

Menstrual function is not completely understood. It is an orchestration of hormones in the hypothalamus, pituitary, ovaries, thyroid, and adrenal glands. Physical stress, emotional stress, weight loss, change in body fat, exercise, and dietary changes can affect the hormones produced by these glands and thereby alter menstrual function.

The pubertal awakening of gonadotropic hormones is thought to be central in origin, genetically controlled and linked to attainment of critical body weight.[46] In the normal cycle, the hypothalamus synthesizes and releases gonadotropin-releasing hormone (luteinizing-hormone-releasing factor, GnRH or LRF). This hormone stimulates the production of two pituitary hormones, follicle-stimulating hormone (FSH) and luteinizing hormone (LH). In the preovulatory phase, FSH stimulates the graafian follicle to grow. The graafian follicle secretes estrogen, which stimulates the growth of the endometrium. The rising estrogen level stimulates the hypothalamic release of more GnRH (LRF), which triggers the surge of FSH and LH, which causes the release of the ovum from the graafian follicle (ovulation). In the postovulatory phase the graafian follicle, without the ovum, undergoes transformation into the corpus luteum. The corpus luteum secretes large amounts of estrogen and progesterone. The estrogen continues to stimulate the endometrium to grow, and progesterone converts an estrogen-stimulated endometrium into a stable structure necessary for the fertilized ovum to implant.

If a fertilized ovum does not implant, the corpus luteum has a life span of approximately 12 days. It then degenerates and stops producing estrogen and progesterone, and shedding of the endometrial lining begins. A normal menstrual cycle is measured from the first day of menstrual flow in one cycle up to, but not including, the onset of menstrual flow of the following cycle. The normal range is generally considered to be 21 to 36 days. The preovulatory (follicular) phase begins with the first day of menstrual flow and ends the day before ovulation (range 10–20 days). The postovulatory (luteal) phase begins at ovulation and ends before the onset of the next menstrual flow (range 10–16 days).

Menarche. Some women who begin exercising before puberty have delayed onset of menses.[19,36,53] Management of delayed menarche depends on age. If a girl is 14 years old and has not started menstruating but is developing breast, axillary and pubic hair, the treatment is reassurance and follow-up. If at age 14 the girl is not developing secondary sexual characteristics, or at age 16, whether she has secondary sexual characteristics or not, a workup for primary amenorrhea should be initiated.[49] Recent studies suggest there should be concern about an increased incidence of scoliosis and decreased bone mass in young women with delayed puberty.[55]

DEFINITIONS. The literature on menstrual cycle abnormalities is often contradictory and confusing. Although the causes of menstrual cycle abnormalities are not always evident, it is important to be aware of the medical consequences.

1. *Menstruation* is the cyclic, physiologic discharge through the vagina of blood and mucosal tissue from the nonpregnant uterus.

2. *A shortened luteal (postovulatory) phase*—less than 8 days may be due to an inadequate corpus luteum. This may be a reason for infertility.[43]

3. *Anovulation* is the absence of egg release. The woman may have cyclic or irregular menstrual periods. It is a hormonal state of unopposed estrogen.[43]

4. *Oligomenorrhea* is a condition in which menstrual cycles occur at intervals longer than 36 days. It may be caused by anovulation.[43]

5. *Amenorrhea* is the absence of a menstrual cycle. Primary amenorrhea is the failure of menstruation to occur at puberty. Secondary amenorrhea means cessation of menstruation after it has once been established at puberty. There are many accepted definitions of how many cycles must be missed to constitute secondary amenorrhea. In this text it is defined as no menstrual cycle in a consecutive 6-month period.[43]

Significance of Menstrual Irregularities. In an anovulatory cycle the hormonal environment of unopposed estrogen has been associated with endometrial hyperplasia and the risk of cancer of the endometrium and breast. In amenorrhea estrogen is low and progesterone is absent. If amenorrhea is long-standing, the woman is at risk for decreased bone density,[17,32,37] atrophic vaginitis, and urethritis.

PREVALENCE. Reported prevalences of secondary amenorrhea range from 3.4 to 43%, depending on the investigator's definition of amenorrhea and the selection of subjects.[17] The prevalence of exercise-related menstrual changes depends on age, previous menstrual cycles, and the exercise status of the women.[43]

Any woman who is concerned about her menstrual cycle should be evaluated, but the extent of the evaluation will depend on the content of the patient's history. The two most common causes of amenorrhea are pregnancy and situational stress. Prolactin-secreting tumors are not uncommon, especially in women with galactorrhea. Hirsutism may suggest hyperandrogenism. Premature ovarian failure is also part of the differential diagnosis. The pathogenesis of exercise-related oligo/amenorrhea correlates with exercise intensity, exercise duration and type (e.g., mileage in runners but not in swimmers or cyclists), weight loss and thinness, body composition (% of body fat), age, previous menstrual irregularity, physical stress, emotional stress, and dietary factors.

PATIENT EVALUATION. The evaluation of the patient should include the following elements:

History:
  (1) Menstrual cycle
  (2) Physical activity—daily frequency, intensity and duration of training, the sport, and any change in the aforementioned.
  (3) Sexual activity
  (4) Nutritional history
  (5) Weight gain/loss 6 months and 12 months prior to onset
  (6) History suggestive of eating disorders
  (7) Pregnancy
  (8) Conflicts and support systems: home, work, and social
  (9) Coping skills

(10) Molimina—the collection of non-distressing symptoms that can be used as a marker of ovulation—breast tenderness, bloating, mood or appetite changes (when severe, the condition is called pre-menstrual tension)

PHYSICAL EXAMINATION. General and gynecologic

(1) General Examination
(2) Tanner stage: breast development, axillary and pubic hair
(3) Vaginal dryness, urethritis (suggest decreased estrogens)
(4) Acne and hirsutism (suggest androgen excess)
(5) Pregnancy (enlarged uterus)
(6) Presence of normal sexual organs

DIAGNOSTIC EXAMINATIONS

(1) Pregnancy test, if indicated
(2) Progesterone challenge—10 mg of medroxy progesterone (Provera) days 16—21 (withdrawal bleeding means adequate levels of estrogen; if there is not withdrawal bleeding, continue workup and consider estrogen and progesterone replacement)
(3) Prolactin level—rule out microadenoma of the pituitary
(4) FSH, LH—rule out ovarian failure

Treatment. See Tables 1 and 2.

Other Gynecologic Concerns

Menstrual-cycle changes related to exercise are associated with lower basal estrogen levels.[6] Low estrogen (hypoestrogenemia) increases calcium resorption from bone and decreases calcium absorption from the intestines and reabsorption from the kidneys. The basic skeleton (calcium deposition in bone) is laid down by age 30–35. Therefore, in order to delay the development of osteoporosis and reduce its severity, one should evaluate and treat menstrual abnormalities in youth.

Menstrual Cramps. Dysmenorrhea is caused by inadequacy of uterine blood flow during myometrial contractions, stimulated by prostaglandin $F_{2\alpha}$ produced in the endometrium.[49] Excellent relief can be obtained from the nonsteroidal anti-inflammatory drugs. An exercise program may also be helpful.

Premenstrual Syndrome. Premenstrual syndrome is real. It is a great source of distress for many women, and it can be treated. The condition is a collection of symptoms that occur cyclically in the week or two before menses (luteal phase), and only in ovulatory cycles. Onset is generally in the mid- to late twenties or early thirties. In more than 30% of women symptoms may be severe enough to interfere with daily life and work and include:[43]

- Mood changes—increased anxiety, anger, and frustration
- Depression
- Breast tenderness and/or enlargement
- Fluid retention and abdominal bloating
- Appetite changes, including cravings for carbohydrates

A diagnostic approach recommended by Severino includes:[47]

- A thorough premenstrual health history
- Psychiatric history, including mental status
- Three-month diary of daily symptoms
- Thorough medical evaluation, including
  General physical examination
  Bimanual pelvic examination
  Pap smear
  Complete blood count
  Chemical screen, including fasting blood glucose

A treatment approach recommended by Prior includes:[43]

- Initiate or increase a conditioning or exercise program
- Decrease stress. If the patient does not have a supportive friend or family member, she should find a professional counselor or peer group

Breast Tenderness

- Avoid caffeine

TABLE 1.   THERAPEUTIC APPROACH TO THE ATHLETE WITH SECONDARY AMENORRHEA

PRESENT OR POTENTIAL PROBLEM	THERAPEUTIC OPTIONS	RATIONALE
Absent menstrual flow[a]	Evaluation to rule out disease	May remove worry-related block
	Explanation and reassurance	
	Medroxyprogesterone 10 mg days 16-25 monthly whether or not withdrawal bleeding occurs	May stimulate cyclic hypothalamic function
Vaginal dryness and atrophy[a]	Conjugated estrogen vaginal cream ½ applicator (1g) 1 night/week	Topical estrogen with little systemic absorption
Risk for osteoporosis[a]	Increase oral calcium to 1.5-2 g/day—4-8 dairy servings and/or supplements—'Tums', 200 mg calcium per tablet	Decrease negative calcium balance associated with low gonadal steroids
	Medroxyprogesterone 10 mg/day for 10 days/month	Positive action on trabecular bone
	Cyclic estrogen and progesterone: i.e. conjugated estrogens 0.3 mg/day, days 1-21 each month Medroxyprogesterone 10 mg/day for days 16-25	Balanced hormonal replacement
Infertility	1. Decrease exercise intensity by 10% 2. Gain 1-2 kg weight 3. Monitor basal temperature for 3 months 4. After 3 months if ovulation has not occurred, give progesterone vaginal suppositories 25 mg bid on days 16-25 of cycle or 10 days/month 5. Further decreases in exercise, additional weight gain, and stress reduction may be necessary 6. Additional therapy may require ovulation induction measures. However, these methods may not work initially	These exercise and diet modifications will allow normal hypothalamic reproductive function to return

[a]Oral contraceptives are not desirable because they suppress cyclic hypothalamic-pituitary function.
From Prior, J.C. and Vigna Y.: Gonadal steroids in athletic women: contraception, complications and performance. Sports Medicine 2:287–295, with permission.

- Vitamin B$_6$ (pyridoxine), 100–200 mg per day while symptomatic
- Bromocriptine, 1.25–2.5 mg b.i.d.

Fluid Retention
- Avoid high-salt foods
- Mild weight-loss program

Food Cravings
- Eat low-caloric foods, e.g., carrots
- Eat complex carbohydrates, e.g., muffins

A number of medications have been used in the treatment of premenstrual syndrome, but their indications and efficacy are still controversial and unproven.

Contraception. It is amazing how little high school and college students know about contraception and reproduction. Contraception for the active woman is generally the same as that for other women. Ideal methods of birth control do not exist. Current methods include barriers, the diaphragm and spermicidal jelly, condoms, oral contraceptives, tubal ligation, and vasectomy of male partners. Women who are taking the newer low-dose oral contraceptives (10/11 or 7-7-7) often ask how they can control when they

TABLE 2. THERAPEUTIC APPROACH TO THE ANOVULATORY MENSTRUATING ATHLETE

PRESENT OR POTENTIAL PROBLEMS	THERAPEUTIC OPTIONS	RATIONALE
Unexpected asymptomatic menses (with or without oligoamenorrhea or metrorrhagia)[a]	Medroxyprogesterone 10 mg (2 tabs) days 16-25	Estrogen-primed endometrium will shed after progesterone withdrawal
Heavy bleeding[a]	Medroxyprogesterone 10-20 mg for 10 days	Medroxyprogesterone will allow complete endometrial shedding
Midcycle spotting[a]	Medroxyprogesterone 10 mg/day taken at first spotting for 10 days	Prevent estrogen withdrawal bleeding after mid-cycle estrogen surge
Infertility	1. Decrease exercise intensity by 10% 2. Gain 1-2 kg weight 3. Monitor basal temperature for 3 months 4. If above don't allow ovulation, or short luteal phase occurs, use progesterone suppositories 25 mg bid days 16-25	If the hypothalamic system is modulated by exercise, this will allow return to ovulation
Risk for osteoporosis[a,b]	Increase calcium intake to 1.5 g/day—4-6 dairy products and/or supplements (2-5 'Tums') Medroxyprogesterone 10 mg days 16-25 cyclically	Decrease negative calcium balance associated with lower gonadal steroids Has positive effect on bone, mechanism not yet known
Androgen excess with hirsutism, acne[a,c]	Spironolactone 100-200 mg/day Medroxyprogesterone 10 mg days 16-25	Antiandrogen medication Medroxyprogesterone will potentiate antiandrogen effect and prevent heavy bleeding
Risk of endometrial and/or breast cancer[b]	Medroxyprogesterone 10 mg days 16-25	Inhibits estrogen's stimulating effect on endometrial and breast tissue

[a]Oral contraceptives could be used but will suppress the desired recovery of the hypothalamic-pituitary axis.
[b]If present in women with lower estradiol levels but high enough to cause menstrual bleeding.
[c]Is a rare temporary transition phase from anovulatory to ovulatory cycles.
 From Prior, J.C. and Vigna, Y.: Gonadal steroids in athletic women: contraception, complications and performance. Sports Medicine 2:287–295, 1985, with permission.

have their menstrual periods. One can recommend a switch to 1/35's; using one of these formulations, they may add a few pills from another cycle to delay menses.

Other concerns about the birth control pill include increased cardiovascular risk, potential thrombotic risk, and decreased exercise performance.[42]

Infertility. With an athletic couple having difficulty conceiving, the first recommendations to the woman include decreasing mileage/training and increasing body fat, if the woman is thin. High-intensity long-distance male runners may have lower sperm counts, and therefore the same recommendations apply to them. It should also be recommended that the woman start recording basal body temperature to help evaluate ovulation. Her partner should have a sperm count. It is estimated that 40% of infertility problems can be attributed to a decrease or absence of spermatogenesis. If this program is not successful after 6 months, the usual infertility workup should be initiated.

Heavy Bleeding. The normal menstrual flow is approximately 40 ml/cycle. One "full tampon or pad" has approximately 3.5 ml of blood. Therefore, if the flow uses more than 8–10 full pads, the individual is at risk for iron-deficiency anemia. Menorrhagia in endurance athletes is usually due to an anovulatory cycle. Treatment is progesterone withdrawal on days 16–25 (medroxyprogesterone—Provera, 10 mg × 10 days). If this is not successful, endometrial curettage is warranted. Metrorrhagia warrants endometrial sampling before initiating progestational therapy to rule out hyperplasia or adenocarcinoma of the endometrium.

Breast Examination. Athletic women (as well as all women) should be encouraged to perform breast examinations monthly just after the menstrual period. A good support bra should generally be recommended. If painful breasts are a problem, a reduction or avoidance of caffeine and salt should be suggested.[48] Vitamin B_6 and body fat reduction are also helpful. Bromocriptine for fibrocystic breast disease is indicated if symptoms are severe.[21]

PREGNANCY AND WOMEN ATHLETES

Exercise and Pregnancy. Women who exercise and are athletes often come to their family physicians with questions about exercise and pregnancy. Their most pressing concern is usually how exercise will affect the fetus. It is very important to take a careful exercise history (type, frequency, duration, and intensity). Is the woman just starting an exercise program? Is she a recreational or a high-performance athlete? What are *her* concerns and desires?

Major areas of concern of the exercising pregnant woman include:

- What is the effect of elevated body temperature on the fetus?
- Will exercise shunt blood from the uterus to the exercising muscle?
- Will the athletic mother's potentially lower body weight and smaller weight gain compromise the fetus?

Lotgering et al., in an exhaustive review of maternal and fetal responses to exercise during pregnancy, conclude that "although the increased demands of pregnancy might compete with those of exercise, under most circumstances the maternal organism can meet the combined demands of gestation and exercise through a remarkable reserve of physiological adjustments."[33] The effects of exercise on pregnancy that must be addressed in counseling the pregnant woman include heat stress, uterine oxygen consumption, and infant size.

HEAT STRESS AND THE FETUS. Some studies show that "fetal temperature lags behind the rapidly changing maternal temperature at the onset and cessation of exercise."[34] Although heat stress has been reported to cause fetal growth retardation,[25] intrauterine death,[18] and central nervous system defects[18] in several species, the effect of heat stress during exercise has not been systematically investigated on a large scale in humans.[7] Jones et al. studied four aerobically conditioned women to characterize the changes in maternal body temperature and heat storage as these women continued to exercise with advancing pregnancy. It was found that maternal core temperature (using rectal and vaginal probes) and heat storage did *not* exceed physiologic limits during exercise. Conditioned maternal thermoregulatory mechanisms appear capable of dissipating the heat production by both the metabolically active fetus and the mother during moderate aerobic exercise. The increased maternal plasma volume during pregnancy helps maintain optimal fetomaternal heat transfer and dissipation.[28] It is important to realize that any large-scale study would be difficult, but more research is necessary before this question can be fully answered.

UTERINE OXYGEN CONSUMPTION. Several human and ovine studies have shown that blood is shunted from the uterus to the exercising muscle. Therefore, another major concern is that the fetus may be compromised. Further studies show that because of increased hemoglobin concentration during pregnancy, and thus increased blood oxygen-carrying capacity, and a flow redistribution within the uterus favoring fetal blood flow at the expense of myometrial flow,[15] the fetus is not compromised. Again, more studies need to be done.

ISSUE OF SMALLER BABIES. In a controlled study, Clapp demonstrated that "women who continued endurance exercise at or above a minimum conditioning level throughout the first, second, and well into the third trimester gained less weight, delivered earlier, and their infants had a consistent reduction in birth weight for gestational age without increased immediate morbidity.[10] The consistent reduction in birth weight was approximately 500 grams. The question is, does being smaller mean being unhealthy? In the past, one criterion used to judge whether a condition had an adverse effect on a pregnancy was to compare the birthweight of the newborn with controls of similar socioeconomic levels. Some authors have used this argument to suggest that exercise (in only those relatively few who continue a prepregnancy training level through the entire gestation) is detrimental. Clapp also noticed that the birth weights of infants born to women who exercised intensively only until the 28th week of pregnancy were not reduced compared with those of infants of nonexercising controls.

The Melpomene study of pregnancy and running provides data based on a questionnaire completed by 195 women.[35] They concluded that only a few health-care providers view running as a positive aspect of a healthy pregnancy, that participants gradually reduce mileage and speed as the pregnancy progresses, and that the average birthweight is 7 lb, 6 oz.

Another indicator of fetal well-being is the non-stress test. In a small study the non-stress test was conducted before and after a 1.5-mile jog in the third trimester of pregnancy. All tests were reactive, with no difference in the mean time to obtain a reactive test before exercise compared with after exercise. Exercise did produce a fetal tachycardia of 155–204 bpm compared with baseline heart rates of 140–155, and a mean of 22 minutes was required for the fetal heart rate to return to the pre-jogging baseline. The authors concluded that moderate exercise in pregnancy does not result in acute fetal distress, but they allowed for the possibility that the fetal tachycardia may be compensatory.[23]

The comments and studies quoted in this section are in reference to healthy pregnancies. Any history of heart disease, diabetes, hypertension, a previous miscarriage, incompetent cervix, anemia, kidney problems, or vaginal bleeding must be evaluated and treated differently. In cardiac patients, especially those with mitral or aortic valve disease, cardiac output *decreases* during pregnancy, making exercise *dangerous*.

The American College of Obstetrics and Gynecology Guidelines for Exercise During Pregnancy and Postpartum are listed in Table 3. They meet the needs of previously

sedentary women and women on a mild exercise program. Some authors have criticized them as being too conservative but logically in an area where the data are thin it is safe to err on the conservative side.

Benefits of exercise in pregnancy include weight control, improved muscle tone, maintenance of self-esteem, decreased varicose veins, decreased backache, better sleep, and a sense of control when so many physiologic changes are occurring that are not under one's control. Possibly, but not yet proven, exercise may result in easier pregnancy, labor and delivery.

EATING DISORDERS AND WOMEN ATHLETES

Anorexia Nervosa. Physicians treating female athletes should be able to recognize patients with eating disorders. The prevalence of anorexia nervosa, a syndrome of self-imposed starvation and distorted body image, has increased over the past 15 years from 0.1% to nearly 1% of the general American population.[14] In certain athletic activities, such as ballet, gymnastics, and running, the prevalence of eating disorders is much greater (ballet, 6.5%).[20]

In appearance some anorexic women are indistinguishable from high-performance athletes.[53] It is essential to make the diagnosis because anorexia nervosa is often fatal.[22]

Anorexia appears to be the product of a complex interaction of biologic, psychologic and socio-cultural factors.[4] The diagnostic criteria for anorexia nervosa are evolving, with the most common thread being a distorted body image. Differentiating athletic anorexic patients from athletes who are striving for low body-fat levels to enhance performance is difficult and often tentative.[9] Twenty-four percent of anorexic women are intensely athletic.[13] Table 4 provides helpful characteristics to distinguish athletes from athletic anorectics.[41] Obtaining a history of disturbed body image, marked feelings of inadequacy, and depression may take time and repeated visits in order to develop a trusting relationship. History should also be obtained from family members.

Treatment must be multifaceted, including

TABLE 3. AMERICAN COLLEGE OF OBSTETRICIANS AND GYNECOLOGISTS GUIDELINES FOR EXERCISE DURING PREGNANCY AND POSTPARTUM

EXERCISE GUIDELINES. The following guidelines are based on the unique physical and physiological conditions that exist during pregnancy and the postpartum period. They outline general criteria for safety to provide direction to patients in the development of home exercise programs.

Pregnancy and Postpartum

1. Regular exercise (at least three times per week) is preferable to intermittent activity. Competitive activities should be discouraged.
2. Vigorous exercise should not be performed in hot, humid weather or during a period of febrile illness.
3. Ballistic movements (jerky, bouncy motions) should be avoided. Exercise should be done on a wooden floor or a tightly carpeted surface to reduce shock and provide a sure footing.
4. Deep flexion or extension of joints should be avoided because of connective tissue laxity. Activities that require jumping, jarring motions or rapid changes in direction should be avoided because of joint instability.
5. Vigorous exercise should be preceded by a 5-minute period of muscle warm-up. This can be accomplished by slow walking or stationary cycling with low resistance.
6. Vigorous exercise should be followed by a period of gradually declining activity that includes gentle stationary stretching. Because connective tissue laxity increases the risk of joint injury, stretches should not be taken to the point of maximum resistance.
7. Heart rate should be measured at times of peak activity. Target heart rates and limits established in consultation with the physician should not be exceeded (see Table 1 for recommended postpartum heart rate limits).
8. Care should be taken to gradually rise from the floor to avoid orthostatic hypotension. Some form of activity involving the legs should be continued for a brief period.
9. Liquids should be taken liberally before and after exercise to prevent dehydration. If necessary, activity should be interrupted to replenish fluids.
10. Women who have led sedentary lifestyles should begin with physical activity of very low intensity and advance activity levels very gradually.
11. Activity should be stopped and the physician consulted if any unusual symptoms appear.

Pregnancy Only

1. Maternal heart rate should not exceed 140 beats per minute.
2. Strenuous activities should not exceed 15 minutes in duration.
3. No exercise should be performed in the supine position after the fourth month of gestation is completed.
4. Exercises that employ the Valsalva maneuver should be avoided.
5. Caloric intake should be adequate to meet not only the extra energy needs of pregnancy, but also of the exercise performed.
6. Maternal core temperature should not exceed 38°C.

American College of Obstetricians and Gynecologists: Exercise During Pregnancy and the Postnatal Period (ACOG Home Exercise Programs). Washington DC, ACOG, 1985, p 4

medical, behavioral and family therapy, as well as personal psychotherapy—with the immediate concern being return of the patient's nutritional status to normal and the long-term goal, the resolution of the behavioral and pschodynamic processes.

Bulimia. Bulimia is a syndrome of secre-tive binge-eating episodes followed by self-induced vomiting, fasting, and purging with laxatives and/or diuretics. The patients are aware that the eating pattern is abnormal and generally maintain weight with frequent fluctuations.[53]

The prevalence among college students

TABLE 4. DIAGNOSIS OF ANOREXIA NERVOSA

SHARED FEATURES (ATHLETE AND ANORECTIC)

Dietary faddism
Controlled calorie consumption
Specific carbohydrate avoidance
Low body weight
Resting bradycardia and hypotension
Increased physical activity
Amenorrhea or oligomenorrhea
Anemia (may or may not be present)

DISTINGUISHED FEATURES

Athlete

Purposeful training
Increased exercise tolerance
Good muscular development
Accurate body image
Body-fat level within defined normal range
Increased plasma volume
Increased O_2 extraction from blood
Efficient energy metabolism
Increased HDL_2

Anorectic

Aimless physical activity
Poor or decreasing exercise performance
Poor muscular development
Flawed body image (believes herself to be overweight)
Body fat level below normal range
Electrolyte abnormalities if abusing laxatives and/or
　diuretics.
Cold intolerance
Dry skin
Cardiac arrhythmias
Lanugo hair
Leucocyte dysfunction

McSherry, J.A.: The diagnostic challenge of anorexia nervosa. American Family Physician 29:144, 1984, with permission.

has been reported to be as high as 10%.[53] Medical complications in bulimics include extreme amounts of weight reduction and losses of dangerous quantities of fluids and electrolytes (hypokalemia). They may also develop dental caries due to erosion of enamel and gums, esophageal tears secondary to vomiting, and acute gastric dilatation.[22]

Weight Loss in Athletes. Excessive weight loss and food aversion in athletes appears to be different from that seen in anorexics and bulimics. In athletes it may be situationally related to athletic performance and/or "making weight." Males and females appear to be at equal risk, affected athletes are recognized

relatively early, and the stresses are usually not deep-seated chronic problems but an accumulation of immediate short-term concerns.[50] Frequent counseling visits as well as instructing the athlete to spend mealtimes in the company of teammates or friends may be helpful. The prognosis is significantly better than that for anorexia nervosa.

MALE ANALOG. A group of compulsive male distance runners was compared to anorectics with the suggestion that they shared basic personality characteristics.[55] The implication was that this form of exercise addiction is a male analog of anorexia nervosa. This view is not universally shared.

MUSCULOSKELETAL PROBLEMS

Are there specific musculoskeletal problems in women and women athletes? Early studies of injuries in women athletes showed a higher incidence of injuries sustained as compared with men, but these studies also reflected the lack of adequate conditioning in women rather than a true physiologic weakness and predisposition to injury. Injuries were more sports-specific than gender-specific; that is, injury types and rates were similar for men and women in the same sport but different for women participating in different sports.[27]

Patellofemoral Pain. Female athletes commonly experience retropatellar knee pain. Symptoms include crepitus, aching, pain going up and down stairs, stiffness after sitting for long periods, and sometimes a subjective feeling of instability. In the recent literature this is referred to as patellofemoral stress syndrome rather than chondromalacia patella, which is an actual pathologic softening and fraying of the retropatellar surface.

In the past, this problem was considered to be a female affliction caused by the influence of the broader gynecoid pelvis on the mechanics of the knee. Several recent studies indicate that it is also common among male athletes.[16,24,44] Retropatellar knee pain is discussed in Walsh's chapter "Tracking Problems of the Kneecap."

Ligamentous Laxity. The issue of increased ligamentous laxity has been raised as a reason women are more predisposed to ligamentous injuries, but this may have been due more to the lack of strengthening of the surrounding muscles from inadequate conditioning than to increased ligamentous laxity.[27] The only time women may be at increased risk for ligamentous and musculoskeletal injuries is during the third trimester of pregnancy, when relaxin, a hormone that makes the pelvic area more flexible in preparation for delivery, is released, and all of the ligaments become more lax.

Stress Fractures. Stress fractures are pathologic fractures, partial or complete, in bone that has been weakened by long-term recurrent microtrauma.[39] The major concerns about stress fractures in women relate to whether conditions such as amenorrhea, anorexia nervosa, low estrogen levels, and reduced calcium intake contribute to the pathologic fractures. Prolonged hypoestrogenism and low calcium intake are suspected to predispose women athletes to stress fractures.

The studies published on amenorrhea and its relation to decreased bone density comment on the increased incidence of stress fractures. Unfortunately, these studies have failed to consider and control for the general causes of stress fractures (a change in frequency, intensity, or duration of training; improper technique; lack of conditioning; environment; anatomy; and equipment).[37,55]

This author studied 50 active women who had had stress fractures, documented by x-ray and/or bone scan, identified retrospectively.[1] There was no difference in the prevalence of amenorrhea in this group compared with a group of college athletes used as a control population. Most of the women were able to attribute their stress fractures to a change in training (frequency, intensity, or duration); anatomy; equipment; environment; improper technique; or lack of conditioning. It is premature to relate stress fracture risk simply to amenorrhea. The duration of the amenorrhea, hypoestrogenemia, anorexia, low calcium intake, and the potential of earlier and more severe osteoporosis are all factors that merit further study.

Osteoporosis

Osteoporosis is characterized by decreased bone mass and increased susceptibility to fracture in the absence of other recognizable causes of bone loss.[11] Clinical features include vertebral compression fractures, hip and wrist fractures (Table 5).

Athletes who have poor nutrition, amenorrhea, and anorexia need calcium supplementation and/or cyclic treatment with estrogen and progesterone. In the menstruating population of active/athletic women, weight-bearing exercise has been shown to delay the onset and decrease the severity of osteoporosis. The issue of whether to treat postmenopausal women prophylactically and therapeutically is still controversial, but it is becoming clearer that treatment is indicated and should include estrogen–progesterone and calcium, or both, especially for those at risk.

Possible causes of osteoporosis include deficiency of estrogen and calcium and problems with absorption of calcium. The mainstay of treatment is prevention and management with estrogen and progesterone, calcium, and vitamin D, and weight-bearing exercise.

Calcium. Bone accretion usually occurs until age 30–35, when peak bone mass is obtained. It has been noted in numerous articles that women's intake of calcium is much lower than the recommended 1000 mg for actively menstruating women and 1500 mg for non-menstruating and postmenopausal women. The best way to obtain calcium is from food (8 oz milk, 4 oz cheese, or 2 oz hard cheese each yields 200 mg calcium), but if this is not possible because of weight restrictions, etc., calcium supplements should be added (TUMS—1 tablet = 200 mg of calcium carbonate). Caffeine, alcohol, cigarette

TABLE 5. RISK FACTORS FOR OSTEOPOROSIS

1. Female
2. Advanced age
3. Menopause (natural or surgical)
4. White or Oriental
5. Small-boned
6. Diet low in calcium
7. Smoking
8. Alcoholism
9. Immobilization
10. Amenorrhea—prolonged, 6 months
11. Anorexia nervosa
12. Prolonged corticosteroid use

smoking, lactose intolerance, and fiber decrease the absorption of calcium, as does a low estrogen level. Vitamin D and estrogens increase the absorption of calcium.

A practical guideline is that athletes who ingest less than 2,000 Kcal of calcium per day should have their diets supplemented with calcium and iron.

Amenorrheic and postmenopausal women should be treated with 0.625 mg estrogen per day on days 1–21 of the menstrual cycle, with the addition of progesterone, 10 mg/day on days 16–25. Amenorrheic young women can be cycled in this way every other month, so if their normal menstrual cycles resume both the doctor and patient will know it.

Vitamin D is obtained from sunlight and milk and, if necessary, may be supplemented with 400–800 units per day.

PSYCHOLOGY

Freud asked: "What does a woman want?" Bernstein and Warner respond: "Women want to be considered as separate, autonomous individuals with their own set of characteristics determined biologically and stemming from their early infantile relationships. They do not want these characteristics to be pejoratively labeled or considered to be merely a compensation for their damaged anatomy, not less good nor less desirable, or less important, merely different."[3]

The Problem. "Assuming the young woman has the opportunity to participate in sports in the first place, the biggest problem she faces is the almost universal stereotype that says women are to be passive, dependent and emotional."[51] Stark states, "The parents' social class can affect how a young girl perceives athletics; sports is rarely seen as a 'way out' even for lower socioeconomic class females, but being stereotypically female to attract a man is."[52]

Corbin notes, "There is considerable evidence that many females lack self confidence in their abilities to perform sports and physical activities, especially in certain situations. This situational lack of confidence is most likely to occur in activities perceived to be sex-role inappropriate, in activities that are evaluative as well as competitive, and in situations in which performance feedback is lacking or unclear."[12] Corbin notes recent research has suggested that Horner's fear of success (females may consciously, or unconsciously, perform less than their best achievement in situations because of the negative consequences associated with this success, i.e., not being feminine) may not be as evident among contemporary females as she originally suggested.[26,52] He further comments that it may be unwise to dismiss this notion entirely, as many females may still feel the need to subvert performances to protect their own feelings of "femininity." Perhaps most important in this regard is helping females to see that physical success is acceptable. *One operational definition of femininity is "whatever females do". If such a definition were universally held, the problem for females seeking achievement in sports would be greatly diminished."*[12]

Possible Solution. To be a success in sports means concentrating, working harder, getting ahead, practicing, and establishing self-confidence.[5] Stark introduces the concept of androgeny—the possession of both traditional male and female qualities. It is generally agreed that persons who are aware of and expressive of both the female and male aspects of their personalities have higher levels of self-esteem than those persons who maintain only male, female or undifferentiated (neither) attitudes and behaviors.[51]

So how do we as physicians help girls and women in all levels of sports, athletics and life? Corbin has suggested guidelines for building self confidence (Table 6). The physician can play a key role in helping the athlete develop this self confidence through following these guidelines.

Women in sports have come a long way. May conducted a pilot study addressing some of the psychological attitudes of 116 elite female athletics who attended training camps at the United States Olympic Training Center in Squaw Valley. He found the female athletes have a positive self-concept about their participation in sports, believe themselves to be at least as feminine as their non-athletic counterparts, and possess a positive body image.[38] King and Chi indicate that "female college athletes are significantly more assertive, more conscientious, and

TABLE 6. GUIDELINES FOR BUILDING SELF-CONFIDENCE

Ensuring Successful Performance:
"Nothing breeds confidence like success"

1. Help establish realistic goals.
2. Establish progressively more difficult tasks.
3. Physically aid performance of progressive tasks.
4. Avoid situational vulnerability (at early stages of learning, avoid competition).
5. Teach proper use of feedback.

Use Positive Reinforcement and Postive Role Models

1. Reward mastery attempts.
2. Be a positive role model (especially female models).
3. Expose girls and women to respected high-skill models.
4. Model approval ("We should be careful to be sure that our actions communicate approval, not just our words").

Use Communication Techniques

1. Help females dream of success.
2. Communicate clearly.
3. Use praise as a reward.
4. Use persuasive techniques.
5. Encourage positive self-talk.

Reduce Anxiety.

Adapted from Corbin C: Self-confidence of females in sports and physical activity. Clinics in Sports Medicine, 3:895–908, 1984, with permission.

more venturesome and independent than their non-athletic counterparts."[29] Challip et al. similarly point out "female athletes have a more positive body image and evidence higher psychological well-being than female non-athletes."[8]

Young female athletes may have a "healthier" approach to sports because they appear to consider the possibilities of positive competitive outcomes more than young men who are motivated more by the avoidance of possible failure.[45] Smith demonstrated that young female athletes exhibit a higher level of sportsmanship than young male athletes, and that young women in general display higher level of sportsmanship than men.[50]

In sports, as in many professions, the attitudes and opportunities for women are changing. It was only during my recent experience as a team physician for a high school football team that I began to understand why my professional training was so arduous. I came to realize that it is very difficult to play the game when you don't know the rules. The rules taught in football (pecking order, team positions, legal plays, what the coach says goes, etc.) apply to all the various professions (including medicine, as typified by morning medical rounds). Women participating in sports (and all the professions) are learning the rules and even changing some of the rules. As a result, the game (and the professions) improves and becomes more reasonable for everyone.

ACKNOWLEDGEMENT. This chapter would not have been possible without the numerous reviews and constructive criticisms of Drs. Morris Mellion, John A. Lombardo, and Jerilynn Prior, M.D. I am also grateful for the editorial assistance of Ms. Sharon O. Sudderth.

REFERENCES

1. Agostini R, Lombardo JA: Stress fractures in active women—Comparison of prevalence of oligo/amenorrhea in women with documented stress fractures, Cleveland Clinic, unpublished.
2. Anderson JL: Women's sports and fitness programs at the U.S. Military Academy. Phys Sportsmed 7:72, 1979.
3. Bernstein AE, Warner GM: Women Treating Women: Case material from women treated by female psychonalysts. New York, International Universities Press, Inc., 1984, p 50.
4. Blumenthal JA, Rose S, Chang JL: Anorexia nervosa and exercise: implications from recent findings. Sports Medicine 2:237–247, 1985.
5. Bostran LC, Gardner I: Achievement motivation and the athlete. Int J Sport Psychol 12:204–215, 1981.
6. Boyden TW, Parmenter RW, Stanforth P, et al: Sex steroids and endurance running in women. Fertil Steril 39:629–632, 1983.
7. Bruser M: Sporting activities during pregnancy. Obstet Gynecol 32:721–725, 1968.
8. Chalip L, Villiger J, Duigan P: Sex-role identity in a select sample of women field hockey players. Int J Sport Psychol 11:240–248, 1980.
9. Chipman JJ, et al: Excessive Weight Loss in the Athletic Adolescent: A Diagnostic Dilemma. Society for Athlete Medicine, 1983, pp 247–252.
10. Clapp III JF, Dickstein S: Endurance exercise and pregnancy outcome. Medicine and Science in Sports and Exercise, Vol 16. 1984, pp 556–562.
11. Consensus Conference on Osteoporosis, National Institutes of Health. JAMA 252:No.6, Aug. 10, 1984.
12. Corbin B: Self-confidence of females in sports and physical activity. Clin Sports Med 3:No. 4, Oct. 1984.

13. Crisp AH, Hsu LKG, Harding, B, Hartshorn J: Clinical features of anorexia nervosa: A study of consecutive series of 102 female patients. J Psychosom Med 24:179–91, 1980.

14. Crisp AH, Palmer RL, Kalucy RS: How common is anorexia nervosa? A prevalence study. Brit J Psychiat 128:549–54, 1976.

15. Curet LB, Orr JA, Rankin JHG, Ungerer T: Effect of exercise on cardiac output and distribution of uterine bloodflow in pregnant ewes. J Appl Physiol 40:725–728, 1976.

16. DeHaven KE, Dolan WA, Mayer PJ: Chondromalacia patella in athletes. Am J Sports Med 7:5–11.

17. Drinkwater BL, Nilson K, Chestnut III GH, et al: Bone mineral content of amenorrheic and eumenorrheic athletes. N Engl J Med 311:277–81, 1984.

18. Edwards MJ: The effects of hyperthermia on brain development. In Nyhan, WL Jones, KJ (eds): Prenatal Diagnosis and Mechanisms of Teratogenesis. New York, Liss, 1982, p 3–11.

19. Frisch RE, Gotz-Welbergen AV, McArthur JW et al: Delayed menarche and amenorrhea of college athletes in relation to age of onset of training. JAMA 246:1559–1563, 1981.

20. Garner DG, Garfinkel PE: Sociocultural factors in the development of anorexia nervosa. Psychol Med 10:647–656, 1980.

21. Greenblatt RB: Fibrocystic breast disease. Clin Obstet Gynecol 25:365, 1982.

22. Halmi KA: Anorexia nervosa. In Kaplan HI, Freedman AM, Sadock BJ (eds): Comprehensive Textbook of Psychiatry III. Baltimore, Williams & Wilkins, 1980, Section 39.2.

23. Hauth JC, et al: Fetal heart rate reactivity before and after maternal jogging during the third trimester. Am J Obstet Gynecol 142:545, 1982.

24. Henry JH, Crosland JW: Conservative treatment of patello-femoral subluxation. Am J Sports Med 7:12–14, 1979.

25. Hensleigh PA, Johnson DC: Heat stress effect during pregnancy. I. Retardation of fetal rat growth. Fertil Steril 22:522–527, 1971.

26. Horner MS: Sex Differences in Achievement Motivation and Performances in Competitive and Non-Competitive Situations. Unpublished doctoral dissertation, University of Michigan, 1968.

27. Hunter LY: Womens' athletics: The orthopedic surgeon's viewpoint. Clin Sports Med 3:809–827, 1984.

28. Jones RL, Botti JJ, Anderson WM, Bennett NL: Thermoregulation during aerobic exercise in pregnancy. Obstet Gynecol 65:340–345, 1985.

29. King JP, Chi PS: Social structure, sex roles and personality: Comparison of male-female athletes-non-athletes. In Goldstein (ed): Sports, Games and Play. Hillsdale, N.J., Lawrence Erlbaum Assoc., 1979.

30. Leduc B: The effect of hyperventilation on maternal placental blood flow in pregnant rabbits. J Physiol, London 225:339–348, 1972.

31. Lenz HW: Women's sports and fitness programs at the U.S. Naval Academy. Phys Sports Med 7:41–50, 1979.

32. Lindberg JS, Fearso WB, et al: Exercise-induced amenorrhea and bone density. Ann Int Med 101:647–648, 1984.

33. Lotgering FK, et al: Maternal and Fetal Responses to Exercise during Pregnancy. Physiol Rev 65:1–36, 1985.

34. Lotgering FK et al: The interaction of exercise and pregnancy: A Review. Am J Obstet Gynecol July 1, 1984, p 560.

35. Lutter JM: Health concerns of women runners. Clin Sports Med 4:671–683, 1985.

36. Malena RM, Haper AB, et al: Age at menarche in athletes and non-athletes. Med Sci Sports 5:11–13, 1973.

37. Marcus R, Cann C, et al: Menstrual function and bone mass in elite women distance runners. Ann Intern Med 102:158–163, 1985.

38. May JR, et al: A preliminary study of elite adolescent women athletes and their attitudes toward training and femininity. In The Elite Athlete, Spectrum Publications, Inc., 1985, pp 163–169.

39. McBryde A: Stress fractures in athletes, J Sports Med Sept./Oct., 1975, pp. 212–217.

40. McElroy MA, Willis JD: Women and the achievement conflict in sports: A preliminary study. J Sports Psychol 1:241–247, 1979.

41. McSherry JA: The diagnostic challenge of anorexia nervosa. Am Fam Physician 29:141–145, 1984.

42. Prior JC, Vigna Y: Gonadal steroids in athletic women: Contraception, complications and performance. Sports Medicine 2:287–295, 1985.

43. Prior JC, Vigna Y: The therapy of reproductive system changes associated with exercise training. In Menstrual Cycle and Physical Activity, pp 105–116.

44. Reider B, et al: Clinical characteristics of patella disorder in young athletes. Am J Sports Med 9:270–273, 1981.

45. Rushall BS, Tox RG: An approach-avoidance motivation scale for sports. Can J Appl Sports Sci 5:39–43, 1980.

46. Rubenstein E, Federman, D: Scientific American Medicine. New York, Scientific American, 1981, pp 1–16.

47. Severino S, et al: Premenstrual syndromes: An update. The Female Patient 12:69–78, 1987.

48. Shade AR: Gynecologic and obstetric problems. Clin Sports Med 2:No. 3, Nov., 1983.

49. Shangold MM: Gynecologic concerns in the woman athlete. Clin Sports Med 3:869–879, 1984.

50. Smith NJ: Excessive weight loss and food aversion in athletes simulating anorexia nervosa. Pediatrics 66:139–142, 1980.

51. Stark JA, Toulouse A: The young female athlete: Psychological considerations. Clin Sports Med 3:909–921, 1984.

52. Tresner D: The cumulative record of research on fear of success. Sex Roles 2:217, 1976.

53. Tucker P (moderator): Eating disorders in young athletes: A round table. Phys Sportsmed 13:98–106, 1985.

54. Warren MP: The effect of exercise on pubertal progression and reproductive function in girls. J Clin Endocrinol Metab 51:1150–1157, 1980.

55. Warren MP, et al: Scoliosis and fracture in young ballet dancers. N Engl J Med 314:1348–53, 1986.

8 Clinical Features of the Athletic Heart Syndrome

TIM P. HUSTON, M.D.
WM. MACMILLAN RODNEY, M.D.

In the last decade the advent of improved noninvasive cardiac imaging has provided new appreciation for the entity known as the "athletic heart syndrome." Although it had long been known that an athletic heart differs in some respects,[1,2] recent imaging improvements yielded new data and insight regarding the details of these differences. Simultaneously, the American public was "rediscovering" the value of health and fitness. The 26-mile marathon metamorphosed from an obscure Olympic race to a major sporting event with up to ten thousand runners participating.

With a popular tune exhorting "Let's Get Physical," physicians encountered the conditioned heart with a greater frequency. Although this new emphasis on health and fitness is a boon to the ultimate goals of the medical profession, some of the desired cardiovascular changes produced physical and laboratory findings that could be considered abnormal. As with all things, interpretation of the findings depends on the context. It is the purpose of this chapter to provide a contextual understanding that allows the clinician to reassure the patient appropriately when these cardiovascular changes are signs of health rather than disease.

CARDIAC CONDITIONING AND EFFICIENCY

Since the ability of the heart to deliver oxygen is generally the limiting factor in the performance of continuing muscular work, the heart must adapt as the athlete strives for greater and greater performance. Several factors that influence cardiac efficiency include:[3] (1) a given stroke volume is ejected with less myocardial muscle cell shortening if contraction starts at a larger ventricular volume; (2) energy losses from friction and tension are minimized with increasing end diastolic diameter; (3) a stretched muscle fiber will, within limits, provide higher tension than a less-stretched fiber; (4) loss of energy is greater when fiber contraction occurs less frequently; and (5) the greater the cardiac volume, the greater is the tension of the myocardial fibers necessary to sustain a given intraventricular pressure. Therefore, the heart would maximize its efficiency via a larger intraventricular volume (to satisfy the first three conditions), a slower heart rate and a thicker ventricular wall (to satisfy the latter). In fact, these changes occur with dynamic ("aerobic") conditioning.

It is interesting to note that a different pattern has been observed in athletes engaging in predominantly static ("anaerobic", e.g., weight lifting) conditioning.[4-8] In these static athletes, one often finds an increase in left ventricular wall thickness unaccompanied by left ventricular dilation. Presumably the reason for this difference is that dynamic athletes adapt to a state of relative "volume overload," in which a large cardiac output must be maintained for prolonged periods in the face of relatively normal vascular resistance. Static athletes, however, adapt to a "pressure overload" and must maintain elevated cardiac outputs for a briefer period of time under greatly elevated vascular resistance. Hence, this adaptation calls for greater wall thickness in order to overcome the wall stress, satisfying Laplace's law:

$$\text{wall stress} = \frac{\text{intraventricular pressure}}{\text{wall thickness} \times 2}$$

Practically speaking, however, most static athletes also engage in dynamic training. Conversely many dynamic athletes do some static training. Hence the clinician often sees a spectrum of changes rather than a strict dichotomy. Furthermore, the clinician is advised to take note of exercise habits during the intake interview or yearly physical review. The conditioning changes described in this chapter usually do not occur with the intermittent exerciser or "weekend warrior." However, we are seeing more and more patients who are finding the time in their daily lives to comply with prescribed aerobic conditioning, a minimum of three to four hours per week regularly. The remainder of this chapter deals with the conditioned athlete's cardiac examination, ECG changes, and morphologic adaptations.

THE CARDIAC EXAMINATION

Frequently, the cardiac examination is entirely normal in athletes. In the dynamic athlete, however, one might note a large pulse amplitude as well as a diffuse left ventricular impulse. Ventricular gallops and soft systolic murmurs are commonly heard. Inter-observer variability is a phenomenon that describes the subjective nature of the auscultatory cardiac examination. With a preconceived notion, the clinician frequently becomes more compulsive in detecting and recording auscultatory findings. This is particularly true for the studies that have been done to record the examinations of well-conditioned athletes. Because of this variability phenomenon, the range of reported findings is quite wide.

For example, midsystolic murmurs have been noted in 30–50% of dynamic athletes. Generally, these murmurs are graded I or II. Similarly, third and fourth heart sounds are common. Third heart sounds are more common than fourth, but even fourth heart sounds have been detected in a range of 20–60%. The chest x-ray occasionally shows modest cardiomegaly (cardiothoracic ratio of 0.5 or greater) with or without a globular appearance. Pulmonary venous engorgement may accompany some of these cases. Nonetheless, the examination alone is likely to neither simulate cardiac illness nor alarm the physician.

Rhythm and Voltage Disturbances. This is not always the case with the rhythm and voltage disturbances that can accompany physical training. The rhythm disturbances seem to be limited to dynamic athletes. The most common abnormality is sinus bradycardia, with the prevalence frequently exceeding 50% in several large studies.[9-11] The degree of bradycardia correlates with the intensity of the training. There is ongoing discussion over the reason for the bradycardia. Some studies indicate that excess vagal predominance ("vagotonia") is responsible, while others claim that there may be an intrinsic cardiac adaptation. ("Vagotonia" could represent either an increase in vagal tone or a decrease in sympathetic tone.)

Sinus dysrhythmia, defined as at least a 10% variation in p-p intervals, is also quite common, having been shown to exist in 13.5%–69% of dynamic athletes.[10,12] Sinus dysrhythmia is likewise known to vary with intensity of training. In controlled studies, wandering atrial pacemaker has been recorded in up to 19% of athletes. Atrial and ventricular tachycardias have been shown to occur in otherwise healthy athletes[14] but not in controlled trials. Hence, it is questionable if these tachycardias are a result of training (i.e., part of the athletic heart syndrome).

After sinus bradycardias and arrhythmias, atrioventricular blocks are the most common rhythm abnormalities seen. Given the vagal influence on AV node conduction, this is not surprising. A prolonged conduction time has been observed in controlled studies and also has been shown to develop *de novo* as athletes embark on training programs.[15] Normalization occurs both after exercise and administration of sympathomimetic drugs.[13,16] In addition, cessation of training results in disappearance of the atrioventricular block. Most common is first degree block, which is detected in 10–37% of resting and ambulatory ECGs. Second degree block (Mobitz I) is clearly related to training.[16] Long term follow-up of these cases reveals no association with evolving cardiac disease.

Prevalence between 2.4 and 10% has been observed for second degree block.[17,18] Mobitz Type II is less frequent, having occurred in only one controlled ambulatory study at a frequency of 8.6%.[19] Similar to previously mentioned arrhythmias, there is no pathologic significance and the prognosis is one of good health. Mobitz Type II block must be quite rare. No cases were reported from a series of 12,000 resting ECGs from the Rome Heart Institute. However, two athletes did have a third degree block that promptly disappeared with cessation on training.[20]

Junctional rhythm might also be anticipated from the theory of excess vagal tone. In fact, junctional rhythm occurs more often than expected in athletes. A 7% prevalence was discovered in one survey of resting ECGs and a 20% occurrence (versus an absence in nonathletes) in a controlled ambulatory study.[13]

Many other disturbances of rhythm and conduction may occur. Examples include anecdotal reports of bundle branch block, pre-excitation, atrial fibrillation, paroxysmal supraventricular tachycardia, ventricular tachycardia, and ventricular fibrillation. Without controlled or prospective studies, they cannot be considered a result of training. Furthermore, the common thread that links documented athletic heart disturbances is a relative increase in vagal tone. This mechanism could not account for these additional abnormalities. A summary of observed rhythm abnormalities is seen in Table 1.

Electrocardiographic Alterations. Alterations in repolarization are also a prominent manifestation of the training effect. ST-segment and T-wave changes again are seen most frequently but not exclusively in dynamic athletes. There are four primary patterns of altered repolarization: (1) ST-segment elevation with peaked T-waves; (2) ST-segment depression with depressed J points; (3) "juvenile" T-wave pattern (right precordial J point elevation with inverted T-waves); and (4) T-wave inversion in the lateral precordium.[21] The frequency of ST-segment elevation varies, but in general the more highly trained the athlete is, the more likely one will find it. Elevation of the ST-segment has been shown to develop and in-

crease in direct relation to training intensity.[22] As with the rhythm changes, it normalizes with exertion and is thought to be due to a change of autonomic input to the heart.

One plausible explanation for St-segment changes is that the mass of myocardial cells has a significant degree of variability regarding the action potential duration of the cells. Sympathetic tone enforces a relative equality of action potential duration upon the myocardial muscle cell masses. The relative decrease in sympathetic input to the heart (which accompanies training) could theoretically unmask an inherent asymmetry. This asymmetry may be associated with ST-segment elevation (or, by the same token, the much less common ST-depression). This is compatible with the observed development of ST-segment changes occurring and increasing with training intensity, obliteration of ST-segment changes during exertion, and disappearance of ST-segment changes with discontinuation of training.

The T-wave changes one sees consist of tall and peaked waves (usually associated with J-point elevation) or of T-wave inversions. Both of these occur in limb and/or precordial leads. These T-wave inversions have been associated with normal arteriograms.[23,24] An increase in left ventricular mass has been

TABLE 1. FREQUENCIES OF RHYTHM DISTURBANCES ON RESTING ELECTROCARDIOGRAMS OF THE GENERAL POPULATION AND ATHLETES*

ARRHYTHMIA	GENERAL POPULATION (%)	ATHLETES (%)
Sinus bradycardia	23.7	50-85
Sinus arrhythmia	2.4-20	13.5-69
Wandering atrial pacemaker	—	7.4-19
First-degree block	0.65	6-33
Second-degree block		
Mobitz I	0.003	0.125-10
Mobitz II	0.003	Not reported
Third-degree block	0.0002	0.017
Nodal rhythm	0.06	0.031-7.0
Ventricular pre-excitation	0.1-0.15	0.15-2.5
Atrial fibrillation	0.004	0-0.63

Reproduced with permission from the New England Journal of Medicine. Huston TP, Puffer JC, Rodney WM: The athletic heart syndrome. N Engl J Med 313:24–32, 1985.

noted when athletes with T-wave inversions are compared to athletes without the inversions.[25] Like the peaked T-waves, inverted T-waves appear as a direct effect of training, and they readily normalize with sympathetic maneuvers. These observations support a probable vagotonic etiology and, therefore, a benign prognosis. A third and less common T-wave change is a biphasic T-wave with terminal negativity in leads V_3 to V_6.[20]

The most striking changes seen in the ECG of the conditioned athlete are the large voltages, which is a manifestation of the physiologic enlargement that occurs as a result of conditioning. Increased P-wave amplitude as well as evidence of right ventricular hypertrophy (RVH) and left ventricular hypertrophy (LVH) are found. The prevalence of LVH has reached up to 85% in various surveys. Right ventricular hypertrophy is slightly less frequent. Ventricular hypertrophy of either chamber occurs less frequently in static athletes when compared to dynamically conditioned athletes. The amplitudes of the voltages have been observed to increase as training progresses. A 25% increase in voltage amplitude was observed during eleven weeks of training in one prospective study.[27] A more detailed analysis of the athlete's ECG has been published by the authors.[28]

The various ECG manifestations of the trained athlete have been observed for many years. More recently, refinements in ultrasound imaging and nuclear isotope imaging have delineated new detailed information regarding the morphologic counterparts of these previously observed electrocardiographic changes. A superb review of this information has been published by Maron.[29]

MORPHOLOGIC ADAPTATIONS

As would be predicted by the need for maximum efficiency as defined earlier, the athlete's heart enlarges in terms of wall thickness and chamber dilation. While there is debate over the degree of change brought about by static versus dynamic training, it seems clear that the changes are not pathological. It is uncommon, though not unheard of, for the clinical presentation and the echo-

cardiographic picture to closely simulate disease such as dilated or hypertrophic cardiomyopathy. The dilation and hypertrophy that occur with the athletic heart syndrome generally fall within accepted ranges of normality. Occasionally values outside the norm are found, but in an asymptomatic highly trained athlete the index of suspicion is justifiably lessened. In these cases the probability of cardiac disease is extremely low, and further invasive testing usually is not indicated.

Left ventricular end diastolic diameter is usually increased and can be observed to change as training progresses. An average increase of 9.8% was found in a compilation of studies.[29] This increase of 9.8% increases ventricular volume by approximately one-third. Since the systolic diameter is not changed, the stroke volume is appreciably increased. And, since cardiac output is the product of heart rate and stroke volume, the athlete's heart substantially increases achievable cardiac output. This is how the athlete's heart contributes to the entire sequence of physiologic adaptation, culminating in an increase in maximal myocardial oxygen uptake (VO_2 max) and, ultimately, athletic performance.

The maximum left ventricular end diastolic diameter (LVEDD) reported is 70 mm, with another study recording an average of 59.8 mm.[30,31] They are both beyond the 57-mm upper range of normal limit as defined by the 1984 UCLA Division of Cardiology standards. Nonetheless, for dynamic athletes most studies in practice report values in the upper part of the normal range. There is evidence that static athletes do not have chamber dilation greater than would be predicted by their increased body mass.[5,6] This is a disputed point, but a difference between the two types of athletes would be physiologically predictable for reasons stated earlier in this chapter.

Right ventricular end diastolic diameter (RVEDD) is generally increased in dynamic athletes.[4,13,32] This has been documented in six of eight studies surveyed by Maron.[29] The average increase in RVEDD, when these studies were summarily tabulated, was 24%. It is not easily to translate the increase in RVEDD into a percent increase in chamber volume, as the right ventricle is more eccentrically shaped than the left. However, it seems logical to assume that right and left ventricles enlarge in a similar qualitative and etiologic fashion. Correlative studies support this proposal.[32] Left atrial enlargement of a mild degree occurred in over half of all studies surveyed.[29] In conditioned athletes, the right atrial transverse axis has been increased by up to 22% when compared to non-athletes.[32]

Clearly, cardiac chamber enlargement of some degree occurs, and it probably occurs to a greater degree in dynamic than static athletes. This allows for an increase in stroke volume and, ultimately, cardiac output. At the same time hypertrophy of the left ventricular free wall and septum has been observed in both static and dynamic athletes.[5,9-11, 13, 32] An average wall thickness increase of 19% and 14%, for dynamic and static athletes respectively, has been reported. Again, the values generally fall within the normal range, but free wall thicknesses greater than 11 mm (up to 15 mm) occasionally have been reported.[10] This physiologic hypertrophy can occur in childhood athletes also.[33]

The ventricular septum hypertrophies with a documented thickness of up to 16 mm.[8] As with the ECG characteristics previously discussed, dilation and hypertrophy of the heart can be seen to develop progressively with conditioning and conversely to reverse with deconditioning. With chamber dilation, the thickening of the myocardium is necessary to reduce the wall strain that would otherwise occur, as dictated by Laplace's law. Sadly, this deconditioning can be observed within four days of rest. Increase and decreases in myocardial oxygen uptake (VO_2 max) closely follow these cardiac changes. A qualitative summary of the changes occurring in athletes utilizing dynamic predominant (isotonic) versus static dominant (isometric) training is portrayed in Table 2. Maron has provided a quantitative tabular description of some of these changes (see Table 3).

SUMMARY OF CHANGES

Hence the five factors that affect myocardial efficiency mentioned in the beginning of this chapter are all dealt with by the athletic heart. There is a slowing of heart rate (for a given cardiac output); there is chamber dilation leading to less myocardial muscle cell shortening and friction; and there is muscular hypertrophy, lessening the tension (and O_2 demand) on myocardial muscle cells.

The clinical significance of this constellation of changes is variable depending upon the clinical context. In a tertiary care context, an individual with a systolic murmur, increased voltage on the ECG, a hypertrophied septum by echocardiogram, and a septal to left ventricular free wall ratio of greater than 1.3 merits consideration of hypertrophic cardiomyopathy. In a primary care context, the athletic heart syndrome is an equally valid consideration. Note that the conditioned athletic heart usually has a normal or enlarged LVEDD and symmetrical myocardial thickening. This is in contrast to the generally encroached-upon ventricular cavity caused by an asymmetric septal hypertrophy in the cardiomyopathic patient. The family history, or lack of it, also helps distinguish the athletic heart. In a similar fashion, a ventricular gallop with an unusual degree of ventricular dilation might simulate a pathologically dilated heart in an older athlete. Yet, in the older athlete, the excellent ventricular function and capacity for physical endeavor would argue against pathology.

The various electrocardiographic changes, especially second and third degree block, ST-segment changes, and T-wave inversions all are potentially pathological. Fortunately, in the athlete, each of them normalizes with adequate exertion or sympathomimetic/vagolytic drugs. Usually it is not difficult to distinguish the athletic from the diseased heart. However, when confronted with an athletic conditioned patient with potentially serious cardiac disease that cannot readily be distinguished from conditioned normality, the clinician should not hesitate to request treadmill testing, Holter monitoring, nuclear imaging studies or angiography.

Jim Fixx, the running expert and well known author died suddenly while engaging in his specialty. Professional tennis player and Wimbledon champion, Arthur Ashe, suffered a myocardial infarction in his early thirties. Sudden death in athletes is occasionally attributable to cardiomyopathy and/or coronary artery disease.[34] The diagnosis of "athletic heart syndrome" can be made premortem. Usually the history and physical examination are sufficient for diagnosis. Occasionally, noninvasive testing will be required for confirmation. Rarely invasive testing will be necessary. A second opinion from a consulting colleague is another useful option in practice.

At least one symptom can be attributable to the athletic heart syndrome (hence justifying the term "syndrome"). Syncope or near syncope was repeatedly reported by four bradycardic athletes, each of whom also manifested large variations in heart rate or second degree block. After cessation of training, all symptoms and abnormalities disappeared.[35] Since the connection would not always be made by the unwary clinician, the appearance of this symptom merits investigation. If athletic heart syndrome is the likely explanation, counseling with the patient should follow. The authors have encountered a "tri-athlete" with several episodes of otherwise unexplained syncope. We suggested a decrease in her training schedule, but she demurred. At the time of this writing, she continues to train and she remains otherwise healthy.

In summary, the process of training induces a state of relatively increased vagal tone that in turn leads to several predictable electrocardiographic rhythm and repolarization changes. Simultaneously, dilation of the cardiac chambers and concomitant myocardial hypertrophy results in voltage changes as well as the corresponding echocardiographic findings. These adaptations allow maximal cardiac output to occur with increased efficiency, enabling the athlete to increase the flow of oxygen and energy producing substrates to the muscles.

With the widespread rediscovery of and continuing emphasis on health and fitness, the primary care physician will encounter more and more patients who are exercising. Regular exercise patterns of sustained activities of greater than four hours per week can lead to a constellation of findings that we have described as the athletic heart syndrome. Much of the recently developed technology in improved diagnostic imaging of the heart has created a new awareness of the electrocardiographic and echocardiographic changes that accompany the athletic heart syndrome. Since much of the initial research

TABLE 2. ECHOCARDIOGRAPHIC CHANGES IN ISOTONIC AND ISOMETRIC ATHLETES*

	ISOTONIC	ISOMETRIC
Left ventricular end-diastolic diameter	↑	↑, no △
Left ventricular end-diastolic diameter per square meter on per square meter or per kilogram	↑	no △
Left ventricular end-systolic diameter	↑, ↓, no △	↑, ↓, no △
Left ventricular end-diastolic volume	↑	no △
Left ventricular posterior-wall thickness	↑	↑
Left ventricular mass	↑	↑
Left ventricular mass, per square meter or per kilogram	↑	no △
Interventricular septal thickness	↑	↑
Interventricular-septum/posterior-wall ratio	↑, no △	↑, no △
Right ventricular diameter	↑	—
Left atrial diameter	↑	—
Ejection fraction	no △	no △
Cardiac output (resting)	no △	no △
Stroke volume	↑	↑, no △
Velocity of circumferential fiber shortening	↑, ↓, no △	no △

*↑ denotes increase, ↓ decrease, and no △ no change.
Reproduced with permission from the New England Journal of Medicine. Huston TP, Puffer JC, Rodney WM: The athletic heart syndrome. N Engl Med 313:24–32, 1985.

TABLE 3. VENTRICULAR DIMENSIONS IN ATHLETES AND NONATHLETES AS ASSESSED BY ECHOCARDIOGRAPHY IN PUBLISHED STUDIES*

ECHOCARDIOGRAPHIC VARIABLE	NONATHLETE CONTROLS		ATHLETES		PERCENT DIFFERENCE
	Mean Value	No. of Subjects	Mean Value	No. of Subjects	
Ventricular septal thickness (mm)	9.1	313	10.4	461	+14.3
Posterior free wall thickness (mm)	9.0	439	10.7	740	+18.9
LV end-diastolic dimension (mm)	49.1	394	53.9	701	+ 9.8
Estimated LV mass (g)	175	252	256	381	+46.3
RV internal transverse dimension (mm)	17.7	146	22.0	147	+24.3

Reprinted with permission from the American College of Cardiology. Maron BJ: Structural features of the athletic heart as defined by echocardiography. J Am Coll Cardiol 7:190–203, 1986.

was done in tertiary care settings, these findings are frequently misinterpreted and/or overemphasized as being correlates of cardiac disease. Primary care physicians have a perspective from which to observe these changes as more frequently correlated with health. The primary care physician should remain vigilant for minor variations that mandate additional investigation. An understanding of the athletic heart syndrome permits reassurance and conservative management to be extended to those in whom this syndrome is encountered.

MANAGEMENT SUMMARY

With the increasing numbers of athletically conditioned patients in practice, a primary care physician is likely to encounter the normal cardiac variance produced by this conditioning. For the practicing physician, the dilemma is a familiar one. The physician must interpret signs and symptoms within the context of the patient's environment. The athlete may have physical findings and electrocardiographic findings that would be considered abnormal in an untrained individual. Simultaneously, the experienced clinician is aware of the fact that disease can occur even in healthy and exceedingly fit individuals.

This chapter was intended to provide an awareness of the variance from normal to be found in the conditioned, healthy, athletic heart. A rational plan for investigation and

management can be more clearly understood once there is such awareness. For the asymptomatic athlete with routine physical findings and an ECG typical of the athletic heart, vigorous reassurance is strongly recommended. In some cases, an exercise treadmill test may be helpful in emphasizing and underlining normalcy. The clinician should be wary of the poor predictive value of a positive result (i.e., false-positive effect).

If the athlete is symptomatic, further investigation may be useful. The first level of this investigation should be an attempt to witness these symptoms. Most frequently, this can be done on an exercise treadmill test. Nevertheless, there are many symptoms that merely require a more thorough history and physical examination. The finding of chest-wall pain or costochondritis does not merit an expensive treadmill investigation.

Each period of history has its unique context. In 1987, the American medical profession is in an extremely cautious posture regarding the underdiagnosis of disease. Nevertheless, when confronted with the physical and electrocardiographic findings previously described, we feel a responsibility to strongly re-emphasize the high probability of health. The message of uncertainty with invasive testing and frequent repeat visits is not in the best interest of the patient or the profession. Our own preference is to categorically state that the athlete is absolutely "super normal" unless we have convincing evidence of possible organic heart disease. With this in in mind, these patients are scheduled for routine adult health maintenance protocols. In ten years, we have seen no cases or read of cases where this strategy has proved harmful. On the other hand, we have encountered multiple cases of cardiac neurosis and/or financial morbidity where this strategy has not been followed.

REFERENCES

1. Osler W: The Principles and Practice of Medicine. New York, Appleton, 1982, p. 635.
2. Blake JB, Larraba RC: Observations upon long distance runners. Boston Med Surg J 148:95, 1903.
3. Astrand P, Rodohl K: Textbook of Work Physiology. New York, McGraw Hill, 1977, p. 176.
4. Zeppilli S, Sandric S, Cecchetti F, et al: Echocardiographic assessments of cardiac arrangements in different sports activities. In Lubich T, Venerando A, (eds): Sports Cardiology. Bologna, Aulo Gaggi, 1980, pp 723–34.
5. Snoeckx LHEH, Abelilng HFM, Lambregts JAC, Schmitz JJF, Verstappen FTJ, Reneman RS: Echocardiographic dimensions in athletes in relation to their training programs. Med Sci Sports Exerc 14:428–34, 1982.
6. Morganroth J, Maron BJ, Henry WL, Epstein SE: Comparative left ventricular dimensions in trained athletes. Ann Intern Med 82:521–24, 1975.
7. Longhurst JC, Kelly AR, Gonyea WJ, Mitchell JH: Chronic training with static dynamic exercise: Cardiovascular adaptation, and response to exercise. Circ Res, 48(6:Part 2):I-171-8, 1981.
8. Keul J, Dickhuth HH, Simon G, Lehmann M: Effect of static and dynamic exercise on heart volume, contractility, and left ventricular dimensions. Circ Res 48(6:Part 2):I-162-70, 1981.
9. Parker BM, Londeree BR, Cupp GV, Dubiel JP: The noninvasive cardiac evaluation of long-distance runners. Chest 73:376–81, 1978.
10. Cohen JL, Gupta PK, Lichstein E, Chadda KD: The heart of a dancer: Noninvasive cardiac evaluation of professional ballet dancers. Am J Cardiol 45:959–65, 1980.
11. Paulsen W, Boughner D, Ko P, et al: Left ventricular function in marathon runner: Echocardiographic assessment. J Appl Physiol 51:881–86, 1981.
12. Minamitani K, Miyagawa M, Konco M, Kitamura K: The electrocardiogram of professional cyclists. In Lubich T, Venerando A (eds): Sports Cardiology. Bologna, Aulo Gaggi, 1980 pp 315–25.
13. Roeske WR, O'Rourke RA, Klein A, et al: Noninvasive evaluation of ventricular hypertrophy in professional athletes. Circulation 53:286–92, 1976.
14. Coelho A, Palileo E, Ashley W: Tachyarrhythmias in young athletes. J Am Coll Cardiol ??
15. Hanne-Paparo N: Long term ECGT monitoring of a sportsman with a second degree A-V block. In Lubich T, Venerando A (eds): Sports Cardiology. Bologna, Aulo Gaggi, 1980 pp 559–67.
16. Zeppilli P, Fenici R, Sassara M, et al: Wenckebach second-degree A-V block in top-ranking athletes: An old problem revisited. Am Heart J 100:281–94, 1980.
17. Meytes I, Kaplinsky E., Yahini JH, et al: Wenckebach A-V block: A frequent problem following heavy physical training. Am Heart J 90:426–30, 1975.
18. Nakamoto K: Electrocardiograms of 25 marathon runners before and after 100 meter dash. Jpn Circ J 33:105–28, 1969.
19. Hanne-Paparo N, Kellermann JJ: Long-term Holter ECG monitoring of athletes. Med Sci Sports Exerc 13:294–8, 1981.
20. Fenici R, Caselli G, Zeppilli P, Piovano G: High degree A-V block in 17 well-trained endurance athletes. In Lubich T, Venerando A (eds): Sports Cardiology. Bologna, Aulo Gaggi, 1980 pp 523–37.
21. Zeppilli P, Pirrami MM, Sassara M, Fenici R: Ventricular repolarization disturbances in athletes: Standardization of terminology, ethiopathogenetic spectrum and pathophysiological mechanism. J Sports Med Phys Fitness 21:322–35, 1981.
22. Kosunen K, Pakarinen A, Kuoppasalmi K, et al: Cardiovascular function and the renin-angiotensin-aldosterone system in long-distance runners during various training periods. Scand J Clin Lab Invest 40:429–35, 1980.
23. Oakley DG, Oakley CM; Significance of abnormal electrocardiograms in highly trained athletes. Am J Cardiol 50:985–9, 1982.
24. Casselli G, Piovano G, Venerando A: A follow-up study of abnormalities of ventricular repolarization in athletes. In Lubich T, Venerando A (eds): Sports Cardiology. Bologna, Aulo Gaggi, 1980, pp 477–99.
25. Nishimura T, Kambara H, Chen C-H, et al: Noninvasive assessment of T-wave abnormalities in precordial electrocardiograms in middle-aged professional bicyclists. J Electrocardiol 14:357–63, 1981.
26. Venerando A, Rulli V: Frequency, morphology and meaning of the electrocardiographic anomalies found in Olympic marathon runners and walkers. J Sports Med 3:135–41, 1964.
27. DeMaria AN, Neumann A, Lee G, Fowler W, Mason DT: Alterations in ventricular mass and performance induced by exercise training in man evaluated by echocardiography. Circulation 57:237–44, 1978.
28. Huston TP, Puffer JC, Rodney WM: The athletic heart syndrome. NEJM 313:24–32, 1985.
29. Maron BJ: Structural features of the athlete heart as defined by echocardiography. J Am Coll Cardiol 7:190–203, 1986.
30. Rost R: The athlete's heart. Eur Heart J 3(Suppl A):193–8), 1982.
31. Sugishita Y, Koseki S, Matsuda M, et al: Myocardial mechanics of athletic hearts in comparison with diseased hearts. Am Heart J 105:273–80, 1983.
32. Hauser AM, Dressendorfer RH, Von M, et al: Symmetric cardiac enlargement in highly trained endurance athletes: A two dimensional echocardiographic study. Am Heart J 109:1038–44, 1985.

33. Cahill NS, O'Brien M, Rodahl A, et al: A pilot study on left ventricular dimensions and wall stress before and after submaximal exercise. Br J Sports Med 13:122–29, 1979.

34. Maron BJ, Roberts WC, McAllister HA, Rosing DR, Epstein SE: Sudden death in young athletes. Circulation 62:218–29, 1980.

35. Rasmussen V, Haunso S, Shagen K: Cerebral attacks due to excessive vagal tone in heavily trained persons. Acta Med Scand 204:401–5, 1978.

9 Exercise and Hypertension

MARK E. MCKINNEY, PH.D.
MORRIS B. MELLION, M.D.

Hypertension afflicts almost 60 million Americans. In daily practice it is one of the most commonly encountered chronic medical problems. Traditionally, hypertension has been managed with salt restriction and a stepped-care drug regimen employing thiazide diuretics as the cornerstone of therapy. Over the past two decades, however, the concept of lifestyle modification as a tool for both prevention and therapy has become popular. Many patients are hoping that routine aerobic exercise will lower their high blood pressure. Those patients who participate in athletics are concerned about the effects of the disease and medications on their performances. Other hypertensive patients have complicating factors such as dietary abnormalities or obesity that affect exercise considerations. The interaction of physical exercise and hypertension may be one of the most complex issues in sports medicine, but it also provides a very fruitful approach to the effective control of blood pressure over the patient's lifespan.

In this chapter, we approach both exercise and hypertension from a hemodynamic point of view. First, the changes in cardiovascular function brought about by both hypertension and exercise are detailed. We then take a hard look at the evidence for using exercise in preventing and treating hypertension. The interaction of exercise and common antihypertensive medications is discussed and some suggestions for treating the exercising hypertensive are offered, with special guidelines for the hypertensive athlete. Finally, we look at the value of exercise stress testing in the diagnosis of hypertension.

Common abbreviations: CO, cardiac output; HR, heart rate; MAP, mean arterial pressure; SV, stroke volume; TPR, total peripheral resistance.

HEMODYNAMICS OF HYPERTENSION

A useful approach to understanding essential hypertension is to approach it hemodynamically, because not all hypertension is the same. Blood pressure is determined grossly by two factors: (1) the amount of blood pumped from the heart, or cardiac output (CO), and (2) the resistance to forward flow from the arterial system, known as total peripheral resistance (TPR). Cardiac output is the amount of blood pumped out of the heart each minute and is calculated by multiplying stroke volume (SV), the amount of blood pumped in a single beat, and heart rate (HR). If BP = CO × TPR, then there are three possible "patterns" of hypertension: elevated CO, elevated TPR, and both elevated CO and TPR.

Most hypertension is idiopathic, or "essential." It is a hemodynamic disorder with characteristic patterns that change with increasing blood pressure level, duration of hypertension, and age. Although the hallmark of well-established essential hypertension is elevated TPR, this alteration is generally not an early finding in the hemodynamic progression. Messerli has illustrated this progression graphically, applying practical terminology to the stages of hypertension (Fig. 1).[73,87,89]

Borderline Hypertension. The earliest stage of the disease is borderline hypertension. Also known as latent or labile hypertension, this stage is generally characterized by an elevated CO and a "normal" TPR.[28] Borderline hypertension is primarily a problem of the young. Typically, both components of CO, stroke volume and heart rate, are increased, as well as left ventricular ejection fraction, serum catecholamines, renin level, and renal blood flow.[30,32] TPR appears to be normal because numerically it is not elevated, but in

NORMOTENSIVE

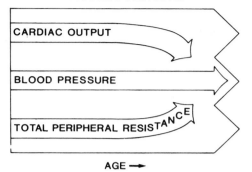

HYPERTENSIVE

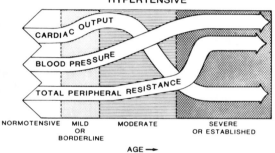

BP = CO X TPR

FIGURE 1A (top). Changes in cardiac output and total peripheral resistance as age increases. Note that blood pressure remains stable.

FIGURE 1B (bottom). Changes in cardiac output, total peripheral resistance, and blood pressure as age increases and hypertension develops.

a normotensive individual TPR would decrease to compensate for the increased CO, due primarily to baroreceptor mechanisms. In the borderline hypertensive, however, TPR remains inappropriately unchanged.[73,87,89] Additionally, borderline hypertensives have an enhanced sensitivity to sympathetic challenge,[89] which rounds out the picture of a hyperkinetic circulatory pattern.[30,75]

Mild Established Hypertension. Borderline hypertension either resolves with time for reasons that are poorly understood, or it gradually progresses to become established, or "fixed," hypertension.[3,66] Lund-Johansen documented this progression when he followed 32 young borderline or mild hypertensives for 10 years. Although the level of their blood pressure did not change appreciably

during this time, the hemodynamic pattern did. Cardiac output, particularly SV, fell, and TPR rose in an almost reciprocal fashion.[66] The change would not have been observable for the clinician monitoring only blood pressure.

There appear to be several factors causing TPR to rise with time in the hypertensive, but we await a complete understanding.[10] When arteries and arterioles are subjected to frequent neurohumoral pressure rises, the media thickens and lumen diameter decreases, thus increasing TPR.[23] Also, local autoregulation of blood blow in the periphery accounts, in part, for increased TPR.

Mild established hypertension is a transitional state. Cardiac output has normalized, although heart rate may still be elevated in some. Renal blood flow also returns to normal levels. In most patients, end organ compromise due to the hypertensive state is not yet evident.

Established Hypertension. As the hypertensive process evolves to more moderate and severe stages, CO continues to decline while TPR progressively rises.[2,29,30] With this increase of vascular resistance comes a parallel increase in afterload on the myocardium, which eventually leads to left ventricular hypertrophy. At the same time, renal vascular changes mark the development of nephrosclerosis as renal blood flow and glomerular filtration rate fall. Serum creatinine and BUN are relatively late indicators of this process, but mild proteinuria or uric acid elevation due to decreased glomerular filtration rate may offer an earlier suggestion of this problem.[44]

Severe Hypertension and Congestive Heart Failure. As the vascular changes of hypertension progress even further, a point is reached where the myocardium can no longer adapt to the increasing afterload. Renal function is markedly impaired by nephrosclerosis. At this stage of hypertension, cardiac output can no longer increase in response to the stress of exercise or emotion; instead, it remains constant or falls.[75] The left ventricle is hypertrophied with attendant loss of myocardial contractility, frequent ventricular ectopy, and increased risk of myocardial infarction and sudden cardiac death.[51] Ultimately, the natural progression of untreated hypertension leads to congestive heart failure where TPR is dramatically elevated and CO has fallen precipitously.

HEMODYNAMICS OF AEROBIC EXERCISE

Physical exercise elicits profound changes in an individual's cardiovascular system, and these responses vary with the type and intensity of exercise. This discussion focuses on the hemodynamics of aerobic endurance exercise, followed by a short mention of isometric strength training effects.

Normotensive Exercisers. Typically, endurance exercise consists of jogging, swimming, bicycling, cross country skiing, or some other form of rhythmic dynamic aerobic exercise at least three times a week for 20 or more minutes each session, plus warm-up and cool-down. Intensity of exercise is measured by the amount of oxygen consumed (VO_2). The Fick principle states that VO_2 equals the cardiac output times the arteriovenous oxygen difference, or the amount of oxygen extracted from the circulating blood (a-v O_2 difference). Since CO equals stroke volume (SV) times heart rate (HR), the relationship can be expressed with the following formula:

$$VO_2 = (SV \times HR) \times \text{a-v } O_2 \text{ diff}$$

The healthy normotensive individual responds to the demands of aerobic exercise with (1) increased SV, (2) increased HR, (3) increased arteriovenous oxygen difference, and (4) peripheral vasodilatation. The pulse pressure (systolic BP minus diastolic BP) increases as systolic BP increases roughly in proportion to CO increase, and diastolic BP decreases in parallel with vasodilatory drop in TPR.[1,63] It appears that the arterial baroreceptors change sensitivity (reset) during dynamic exercise to allow homeostatic control of blood pressure about a higher than normal level.[101] Systolic BP and diastolic BP eventually plateau, but HR continues to increase to supply oxygen to the muscles, until maximum HR is attained.[63] The increased systolic BP is due to increased CO and reflex vasoconstriction in the splanchnic and renal vascular beds. However, if CO cannot increase enough to meet exercise demands owing to disease or drug effects, TPR will adjust in order to maintain adequate pressure levels.[101] As the pulse pressure widens during exercise in the normotensive, the rise in systolic BP is generally much greater than the fall in diastolic BP; therefore, mean arterial pressure (MAP) rises with increased oxygen consumption. Figure 2 shows the blood pressure response to increased oxygen demands.

Hypertensive Individuals. Both normotensive and hypertensive subjects respond to acute exercise demand with increases in CO, but in the normotensive this is due to a greater increase in SV, while the major component of the increase in the hypertensive is increased HR.[64,87] The difference is likely due to the increased afterload experienced in hypertension and the myocardial changes that result. Both normotensives and hypertensives respond to acute exercise with a reduction in TPR, but the decrement is less in hypertensives, particularly older hypertensives, who have presumably had the disease for a longer period of time.[64] As a result of these alterations in CO and TPR during exercise, the hypertensive individual has an exaggerated blood pressure response to exercise when compared to the normotensive.[35] Figure 3 illustrates these different patterns of response. It is important to recognize that an exaggerated systolic BP response to acute exercise in normotensives indicates an increased risk for developing hypertension.[14]

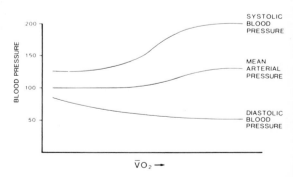

FIGURE 2. Changes in blood pressure as workload increases.

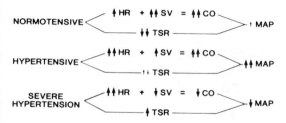

FIGURE 3. Hemodynamic responses to acute exercise in normotensives, hypertensives, and persons with severe hypertension and cardiac failure.

ISOMETRIC EXERCISE

Intensive weight training has been associated with higher blood pressure,[100] and researchers have reported higher blood pressures in weight lifters[40] and college football players.[71] During typical isometric exercise, MAP can increase 40 mmHg due to elevated CO with "normal" TPR.[19,63] Note that this pattern mimics the natural development of hypertension. In addition, isometric exercise leads to left ventricular hypertrophy (LVH) and should be avoided in patients with existing LVH.[21] Because of the large increases in blood pressure during isometric exercise, and the abnormal underlying hemodynamics of this increase, care should be taken in recommending such exercise to the hypertensive patient.

EXERCISE AS A TREATMENT FOR HYPERTENSION

Epidemiologic Evidence. Several large epidemiologic studies have shown that routine vigorous exercise correlates with a lower risk of developing hypertension.[5,6,77,80,90] Although epidemiologic research designs limit the conclusions the clinician can draw about an individual patient, it appears safe to say that these studies suggest a preventive role for exercise. Exercise may be useful as a prophylactic measure for persons at risk for developing hypertension, such as those with a positive family history, obese patients, and persons whose blood pressure is labile under stress. These conclusions are reinforced by a report from the Institute for Aerobics Research, which demonstrates that fitness level,

as determined by treadmill performance, correlates with concurrently measured blood pressure, suggesting that, even within the normal population, exercise may aid in keeping blood pressure low.[11]

Clinical Evidence. Can exercise be used to treat existing hypertension? As Kaplan has noted, "Some other practices have been advocated as effective ways to lower the blood pressure, but none more fervently than physical exercise."[52] The literature includes several recent reviews of the evidence for the exercise/hypertension hypothesis.[27,70,84,96] The general consensus is that exercise aids in lowering resting blood pressure, particularly in borderline hypertensives. Longitudinal studies in hypertensives demonstrate drops in systolic BP of 5–25 mmHg and in diastolic BP of 3–15 mmHg in response to aerobic exercise training. These changes are more prominent in, but not limited to, young borderline hypertensives. Unfortunately, many of these studies have experimental design problems, such as small numbers of subjects, lack of a nonexercising hypertensive control population, or evaluating heterogeneous populations of hypertensives as a single group.[70,96]

Still, the overall evidence indicates that exercise can aid in the reduction of resting blood pressure, and a variety of mechanisms have been suggested. Exercise may normalize renal function,[97] or it may affect the body's processing of sodium by blocking BP increases stimulated by salt loading.[91] Exercise may also reduce the increases in plasma renin activity and plasma aldosterone concentration that follow salt restriction,[78] and may lower insulin levels, causing less sodium reabsorption in the kidney.[4]

Exercise may also decrease sympathetic activity and increase parasympathetic activity, as evidenced by lower resting HR, lower TPR,[43] lower resting catecholamine levels,[16,34] and lowered responsivity to circulating catecholamines.[81] However, exercise must decrease TPR in order to improve both hemodynamic functioning and long-term prognosis.[53] Exercise may reduce peripheral sensitivity to circulating catecholamines or even induce changes in the receptor population. Both of these factors are thought to be abnormal in hypertensive animals and humans.[24,37,83] Also, both hypertensives and children of hypertensives who do not yet have high blood pressure show increased cardiovascular reactivity to mental stress,[13,36,89] a process thought to be mediated by increased sympathetic nervous system activity. Persons who show such excessive reactions may be candidates for preventive exercise prescription, although the jury is still out on whether exercise can mitigate cardiovascular reactivity directly.[15]

Prescribing Exercise.   In prescribing exercise for hypertensive patients, there are some special considerations. Exercise seems to be most successful for persons with borderline hypertension.[84,88] Since exercise appears to lower sympathetic tone, this form of hypertension is more likely to respond to exercise intervention. In addition, the patient's sex, age at initiation of the exercise program, and intensity of exercise may influence the eventual success of the treatment regimen. Younger persons show training effects more easily, and initiating regular exercise at younger ages would serve as a preventive measure as well. Also, isometric exercise has different hemodynamic, anatomical, and biochemical effects from aerobic exercise; most physicians agree that the hemodynamic effects of isometric exercise may be more harmful than helpful in controlling blood pressure.[27]

Exercise regimens will have the same compliance problems as other hypertension treatments. In addition, self-reported level of activity does not correlate with objective measures of fitness in the laboratory.[79] Therefore, if a physician is going to recommend exercise as antihypertensive therapy, it is important to plan a training program that is well suited to the individual patient. This probably means an evaluation of exercise capacity and individual preferences prior to structuring an exercise program, rather than a simple admonition to get a program started. It also means monitoring the exercise effort for appropriate intensity, perhaps by recording resting and exercise pulse rates.

OBESITY, HYPERTENSION, AND EXERCISE

Hemodynamics of Obesity and Left Ventricular Hypertrophy.   The increased body mass of the obese individual requires a higher CO and increased intravascular volume to meet its metabolic needs. The actual increase in intravascular volume, however, exceeds these needs. As long as the blood pressure remains unchanged, the obese patient will have a reduced TPR.[59,73] Indeed, it has been suggested that mild obesity may be somewhat protective against the end-organ damage caused by hypertension because of this reduced vascular resistance.[59]

In obesity the increase in CO noted results primarily from expanded SV rather than HR elevation. With expanded intravascular volume and increased SV comes increased left ventricular preload. Over time, the heart adapts to elevated preload with peripheral dilatation and eccentric left ventricular hypertrophy. Conversely, hypertension causes increased afterload with ensuing concentric left ventricular hypertrophy. The obese hypertensive with both preload and afterload elevation is subject to a much more accelerated form of left ventricular hypertrophy that often leads to early congestive heart failure.[73,76]

Exercise and Weight Reduction.   Exercise lowers blood pressure through weight loss, but there is evidence suggesting that exercise acts independently on blood pressure, as well. Furthermore, the combination of weight reduction and exercise may lower blood pressure more than either alone.[39] Both aerobic fitness training and weight reduction lower the central norepinephrine output that characterizes obesity,[39,42,92] thus reducing sympathetic cardiovascular drive. Additionally, this reduced adrenergic activity is associated with reductions in plasma renin activity and sodium retention.[92] Also, weight reduction has been shown to reduce left ventricular mass in obese hypertensives.[69]

TREATING THE EXERCISING HYPERTENSIVE

Traditionally, the standard treatment of hypertension has been the stepped-care approach: a trial of a diuretic, usually followed by the addition or substitution of a beta-blocker, and, if that is not effective, the use of a third-step drug such as a vasodilator or a central alpha agonist. Recently, other drugs have been recommended as step one therapy, as well. The addition of new categories of drugs, such as central alpha blockers, vasodilators, ACE inhibitors, and calcium slow-channel blockers, has led to some modification of this scheme, but, for the most part, stepped care is still the usual approach to treating hypertension.[44]

Behavioral Therapy. Advances in the detection of underlying hemodynamic states contributing to hypertension, recognition of the apparent value of exercise in the treatment of labile hypertension, and the advent of exercise programs with widespread participation make modifications to the standard stepped-care approach necessary. Let us take the easiest case first. The literature suggests a trial of behavioral intervention in patients with mild to moderate hypertension and without end organ damage or other complications. This would include sodium intake restriction, weight loss, relaxation training, and, most definitely, an aerobic exercise program. Like the other behavioral interventions, the exercise prescription cannot be a simple admonition; it must be a thoughtful, tailored plan. Otherwise, no benefits will accrue, because chances are the patient will not comply. In addition, the physician must conduct follow-up with behavioral therapy just as thoroughly as he or she would with pharmacotherapy. This means repeated blood pressure checks *and* monitoring of the treatment regimen, perhaps even through periodic assessment of aerobic capacity. The patients who will probably respond best to this kind of treatment are young, labile hypertensives.

Pharmacotherapy. A big challenge for the physician is choosing antihypertensive medication for the athlete or regular exerciser. Some medications produce unwanted side-effects; others may endanger the patient. Care must be taken in treating this population to ensure better compliance rates than the 40-50% usually reported.[20] In treating both recreational and competitive hypertensive athletes, the physician is well-advised to consider the hemodynamic demands of the sport in selecting appropriate medications.

Virtually all currently used antihypertensive medications permit an essentially normal exercise response, except beta-blockers, and even this class of medication has a role

in the exercising hypertensive. If the hypertensive is involved in a mildy or moderately intensive sport with periodic interruptions in activity, such as softball, volleyball, football, or downhill skiing, then the choice of agent may be made on a hemodynamic basis. Consideration should be given to choosing agents that control the hyperkinetic CO in the younger, borderline hypertensive, whereas agents that lower TPR might be more effective in the older, well-established hypertensive.

In the endurance athlete, the situation is not as simple. Hypertensive runners, swimmers, cyclists, and cross-country skiers will not comply with a regimen that lowers CO or in other ways inhibits participation. In this group of hypertensives, the physician must choose agents that reduce blood pressure but not performance.

Diuretics. Thiazide diuretics have been the traditional cornerstone of hypertension pharmacotherapy. They reduce blood pressure acutely by depleting plasma volume and decreasing CO. The hemodynamic effects of diuretics change with time, and their long-term antihypertensive effect is achieved by lowering TPR.[65]

Diuretics present several problems for the endurance athlete performing intensive exercise. The most serious limitations are fluid and potassium depletion, which become of particular concern when one exercises in heat or humidity. The importance of intravascular fluid volume for exercise in the heat is discussed in Chapter 5. Exercise stimulates potassium loss through increased epinephrine production,[8] and thiazide diuretics can exacerbate this loss by promoting increased sweating and renal wasting of potassium.[54,55,93] Exercise in the heat, when the patient is potassium depleted, may lead to rhabdomyolysis.[54,55]

Thiazide diuretics may produce widespread, exercise-induced muscle cramping in endurance athletes during the first few weeks of therapy. These cramps may involve intercostal and abdominal wall muscles, as well as limb muscles. Previously unpublished personal experience of the second author and anecdotal reports from other physicians indicate that these cramps are usually not accompanied by abnormally low serum potassium levels; the etiology of the cramping is not known. If such cramps appear, the athletes could be "weaned onto" the drug by starting with low doses every other day and gradually increasing administrations and dose.

Beta-blockers. Beta-blockers are extremely useful antihypertensive agents that are currently first-line therapy, especially for exercising hypertensives who (1) are participating in intermittent exertion sports, (2) have little or no conditioning training and are just beginning an exercise program, and (3) have coronary artery disease. In otherwise healthy hypertensives wishing to perform prolonged intense endurance exercise, they can be problematic, although they may be effective in those patients wishing only to engage in moderate endurance exercise such as brisk walking.

Although there are significant differences among individual beta-blockers, as a group these agents reduce HR and CO at rest and during exercise, increase TPR, increase muscle fatigue, reduce endurance time, and expose the athlete to a risk of hypoglycemia. The ensuing discussion will attempt to clarify the action of these drugs and identify which beta-blockers are more or less likely to affect performance.

Beta-blockers lower CO, and HR may fall by as much as one third of the pretreatment resting rate. The body partially compensates for the bradycardia with increased SV and increased oxygen extraction, but VO$_2$ still falls.[17,82,86,94] Figure 4 shows these effects.

In the otherwise healthy hypertensive these changes tend to blunt exercise performance. In the coronary artery patient, however, the hemodynamic response to beta blockade may actually increase the tolerance of exercise. By reducing HR, they increase diastole and thus improve myocardial perfusion.[58,85,99] While reports conflict about whether individuals without coronary artery disease can attain a significant training effect from aerobic exercise while on beta-blockers, it is evident that these patients increase both workload and duration of exercise while taking these drugs.[62] Wilmore and colleagues present a more comprehensive view of the relationship between beta-blockers and training effect. They contend that beta blockade increases the exercise capacity of patients with angina, decreases the capacity of well-conditioned individuals, and has little or no effect on the capacity of healthy, untrained subjects. They further suggest that untrained individuals have more hemodynamic capacity to compensate for decreased HR by increasing SV and oxygen extraction. The more highly trained athletes have generally already achieved maximal potential in both of these parameters and cannot compensate further for the bradycardic effect of beta-blockers.[103]

Beta-blockers increase the perceived exertion of exercise,[82] and this effect is muscular rather than cardiorespiratory.[95] Indeed, several factors may contribute to this prominent side effect experienced while performing endurance exercise during beta blockade. First, the lower maximum CO already noted will reduce peripheral oxygen carrying capacity. Second, beta-blockers, particularly noncardioselective agents without intrinsic sympathomimetic activity, reduce the vasodilatory beta stimulus to peripheral blood vessels. The alpha vasoconstrictive stimulus dominates, and TPR increases.[31] Consequently, blood flow to exercising muscles may be diminished. Third, metabolic changes induced by beta blockade may limit the energy producing substrate available to the working muscle.

Metabolically, beta-blockers have several effects that may limit dynamic exercise performance and increase the awareness of fatigue. Catecholamines stimulate the mobilization and utilization of free fatty acids as an energy source in exercise, and both selective and nonselective beta-blockers inhibit this process.[46,56,60] Nonselective beta-blockers also attenuate glycogenolysis, further reducing available energy substrates. This effect is negligible during short periods of submaximal endurance exercise,[47,50] but gains significance with increasing exercise duration and intensity.[56] The decreased availibility of both free fatty acids and muscle glycogen for en-

$$\overline{V}O_2 = (HR \times SV) (a - v \ O_2 \ DIFF)$$
$$\downarrow \quad \downarrow\downarrow\downarrow \quad \uparrow \quad \quad \uparrow$$

FIGURE 4.   The effect of beta blockade on the hemodynamic response to exercise.

ergy causes increased dependence on blood glucose and may lead to hypoglycemia during exercise.[46,56] Lactate production, a good indicator of energy metabolism, is also attenuated during nonselective beta blockade,[38,72] demonstrating that the above-described process is taking place. Muscle biopsy research has shown that serious distance runners with a high percentage of slow-twitch muscle fibers are more likely to experience a marked effect of beta blockade, especially noncardioselective blockade, on muscle metabolism.[49] In addition to their effects on metabolism during exercise, some beta-blockers also eliminate the favorable changes in serum lipid levels that usually result from an exercise conditioning program.[7,60]

Beta-blockers tend to increase sweating in response to exercise in the heat, as well. This effect appears greater, at least initially, with propranolol than with noncardioselective agents, but the long-term effects of cardioselective blocker use on sweating are not yet clear.[33,102] The hypertensive athlete on beta blockade must pay special attention to fluid replacement during exercise in the heat.

Beta-blockers with intrinsic sympathomimetic activity (ISA) provide much of their antihypertensive effect by reducing TPR while HR is maintained at normal levels through the ISA effect. This description is valid at rest, but research has produced conflicting results concerning the HR response to these drugs during exercise.[22,25,26] At the present time, it is difficult to say that they possess an advantage compared to beta-blockers without ISA for the hypertensive patient performing dynamic endurance exercise.

In summary, beta-blockers limit dynamic endurance exercise through muscle fatigue and the underlying metabolic etiologies. Although beta blockade reduces HR during exercise, compensatory increases in stroke volume and oxygen extraction allow performance of submaximal endurance exercise with no marked hemodynamic limitation. Cardioselective beta-blockers produce less perceived exertion by the patient,[48,102] less metabolic limitation as indicated by decreased lactate production,[38,72] less hypoglycemia, and less functional limitation on slow twitch

muscle fibers,[49] when compared with non-selective agents. Therefore, they are more likely to be tolerated by the exercising hypertensive.

Central Alpha Antagonists. The central alpha antagonists, clonidine and guanabenz, act on alpha receptors in the brainstem to block central, sympathetically mediated increases in HR and CO, thereby reducing blood pressure at rest. Since the baroreflexes are left intact, these drugs permit a normal but mildly attenuated hemodynamic response to exercise.[18,61] Because the hypertensive performing endurance exercise experiences only a minimal drop in CO during submaximal exercise on central alpha antagonists, they are unlikely to affect performance.

Alpha₁ Blockade. For the dynamic endurance athlete, prazosin is the only vasodilator to be considered as primary antihypertensive therapy. Prazosin acts by blocking postsynaptic alpha₁ receptors and normalizes blood pressure both at rest and during exercise. Hemodynamically, it reduces TPR with negligible effects on HR and CO.[67] Were it not for concern over the frequent hypotensive effect of the first dose of prazosin, this drug would probably be universal therapy for exercising mild to moderate established hypertensives.

Combined Beta and Alpha₁ Blockade. In the severe hypertensive a single hemodynamic approach to therapy is often inadequate. The combined adrenergic blocker labetolol acts on the heart to reduce CO and on the peripheral vasculature to lower TPR. It actually appears to have three mechanisms of action: (1) nonselective beta blockade reduces HR and thereby lowers CO, (2) postsynaptic alpha₁ blockade reduces peripheral vasoconstriction, thus lowering TPR, and (3) beta₂ agonist effects increase peripheral vasodilatation, further lowering TPR. Labetolol lowers blood pressure initially by lowering both CO and TPR, but over several years the CO returns to baseline levels due to increased SV.[48] It is a good choice for the more severe hypertensive wishing to exercise, where a mild diminution in CO is worth the major therapeutic gains.

Angiotension Converting Enzyme (ACE) Inhibitors. ACE inhibitors block the conversion of angiotension I to angiotensin II and thus inhibit the peripheral vasoconstriction and sodium retention caused by angiotension II. Hemodynamically, they work by decreasing TPR with little or no effect on HR and an increase in SV of patients with hypertension or congestive heart failure.[12,41,45] These are well-proven agents for the exercising hypertensive, but please note that the present data are generally from persons with more severe, established hypertension or congestive heart failure.

The choice of medication for treating hypertension in the exerciser must take into account the underlying hemodynamic disorder, the severity of the disease, the type of exercise to be performed, and the individual reaction to the medication. As a practicing physician, the reader should be aware that it may take some time to match the patient and the appropriate drug regimen, but hypertension therapy should not be a limitation on exercise, if prescribed properly.

EXERCISE TESTING AND THE DIAGNOSIS OF HYPERTENSION

Hypertensives respond differently to exercise from normotensive individuals. Knowledge of these differences may be useful in diagnosing hypertension and even in dividing hypertensives into subsets based upon hemodynamic performance. Persons who are normotensive at rest, but who show elevated maximal exercise blood pressure have over twice the risk of developing hypertension as normotensives with a normal exercise BP response.[41,104] Furthermore, differences in hemodynamic performance during exercise may aid in separating patients into established or borderline categories. Established hypertensives usually show higher diastolic pressures during exercise, and a rapid increase of SBP to very high levels.[9,98] Borderline hypertensives, on the other hand, start off at elevated levels but do not increase dramatically, so that their SBPs are "normal" at high performance levels. This information may be useful in determining the underlying hemodynamic causes of the hypertension and may aid in directing therapeutic approach.

SUMMARY AND CONCLUSIONS

Both exercise and hypertension have dramatic impact upon the biochemical and physiological systems governing cardiovascular functioning. When they are encountered in tandem, the results can be positive, negative, or both. The careful physician must attempt to sort out these interrelationships and guide his or her patient in making decisions about exercise and therapy. The following statements may help the reader in pulling together this information:

(1) The underlying hemodynamics of borderline hypertension differ from those of established hypertension. The latter is almost always marked by increased TPR; the former by increased CO. Treatment should proceed accordingly.

(2) Dynamic exercise increases SV and lowers HR, whereas isometric exercise does not have as dramatic an effect on these variables. However, intense isometric exercise does lead to extremely elevated blood pressure (due to increased TPR) and should be avoided in patients with very high levels of blood pressure or with left ventricular hypertrophy.

(3) Traditional stepped-care approaches to the treatment of hypertension need to be modified. In borderline hypertensives, and even hypertensives with mild or moderate disease without severe end organ damage, try behavioral intervention first, including exercise prescription for aerobic conditioning.

(4) To maximize compliance among exercising hypertensives, take into account the fact that certain medications are more likely to produce side-effects that can interfere with athletic performance. This is of particular concern when using beta-blockers with endurance athletes.

(5) Exercise stress testing differentiates hypertensives from normals, and even borderline from established hypertensives. In patients who have occasional elevated readings or who are concerned about blood pressure during exercise performance, such testing is warranted.

REFERENCES

1. Bezucha GR, Lenser MC, Hanson PG, Nagle FJ: Comparison of hemodynamic responses to static and dynamic exercise. J Appl Physiol 53:1589, 1982.
2. Birkenhager WH, Kho TL, Kolsters G, et al: Hemodynamic setting of essential hypertension as a guide to management. Lancet 1:386, 1975.
3. Birkenhager WH, Schalekamp MADH, Krauss XH, et al: Consecutive haemodynamic patterns in essential hypertension. Lancet 1:560, 1972.
4. Bjorntorp P: Hypertension and exercise. Hypertension 4(Suppl III):III–56, 1982.
5. Blair SN, Cooper KH, Gibbons LW, et al: Changes in coronary heart disease risk factors associated with increased physical fitness. Am J Epidemiol 118:352, 1983.
6. Blair SN, Goodyear NN, Gibbons LW, Cooper KH: Physical fitness and incidence of hypertension in healthy normotensive men and women. JAMA 252:487, 1984.
7. Brammell HL, Sable DL, Horwitz LD: Beta-adrenergic blockade prevents effects of aerobic conditioning on blood lipids. Circulation 62(Suppl. III):III–122, 1980.
8. Brown MJ, Brown DC, Murphy MB: Hypokalemia from beta-2-receptor stimulation by circulating epinephrine. N Engl J Med 309:1414, 1983.
9. Chaix RL, Dimitriu VM, Wagniart PR, Safar ME: A simple exercise test in borderline and sustained essential hypertension. Int J Cardiol 1:371, 1982.
10. Coleman TG, Smar RE, Murphy WR: Autoregulation versus other vasoconstrictors in hypertension: A critical review. Hypertension 1:324, 1979.
11. Cooper KH, Pollock ML, Martin RP, et al: Physical fitness levels vs. selected coronary risk factors. JAMA 236:166, 1976.
12. Creager MA, Massie BM, Faxon DP, et al: Acute and long-term effects of enalapril on the cardiovascular response to exercise and exercise tolerance in patients with congestive heart failure. J Am Coll Cardiol 6:163, 1985.
13. Ditto B: Parental history of essential hypertension, active coping, and cardiovascular reactivity. Psychophysiology 23:62, 1986.
14. Dlin RA, Hanne N, Silverberg DS, Oded B: Follow-up of normotensive men with exaggerated blood pressure response to exercise. Am Heart J 106:316, 1983.
15. Dorheim TA, Ruddel H, McKinney ME, et al: Cardiovascular response of marathoners to mental challenge. J Cardiac Rehabil 4:476, 1984.
16. Duncan JJ, Hagan RD, Upton J, et al: The effects of an aerobic exercise program on sympathetic neural activity and blood pressure in mild hypertensive patients. Circulation 68:III–285, 1983.
17. Epstein SE, Robinson BF, Kahlor RL, Braunwald E: Effects of beta-adrenergic blockade on the cardiac response to maximal and submaximal exercise in man. J Clin Invest 44:1745, 1965.
18. Fagard R, Lijnen P, Vanhees L, Amery A: Hemodynamic response to converting enzyme inhibition at rest and exercise in humans. J Appl Physiol 53:576, 1982.
19. Fardy PS: Isometric exercise and the cardiovascular system. Phys Sportsmed 9:43, 1981.
20. Fleming DS, Finkelstein S, Papra JC, Twogood GR: Hypertension control. Minn Med 58:895, 1975.
21. Fletcher GF: Exercise in the management of high blood pressure and peripheral vascular disease. *In* Fletcher GF (ed): Exercise in the Practice of Medicine. Mount Kisco, NY, Futura Publishing Co., 1982, pp 285–296.
22. Floras JS, Hassan MO, Jones JV, Sleight P: Cardioselective and nonselective beta-adrenergic blocking drugs in hypertension: A comparison of their effect on blood pressure during mental and physical activity. J Am Coll Cardiol 6:186, 1985.
23. Folkow B, Hallback M, Lundgen Y, et al: Importance of adaptive changes in vascular design for establishment of primary hypertension, studied in man and in spontaneously hypertensive rats. Circ Res 33(Suppl 1):I2, 1973.
24. Folkow B: Physiological aspects of primary hypertension. Physiol Rev 62:347, 1982.
25. Franciosa JA, Johnson SM, Tobian LJ: Exercise performance in mildly hypertensive patients. Chest 78:291, 1980.
26. Franz IW, Lohmann FW, Koch G: Effects of chronic antihypertensive treatment with acebutolol and pindolol on blood pressure, plasma catecholamines, and oxygen uptake at rest and during submaximal and maximal exercise. J Cardiovas Pharmacol 4:180, 1982.
27. Fraser GE: Can exercise prevent or reduce hypertension? Primary Cardiol 159, 1985.
28. Frolich ED: Hemodynamic factors in the pathogenesis and maintenance of hypertension. Fed Proc 41:2400, 1982.
29. Frolich ED, Kozul VJ, Tarazi RC, Dustan HP: Physiological comparison of labile and essential hypertension. Circ Res 26–27(Suppl. I):I–55, 1970.
30. Frolich ED, Tarazi RC, Dustan HP: Re-examination of the hemodynamics of hypertension. Am J Med Sci 257:9, 1969.
31. Frolich ED, Tarazi RC, Dustan HP, Page IH: The paradox of beta-adrenergic blockade in hypertension. Circulation 37:417, 1968.
32. Goldstein DS: Plasma catecholamines and essential hypertension: an analytical review. Hypertension 5:86, 1983.
33. Gordon NF: Effect of selective and nonselective beta-adrenoceptor blockade on thermoregulation during prolonged exercise in heat. Am J Cardiol 55:74D, 1985.
34. Hartley LH, Mason JW, Hogan RP, et al: Multiple hormonal responses to prolonged exercise in relation to physical training. J Appl Physiol 33:607, 1972.
35. Haskell WL: The influence of exercise on the concentrations of triglyceride and cholesterol in human plasma. Exerc Sports Sci Rev 12:205, 1984.

36. Hastrup JL, Light KC, Obrist PA: Parental hypertension and cardiovascular response to stress in healthy young adults. Psychophysiology 19:615, 1982.

37. Henquet JW, van Baak M, Schols M, Rahn KH: Studies on the autonomic nervous system in borderline hypertension. Eur J Clin Pharmacol 22:285, 1982.

38. Hespel P, Lijnen P, VanHees L, et al: Differentiation of exercise-induced metabolic responses during selective beta-1 and beta-2 antagonism. Med Sci Sports Exerc 18:186, 1986.

39. Horton ES: The role of exercise in the treatment of hypertension in obesity. Int Obesity 5(Suppl. I):165, 1981.

40. Hunter GR: Overtraining and systolic blood pressure. Int Olympic Lifters 7:30, 1980.

41. Ibsen H, Egan B, Osterziel K, et al: Reflex-hemodynamic adjustments and baroreflex sensitivity during converting enzyme inhibition with MK-421 in normal humans. Hypertension 5(Suppl I):I–184, 1983.

42. James WPT, Haraldsdottir J, Liddell F, et al: Autonomic responsiveness in obesity with and without hypertension. Int J Obesity 5:73, 1981.

43. Johnson WP, Grover JA: Hemodynamic and metabolic effects of physical training in four patients with essential hypertension. Can Med Assoc J 96:842, 1967.

44. Joint National Committee on Detection, Evaluation, and Treatment of High Blood Pressure. The 1984 report of the joint national committee on detection, evaluation, and treatment of high blood pressure. Arch Intern Med 144:1045, 1984.

45. Jones RI, Hornung RS, Cashman PMM, Raftery EB: Effect of enalapril at rest, during tilt, static and dynamic exercise in systemic hypertension. Am J Cardiol 55:1534, 1985.

46. Juhlin-Dannfelt A: Beta-adrenoceptor blockade and exercise: effects on endurance and physical training. Acta Med Scand (Suppl 672):49, 1983.

47. Juhlin-Dannfelt AC, Terrianche SE, Fell RD, et al: Effects of beta-adrenergic receptor blockade on glycogenolysis during exercise. J Appl Physiol 53:549, 1982.

48. Kaiser P, Hylander B, Eliasson K, Kaiser L: Effect of beta-1-selective and nonselective beta blockade on blood pressure relative to physical performance in men with systemic hypertension. Am J Cardiol 55:79D, 1985.

49. Kaiser P, Rossner S, Karlsson J: Effects of beta-adrenergic blockade on endurance and short-time performance in respect to individual muscle fiber composition. Int J Sports Med 2:37, 1981.

50. Kaiser P, Tesch PA, Thorsson A, et al: Skeletal muscle glycogonolysis during submaximal exercise following acute beta-adrenergic blockade in man. Acta Physiol Scand 123:285, 1985.

51. Kannel WB, Dawber TR: Hypertension as an ingredient of a cardiovascular risk profile. Br J Hosp Med 10:508, 1974.

52. Kaplan NM: Non-drug treatment of hypertension. Ann Intern Med 102:359, 1985.

53. Kenney WL, Zambraski EJ: Physical activity in human hypertension: A mechanisms approach. Sports Med 1:459, 1984.

54. Knochel JP, Dotin LN, Hamburger RJ: Pathophysiology of intense physical conditioning in a hot climate. I. Mechanisms of potassium depletion. J Clin Invest 51:242, 1972.

55. Knochel JP, Vertel RM: Salt loading as a possible factor in the production of potassium depletion, rhabdomyolysis, and heat injury. Lancet 1:659, 1967.

56. Koch G, Franz I, Gubba A, Lohmann FW: Beta-adrenoceptor blockade and physical activity: Cardiovascular and metabolic aspects. Acta Med Scand (Suppl 672):55, 1983.

57. Landsberg L, Young JB: Fasting, feeding and regulation of the sympathetic nervous system. N Engl J Med 298:1295, 1978.

58. Laslett LJ, Paumer L, Scott-Baier P, Amsterdam EA: Efficacy of exercise training in patients with coronary artery disease who are taking propranolol. Circulation 68:1029, 1983.

59. Lavie CJ, Messerli FH: Cardiovascular adaptation to obesity and hypertension. Chest 90:275, 1986.

60. Lawlor MR, Thomas DP, Michele JJ, et al: Effects of chronic beta-adrenergic blockade on hemodynamic and metabolic responses to endurance training. Med Sci Sports Exerc 17:393, 1985.

61. Lowenthal DT, Affrime MB, Rosenthal L: Dynamic and biochemical responses to single and repeated doses of clonidine during dynamic physical activity. Clin Pharmacol Ther 32:18, 1982.

62. Lowenthal DT, Saris SD, Pachor J, et al: Mechanisms of acting and the clinical pharmacology of beta-adrenergic blocking drugs. Am J Med 77:119, 1984.

63. Ludbrook J: Reflex control of blood pressure during exercise. Ann Rev Physiol 45:155, 1983.

64. Lund-Johansen P: Hemodynamic in early essential hypertension. Acta Med Scand 482(Suppl): 1, 1967.

65. Lund-Johansen P: Hemodynamic changes in long-term diuretic therapy of essential hypertension. Acta Med Scand 187:509, 1970.

66. Lund-Johansen P: Spontaneous changes in central hemodynamics in essential hypertension—a 10-year follow-up study. In Onesti G, Klimt TR (eds): Hypertension: Determinants, Complications and Intervention. New York, Grune and Stratton, 1979, p 201.

67. Lund-Johansen P: Hemodynamic changes at rest and during exercise in long-term prazosin therapy of essential hypertension. In Cotton DWK (ed): Prazosin—A New Antihypertensive Agent. Excerpta Medica, 1974, p. 43.

68. Lund-Johansen P: Short- and long-term (six-year) hemodynamic effects of labetolol in essential hypertension. Am J Med 75:24, 1983.

69. MacMahon SW, Wilcken DEL, MacDonald GJ: The effect of weight reduction on left ventricular mass: A randomized controlled trial in young, overweight hypertensive patients. N Engl J Med 314:334, 1986.

70. Martin JE, Dubbert PM: Exercise in hypertension. Ann Behav Med 7:13, 1985.

71. McKeag D, Hough D, Thompson C: Increased incidence of elevated blood pressure in an intercollegiate football team: A screening and follow-up study, abstracted. Med Sci Sports Exerc 10:39, 1978.

72. McLeod AA, Brown JE, Kuhn C, et al: Differentiation of hemodynamic, humoral and metabolic responses to beta-1 and beta-2-adrenergic stimulation in man using atenolol and propranolol. Circulation 67:1076, 1983.

73. Messerli FH: Cardiovascular effects of obesity and hypertension. Lancet 1:1165, 1982.

74. Messerli FH: The age factor in hypertension. Hosp Pract 21:103, 1986.

75. Messerli FH, Carvalho JGR: Management of mild hypertension. Drug Ther 63, 1979.

76. Messerli FH, Ventura HO: Cardiovascular pathophysiology of essential hypertension: A clue to therapy. Drugs 30(Suppl 1):25, 1985.

77. Montoye HJ, Metzner HL, Keller JB, et al: Habitual physical activity and blood pressure. Med Sci Sports Exerc 4:175, 1972.

78. Nomura G, Eiichiro K, Midorikawa K, et al: Physical training in essential hypertension: Alone and in combination with dietary salt restriction. J Cardiac Rehabil 4:469, 1984.

79. Optenberg SA, Lairson DR, Slater CH, Russell ML: Agreement of self-reported and physiologically estimated fitness status in a symptom-free population. Prevent Med 13:349, 1984.

80. Paffenbarger RS Jr, Wing AL, Hyde RT, Jung DL: Physical activity and incidence of hypertension in college alumni. Am J Epidemiol 117:245, 1983.

81. Pavlik G, Frenkl R: Sensitivity to catecholamines and histamine in the trained and untrained human organism and sensitivity changes during digestion. Eur J Appl Physiol 34:199, 1975.

82. Pearson SB, Banks DC, Patrick JM: The effect of beta-adrenoceptor blockade on factors affecting exercise tolerance in normal man. Br J Clin Pharmacol 8:143, 1979.

83. Pettinger WA: Dietary sodium and renal alpha-2 adrenergic receptors in Dahl hypertensive rats. Clin Exper Hypertens 4:819, 1982.

84. Pickering TG: Dietary and behavioral treatments of hypertension—Do they work? Primary Cardiol 59, 1986.

85. Pratt CM, Welton DE, Squires WG, et al: Demonstration of training effect during chronic beta-adrenergic blockade in patients with coronary artery disease. Circulation 64:1125, 1981.

86. Reybrouck T, Amery A, Billiet L: Hemodynamic response to graded exercise after chronic beta-adrenergic blockade. J Appl Physiol 42:133, 1977.

87. Sannerstedt R: Hemodynamic findings at rest and during exercise in mild arterial hypertension. Am J Med Sci 258:70, 1969.

88. Sannerstedt R, Wasir H, Henning R, Worko L: Systemic hemodynamics in mild arterial hypertension before and after physical training. Clin Sci Molec Med 45:145, 1973.

89. Schulte W, Neus H, Thones M, von Eiff AW: Basal blood pressure variability and reactivity of blood pressure to emotional stress in hypertension. Basic Res Cardiol 79:9, 1984.

90. Sedgwick AW, Brotherhood JR, Harrison-Davidson A, et al: Long-term effects of physical training program on risk factors for coronary heart disease in otherwise sedentary men. Br Med J 2:7, 1980.

91. Sheperd RE, Kuehne ML, Kenno KA, et al: Attenuation of blood pressure increases in Dahl salt-sensitive rats by exercise. J Appl Physiol 52:1608, 1982.

92. Sowers JR, Nyby M, Stern N, et al: Blood pressure and hormone changes associated with weight reduction in the obese. Hypertension 4:686, 1982.

93. Struthers AD, Whitesmith R, Reid JL: Prior thiazide diuretic treatment increases adrenaline-induced hypokalemia. Lancet 1:1358, 1983.

94. Tesch PA: Exercise and beta-blockade. Sports Med 2:389, 1985.

95. Tesch PA, Kaiser P: Effects of beta-adrenergic blockade on O_2 uptake during submaximal and maximal exercise. J Appl Physiol 54:901, 1983.

96. Tipton CH: Exercise, training, and hypertension. Exerc Sports Sci Rev 12:245, 1984.

97. Tipton CM, Matthes RD, Marcus KD, et al: Influences of exercise intensity, age, and medication on resting systolic blood pressure of SHR populations. J Appl Physiol 55:1305, 1983.

98. Toto-Moukouo J, Asmar RG, Safar ME: Use of exercise testing in the evaluation of patients with borderline hypertension. Pract Cardiol 10:61, 1984.

99. VanHees L, Fagard R, Amery A: Influence of beta adrenergic blockade on effects of physical training in patients with ischaemic heart disease. Br Heart J 48:33, 1982.

100. Viitasalo JT, Komi PV, Karvonen MJ: Muscle strength and body composition as determinants of blood pressure in young men. Eur J Appl Physiol 42:165, 1979.

101. Walgenbach SC, Sheperd JT: Role of arterial and cardiopulmonary mechanoreceptors in the regulation of arterial pressure during rest and exercise in conscious dogs. Mayo Clin Proc 59:467, 1984.

102. Wilcox RG, Bennett T, MacDonald IA, et al: The effects of acute or chronic ingestion of propranolol or metoprolol on the physiologic responses to prolonged, submaximal exercise in hypertensive men. Br J Clin Pharmacol 17:273, 1984.

103. Wilmore JH, Ewy GA, Freund BJ, et al: Cardiorespiratory alterations consequent to endurance exercise training during chronic beta-adrenergic blockade with atenolol and propranolol. Am J Cardiol 55:142D, 1985.

104. Wilson NV, Meyer BM: Early prediction of hypertension using exercise blood pressure. Prevent Med 10:62, 1981.

10 Guidelines for Physically Active Diabetics

KRIS BERG, ED.D.

Exercise has been a part of diabetic management for many years. However, in comparison to insulin, oral hypoglycemic medications and diet, exercise has typically received little emphasis. It is only recently that diabetes education has included detailed information regarding exercise.

Although the acute effects of exercise on diabetics are well understood, the chronic effects have not been investigated thoroughly.[6] In theory, physical activity can have a number of benefits for people with type 1 and type 2 diabetes, and probably for this reason current medical expertise supports the role of exercise in the management of diabetes.[7,17]

TYPES OF DIABETES

Characteristics of the two types of diabetes are summarized in Table 1[5]. Approximately 90 percent of the some 10 million American diabetics have type 2 or non-insulin dependent diabetes mellitus. Exercise probably has a more consistent effect in improving the medical status of this majority group than with type 1. Although this group is prone to hypoglycemia, it is not prone to ketosis. Also, with exercise some type 2 diabetics may be able to control their blood sugar without oral medication or insulin, particularly if they lose weight.

BENEFITS OF EXERCISE

Consistent maintenance of blood glucose levels reasonably close to normal may reverse the sequelae of poorly controlled diabetes such as retinopathy, nephropathy, microangiopathy, and neuropathy. Furthermore, current research data suggest that the state of the blood sugar is probably a key determinant of when and how severely these sequelae occur. Because exercise will cause the blood sugar to drop in controlled diabetics of both types, it is a useful adjunct to the insulin- or medication-diet regimen.

Exercise of the proper type, intensity, duration and frequency will provide the same training effect in diabetics as nondiabetics, if reasonable blood sugar control is maintained and if a reasonable level of health exists so that the vigor and duration of exercise sessions are comparable.[9,15] For these reasons, exercise appears to offer a number of advantages for people with diabetes in terms of general health as well as in diabetes management specifically.

Today with the availability of equipment to measure blood sugar at home, diabetics should find it easier and safer to exercise. A daily record of blood sugar test results will allow both the patient and physician to keep track of progress in blood sugar control. Periodic measures of glycosylated hemoglobin (Hb^{AIC}) can also substantiate blood-sugar control for the previous 4 to 6 weeks. With such indices of diabetic management, the value of exercise in glucose control can be determined in patients.

Table 2 summarizes the physical, physiological, and psychological benefits that can occur in properly regulated and properly exercised diabetics. Details are available elsewhere in the literature.[4]

EXERCISE GUIDELINES

When starting a fitness program, the blood glucose should be measured before exercise. Diabetics perform best during exercise when the blood glucose is fairly normal and an

TABLE 1. CHARACTERISTICS OF TYPE 1 AND TYPE 2 DIABETES

CHARACTER-ISTICS	TYPE 1 OR INSULIN-DEPENDENT	TYPE 2 OR NONINSULIN-DEPENDENT
Former terminology	Juvenile-onset	Adult-onset
Age at onset	Usually before 20	Usually after 40
Family history	Infrequent	Frequent
Appearance of symptoms	Rapid	Slow
Use of insulin	Always	Common but not always required
Production of insulin by pancreas	Absent or greatly reduced	Usually normal or elevated
Proneness to ketoacidosis	Prone	Not prone; rarely occurs
Body fatness	Usually normal or lean	Often obese

From Berg, K: Diabetic's Guide to Health and Fitness. Champaign, IL, Human Kinetics, 1986, p. 16, with permission.

adequate level of insulin is in the blood. Exercising when the blood glucose is below normal is dangerous, and a reasonable intensity of effort cannot be maintained long enough to provide a training effect. Conversely, exercise with blood glucose levels above about 250 mg/dl will tend to further elevate the blood sugar as well as possibly lead to ketosis. When the blood glucose reaches this threshold level, the lack of insulin stimulates the liver to release glucose via glycogenolysis. However, the tissues have a limited capacity to take in glucose and, consequently, the longer the relative lack of insulin occurs, the greater the rise in blood sugar.

Low blood insulin levels also stimulate the breakdown of fat through lipolysis. A rise in several hormones including the catecholamines, cortisol, growth hormone, and glucagon add to the effects of insulin shortage and enhance the rise in ketones and glucose. Type 1 diabetics are particularly prone to these effects. The liver converts some of the fatty acids to ketones, leading to ketoacidosis.

TABLE 2. SUMMARY OF CHRONIC TRAINING EFFECTS IN HEALTHY, WELL-CONTROLLED DIABETICS

1. Improved circulorespiratory fitness
   - Greater maximal minute ventilation and frequency
   - Capacity for greater work load before heavy breathing occurs (i.e., a rise in ventilation or anaerobic threshold)
   - Greater maximal stroke volume, cardiac output, and oxygen pulse
   - Greater capacity of blood to carry oxygen
   - Greater dissociation of oxygen from hemoglobin so that more oxygen is dumped into active muscles
   - Greater capillarization of heart, lungs, and skeletal muscle
   - Greater maximum oxygen uptake
   - Less strain on heart at the same submaximal work load (i.e., lower pressure—rate product due to reduction in exercise heart rate and blood pressure)

2. Improved ability for tissues to use oxygen
   - Greater number and size of mitochondria
   - Greater activity of mitochondrial enzymes
   - More myoglobin
   - Enhanced use of fat vs. glycogen as a source of muscular energy, which increases the capacity for prolonged exercise and allows a more vigorous work pace to be sustained

3. Greater muscular fitness
   Increased strength, muscle mass, muscle endurance, and power

4. Increased joint range of motion

5. Reduced risk factors for cardiovascular disease
   - Less body fat
   - Drop in blood pressure
   - Reduced cholesterol and triglyceride
   - Improved lipoprotein profile: greater HDL, greater HDL to total cholesterol ratio, less LDL
   - Increased maximum oxygen uptake
   - Increased fibrinolysis
   - Reduced clotting
   - Reduced uric acid
   - Better ability to tolerate stress
   - Increased joie de vivre

6. Improved blood sugar control

7. Reduced likelihood of hypoglycemia during exercise due to greater fat utilization and increased liver and muscle glycogen

8. Reduced insulin or oral medication to regulate blood sugar

9. Increased self-concept and self-image

The severe disturbance in acid-base balance, dehydration and loss of electrolytes is a serious state that may necessitate hospitalization. Consequently, exercising diabetics should have a functional level of insulin in the blood to prevent these changes.

It is obvious that diabetics who are beginning an exercise program or those with limited blood sugar control should measure their blood sugar before exercising. Once a diabetic has established good control and has successfully been exercising for several months, blood sugar determination before exercise may not always be essential. However, experienced diabetic athletes and exercisers also realize that on occasions when one suspects elevated glucose it is better to check. For example, when an unusual amount of exercise is to be performed or when activity has been increased (or reduced) much beyond normal (e.g., backpacking or driving all day), a diabetic should realize that the blood sugar will tend to vary considerably, even though insulin or medication and diet have been identical with that of more typical days.

Table 3 describes a plan for type 1 diabetics for handling an elevated blood glucose taken before exercise. Such a plan should be developed for active diabetics, as many, particularly IDDMs, will frequently experience elevated blood sugar. The exact amount of insulin to be administered when the pre-exercise blood glucose is elevated can only be determined by trial and error, but it is better to be conservative so that the likelihood of insulin reaction is minimized. Patients should understand that under no condition should they exercise when the blood glucose exceeds 250 mg/dl.

Skyler and associates[16] recommend striving to keep blood glucose in a range of 60 to 130 mg/dl before meals, 140 to 180 mg/dl one hour after meals, and 120 to 150 mg/dl two hours after meals. If the blood sugar remains reasonably close to these values, a diabetic can be considered well-controlled and infrequently will need supplemental insulin or medication before exercise.

Exercise should be done about an hour after a meal whenever possible. This will minimize the occurrence of insulin reactions. Insulin reactions are most likely to occur late in the interval between meals or at the time of a scheduled snack. If one's schedule dictates exercise at such times, a snack before exercise can provide the energy needed. As stated previously, a blood-sugar test before exercise followed by one after the exercise session will indicate if enough or too many calories of the right type were consumed. The snack should be composed largely of carbohydrates, which can be digested and assimilated rapidly. These processes take 2 to 3 hours for fats and proteins, and they are therefore of no value in a typical 30–40 minute exercise bout. Furthermore, the rise in blood sugar from fat and protein will not occur until well after the exercise is completed, which may produce an unexplained or unanticipated rise in the post-exercise blood glucose.

Insulin or oral medication will typically need to be reduced when starting an exercise program. In the first several months of an exercise program, a 20 to 40 percent reduction is typical.[2] Additional reductions may not be needed, because one result of aerobic or endurance training is an increased utilization of fat[11,14] as well as increased storage of muscle and liver glycogen.[8] Furthermore, because exercise and fat loss increase insulin sensitivity, less insulin or medication is needed. Consequently, while increased energy expenditure from exercise and increased insulin sensitivity reduce the requirement for insulin or medication, the increased fat utilization dur-

TABLE 3.   PLAN FOR TAKING SUPPLEMENTAL INSULIN BEFORE EXERCISE

If the blood sugar exceeds 250 mg/dl, do not exercise; take _____ units of rapid-acting insulin and postpone exercise until later in the day.

If 200–250 mg/dl, take _____ units of rapid-acting insulin and exercise. If planning on exercising beyond 30 minutes, be alert for symptoms of low blood sugar. Check blood sugar again an hour or two later.

If 130–200 mg/dl, take no insulin before exercising. If exercising for longer than 30 minutes, consume one carbohydrate exchange per 20 to 30 minutes of additional exercise.

If less than 130 mg/dl and planning to exercise for 20 to 30 minutes, consume one carbohydrate exhange before exercise and one additional exchange for each additional 20 to 30 minutes of exercise.

ing exercise maintains the need for some medication. Thus, an exercise program has a limited effect in reducing the insulin or medication requirement.

Skyler et al.[16] suggest an insulin dosage for type 1 diabetics in the range of .5 to 1.0 units per kilogram of body weight. However, highly active diabetics are often below this range, particularly during days of prolonged activity.[3]

On days of normal activity, most diabetics do not reduce their insulin.[12] This would be expected if the activity has been performed consistently for several months. Also, if exercise is a customary part of each day, no alteration in insulin or oral medication is needed.

The degree that a typical exercise session reduces blood sugar should be tested. If diabetics err, it is all too common to allow the blood sugar to be elevated too high. Most diabetics starting an exercise program fear insulin reaction and so will exaggerate the amount of food eaten in a pre-exercise snack or they will reduce their insulin or medication excessively. By measuring blood sugar before and after exercise, diabetics may realize that while activity reduces blood glucose if an adequate amount of insulin or medication has been taken, it will not commonly drop the glucose to the point of hypoglycemia. Fear of this occurrence may be alleviated by having the patient carry several hard candies during exercise.

During prolonged exercise such as running a marathon, backpacking, or playing in a daylong athletic tournament, carbohydrate should be consumed every 20 to 30 minutes. In addition, insulin dosage should be decreased about 50 percent,[10] but some insulin or oral medication will be needed to enhance peripheral glucose uptake.[7]

Athletes should measure their blood sugar before practice and particularly before games. All athletes get anxious and nervous before competition and the symptoms mimic those of insulin reaction (e.g., tremor, perspiration, nervousness). Checking the blood sugar will allow distinguishing between nervousness and insulin reaction. Also, the stress associated with the pregame conditions will elevate the blood sugar. If the athlete eats as a treatment for symptoms of "false" insulin reaction, blood sugar may rise to the point where optimal performance is compromised. Ketosis may be produced in a type 1 diabetic.

The insulin injection site should be selected according to the type of exercise performed. The absorption of insulin into the blood is enhanced by an increase in local circulation.[17] This will bring the injected insulin(s) to a peak effect sooner than normal, which would tend to lower the blood sugar faster. To avoid the hypoglycemia possibly produced from this effect, diabetics using insulin should not use the thigh as an injection site before walking, running, cycling, aerobic dance or other leg-predominant forms of exercise. Similarly, the arm or shoulder should not be used as an injection site before activities such as rowing, weight training, and calisthenics. Because many physical activities involve both the arms and legs (e.g., weight training, aerobic dance, swimming, cross-country skiing), the abdomen or gluteal region are good sites, because most people have a thick enough fat pad at these sites, which, due to limited capillarization, will delay the absorption of insulin.

Diabetics should be wary of insulin reaction the day after extensive exercise. Following one or more days of high energy expenditure, the glycogen level in the active muscles can be very low and possibly even depleted. Many of the carbohydrate calories ingested on the following day will be taken up by the skeletal muscles to synthesize glycogen. Furthermore, the rate of metabolism is elevated for hours after vigorous, prolonged exercise.[13] Consequently, the blood sugar may have a tendency to be lower than expected the day after extensive exercise. There is also a tendency for night-time insulin reactions to occur for the same reasons. If the blood sugar is not normally measured before retiring, it should be done in times of unusual physical activity as well as the day after.

The main goal of people with type 2 diabetes should be to lose weight. Reduction of body fat and increased physical activity improve insulin sensitivity. Consequently, in some type 2 diabetics, insulin production may become adequate to normalize their metabolism without oral medication or with less medication.

Research indicates that exercise can be effective in fat loss if two criteria are met. One, exercise must be taken at least three times weekly; secondly, in each session at least 300 kcal must be expended.[1] To achieve this energy expenditure, the intensity of the exercise for most people should be moderate, often just meeting or even below the level that is necessary for a cardiorespiratory training effect to occur. Inactivity and an associated obesity typify the majority of people with type 2 diabetes, so their relative lack of fitness will typically not allow burning 300 kcal per session unless the exercise intensity is low to moderate.

A cardiorespiratory or aerobic training effect threshold occurs at 40–50 percent of a person's maximum oxygen uptake. This is equivalent to about 55 to 65 percent of the maximum heart rate (maximum heart rate can be estimated by the equation 220 minus the age). This threshold heart rate can be a training goal for the inactive, overweight diabetic, but if used at the onset of an exercise program, the intensity of the work may be perceived by the patient as too high. A useful adjunct to the heart rate concept and perhaps a more valid indicator regarding the physiological strain imposed by exercise is the concept of the "talk test." When breathing is moderate and not labored, most people perceive the work load to be acceptable and are able to sustain continuous exercise for at least 15 to 20 minutes. Over several weeks of increasing the duration of each exercise session, most people will be able to tolerate a duration of exercise that allows expending 300 or more kcal.

Thus, exercise duration is the key training variable for each exercise session rather than intensity. Nearly any activity that uses the legs predominantly will involve adequate muscle mass to expend the required 300 kcal. Depending on the work rate and body weight, approximately 30 to 60 minutes of exercise are needed by people of low to moderate fitness levels to expend this amount of energy. However, as the level of fitness improves and body weight is slowly decreased, the speed of exercise will increase and more kcal can be expended each minute. For example, a person weighing 160 pounds expends about 3 kcal per minute when walking one mile in 30 minutes. Walking the mile in 15 minutes, however, would expend about 7.9 kcal per minute. If this 160 pound individual walked 30 minutes at this rate, 237 kcal would be burned. A 10 min per mile jog pace, however, expends 10 kcal each minute or 300 for a 30 minute session.[18]

Type 1 diabetics can gain weight with improved glucose control and exercise. When blood glucose is elevated, it indicates an inadequate level of insulin or medication. This retards glucose uptake by the tissues and the synthesis of glycogen. Because glycogen formation is accompanied by water storage, the poorly regulated diabetic stores less glycogen and water, and may be chronically dehydrated. Inadequate insulin also slows the uptake of amino acids. This may interfere with the normal rate of protein synthesis and maintenance of skeletal muscle mass.

A shortage of insulin stimulates lipolysis or the breakdown of fat and inhibits fat synthesis by decreasing the rate of glucose uptake into the adipose tissue to produce triglyceride. Consequently, the sum of these effects is that the diabetic with chronically elevated blood glucose loses glycogen, body water, protein, and fat. For type 2 diabetics, this weight loss coincides with their most important exercise goal, to lose weight. However, it occurs at the expense of healthy tissue and body water. Some diabetics may purposely overeat, recognizing that a weight loss rather than a weight gain ensues. Obviously, this practice should be discouraged.

Most type 1 diabetics are lean or of normal body weight and commonly wish to gain lean tissue. Progressive resistance exercise is effective in producing muscle hypertrophy in diabetics as well as nondiabetics, but a second factor promoting weight gain for diabetics is blood sugar. Tight control will minimize water, fat, and protein loss and will help to maximize the building and maintenance of muscle weight. For some diabetics, particularly young males, this realization may help them maintain stricter dietary management and blood sugar control.

CONTRAINDICATIONS FOR EXERCISE

Metabolic control must be established before an exercise program is started. As previously stated, if exercise occurs with a lack of insulin in the blood, the blood sugar will rise during exercise and ketosis may develop. Newly diagnosed diabetics or those who are not reasonably well controlled should not begin an exercise program. First priority should be to achieve a fairly stable relationship between food intake and insulin or medication. Once a balance is demonstrated by acceptable blood glucose data, only then should the third variable, exercise, be introduced. For some diabetics this special clearance for exercise may aid motivation to use a home glucose monitoring kit and to discipline their eating habits to achieve good blood-sugar control.

An exercise EKG is usually warranted for diabetics past age 40 or if the duration of diabetes exceeds 25 years. Diabetics are at two to three times the risk for heart and large artery disease than non-diabetics. Consequently, a functional test of their circulation and exercise capacity should be administered. The results of the test are useful in deciding if their exercise program should be supervised and for the writing of an exercise prescription.

Exercise that causes trauma to the feet should be avoided in patients with limited peripheral nerve and blood vessel function. One of the common sites of vascular insufficiency and peripheral sensory neuropathy is the feet. Patients with these disabilities may injure their feet without realizing the damage. With limited peripheral circulation, injuries are slow to heal and infection is more likely to be a problem. Activities such as jogging, martial arts, and diving place considerable trauma on the feet. For the same reasons, diabetics are advised to avoid not wearing shoes and socks; to examine their feet for blisters, corns, and bunions regularly; and to keep the feet well lubricated.

Patients with retinopathy should avoid strenuous activity which may induce hemorrhage. Contact sports, jumping, scuba diving, weight training and hanging inverted are not recommended for this reason.

SUMMARY

People with diabetes should consistently use exercise in a judicious manner as a basic part of their overall management program.

Exercise has a number of physical, physiological, and psychological benefits, many of which may directly or indirectly affect blood sugar and consequently their long-term health. With appropriate use of home/field glucose monitoring devices, most diabetics can and should be regularly active. Pubescent and adolescent diabetics can be active in competitive sports. As a matter of fact, for many adolescent diabetics, participation in sports may reduce the common stigma that they are physically limited. Furthermore, regular exercise may motivate some diabetics to maintain better blood sugar control because of the impact on their self-esteem and confidence.

REFERENCES

1. American College of Sports Medicine: Guidelines for Exercise Testing and Prescription, 3rd ed. Philadelphia, Lea and Febiger, 1986.
2. A Round Table: Diabetes and exercise. Phys Sportsmed 7:49–64, 1979.
3. Berg K: Blood glucose regulation in an insulin-dependent diabetic backpacker. Phys Sportsmed 11:101–104, 1983.
4. Berg K: Metabolic disease: diabetes mellitus. *In* Seefeldt V (ed): Physical Activity and Human Well Being. Reston, VA, American Alliance of Health, Physical Education, Recreation and Dance, 1986.
5. Berg, K: Diabetic's Guide to Health and Fitness. Champaign, IL, Human Kinetics, 1986.
6. Berger, M: Metabolic diseases and exercise performance. *In* Vol 13. Knuttgen HG, Voge JA, Poortman J (eds): Biochemistry of Exercise: International Series on Sports Sciences. Champaign, IL, Human Kinetics, 1983.
7. Berger M, Berchtold P, Cuppers JJ, et al: Metabolic and hormonal effects of muscular exercise in juvenile type diabetics. Diabetologica 13:355–65, 1977.
8. Bergstrom J, Hermansen L, Saltin B: Diet, muscle glycogen and physical performance. Acta Physiol Scand 71:140–150, 1967.
9. Costill DL, Cleary P, Fink WJ, et al: Training adaptations in skeletal muscle of juvenile diabetics. Diabetes 28:812–822, 1979.
10. Etzwiler DD: When the diabetic wants to be an athlete. Phys Sportsmed 2:45–50, 1974.
11. Felig P, J Wahren : Amino acid metabolism in exercising man. J Clin Invest 50:2703–2714, 1971.
12. Flood T: Who's running? Forecast, March–April, 22, 1979.
13. Hagberg JM, Mullin JP, Nagle FJ: Effect of work intensity and duration in recovery O_2. J Appl Physiol 48:540–544, 1980.
14. Hagenfeldt L, Wahren J: Metabolism of free fatty acids and ketone bodies in skeletal muscle. *In* Per-

now B, Saltin B (eds): Muscle metabolism during exercise. New York City, Plenum Press, 1971.

15. Larsson Y, Persson B, Sterky G, Thoren C: Functional adaptation to vigorous training and exercise in diabetic and nondiabetic adolescents. J Appl Physiol 19:629–635, 1964.

16. Skyler J, Skyler D, O'Sullivan M: Algorithms for adjustment of insulin dosage by patients who monitor blood glucose. Diabetes Care 4:311–318, 1981.

17. Vranic M, Berger M: Exercise and diabetes mellitus. Diabetes 28:147–163, 1979.

18. Wilmore, JH: Sensible Fitness. Champaign, IL, Leisure Press, 1986.

11 Exercise-Induced Asthma and Related Problems

ROGER H. KOBAYASHI, M.D.
MORRIS B. MELLION, M.D.

In the 1972 Summer Olympic Games, United States swimmer Rick DeMont had his gold medal award rescinded as a result of disqualification. This asthmatic young man had traces of ephedrine, an anti-asthmatic drug, detected in his urine following the race. Despite this setback, asthmatic athletes continued to persevere and in the XXIII Summer Olympic Games in Los Angeles, California, in 1984, 41 out of 67 American athletes with asthma won medals. That asthmatic athletes did well in the heat, humidity and significant air pollution encountered in Los Angeles should serve to encourage all individuals with asthma who would like to participate in physical activity.

It has been known since antiquity that exercise could bring about an asthma attack. Aretaeus the Cappadocian described this phenomenon in the second century AD and the English physician Willis in the 17th century provided a classical description of exercise-induced asthma. Nevertheless, despite awareness of this condition for nearly 20 centuries, the mechanisms of asthma and particularly exercise-induced asthma remain unknown.[48,28]

During exercise, in normal and asthmatic individuals the brochioles dilate causing an increase in pulmonary function. However, in the post-exercise period, pulmonary function decreases mildly in normal individuals and significantly in many asthmatics. Usually after exercising for five to ten minutes, patients with exercise-induced asthma experience a decrease of 15% or more in their lung function tests.[5,68] Not infrequently, these individuals are unaware of bronchospasm, since they may experience only shortness of breath, coughing, chest pain or tightness. Older individuals may think they are "out of shape." In children, coughing and lack of endurance may be the common presenting features; as a result, these children tend to avoid vigorous play. This situation may go on for months or years before being properly recognized. Frequently, when the examining physician suggests the diagnosis of asthma, there is denial or rejection of the condition by the patient or parents. Nevertheless, exercise-induced asthma is very common, occurring in as many as 80–90% of asthmatics[28,1] and in 40–50% of persons with allergic rhinitis without any previous history of asthma.[19] Surprisingly, in a random testing of athletes, 10% have exercise-induced asthma (Fig. 1).

Definition. Exercise-induced asthma may be clinically described as a transient increase in airway resistance following 6–8 minutes of vigorous exercise.[29,13,6] More precisely it is defined as a 15% or more decrease in FEV_1 or PEFR occurring maximally at 3–15 minutes (usually 10 minutes) after vigorous exercise.[1,19] Generally a decrease of 20% or less in FEV_1 is considered mild, 20–40% decrease is moderately severe, and 40% or more is considered severe.[21]

Several important factors determine the severity of EIB: (1) the kind of exercise, (2) the severity of exercise, (3) the conditions under which the exercise is occurring, and (4) the duration of the exercise. Generally, the more vigorous and prolonged the exercise, the more severe the bronchospasm will be. In addition, exercising in cold, dry air or where

ABBREVIATIONS:
EIB   Exercise-induced bronchospasm
PFT   Pulmonary function test
FEV_1 Forced expiratory volumn in one second
PEFR   Peak expiratory flow rare

117

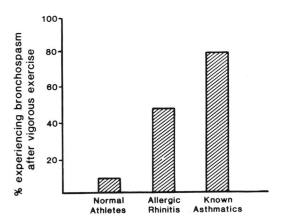

FIGURE 1. Incidence of exercise-induced bronchospasm.

allergens, irritants or air pollutants are present will aggravate exercise-induced asthma. Often, a concurrent viral infection will also increase the likelihood of inducing exercise-related asthma (Fig. 2).

MECHANISM

In the early 1970s, it was generally believed that exercise-induced bronchospasm (EIB) was caused from mediator-release through a mechanism provoked by exercise. This view was particularly attractive, since cromolyn sodium, an inhibitor of mediator-release, attenuated EIB if given before exercise but was ineffectual if given after exercise, when the patient was wheezing (presumably after mediators had been released). However, it was difficult to explain how certain kinds of strenuous exercise, such as swimming, failed to cause asthma. Early studies suggested that breathing humidified air decreased the severity of EIB,[5,2] thus helping to explain how swimming might be less likely to cause bronchospasm. Subsequently, Dr. E. R. McFadden and his colleagues published a series of artilces indicating a correlation between the amount of respiratory heat loss and the severity of asthma. It appeared that heat loss was the important factor, whether it was induced by hyperventilation from exercise or by hyperventilation alone.[17,18] Recently studies have indicated that EIB can occur even when there is no respiratory heat loss.[8,31] Careful studies by Dr. Sandra Anderson and associates have shown that it may be relative water loss with resultant hyperosmolarity in the respiratory epithelial fluid that initiates bronchospasm[3,4] rather than heat loss. The evidence for this theory is nicely summarized by Dr. Anderson[2] and Dr. Sheppard's group.[64]

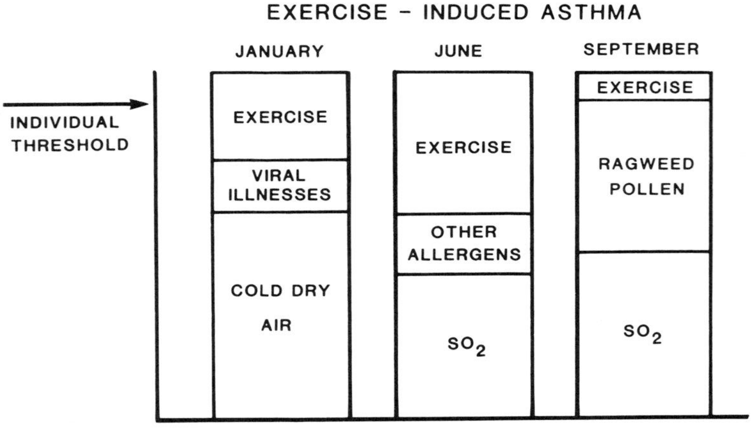

EXERCISE – INDUCED ASTHMA

	JANUARY	JUNE	SEPTEMBER
INDIVIDUAL THRESHOLD →	EXERCISE	EXERCISE	EXERCISE
	VIRAL ILLNESSES		RAGWEED POLLEN
		OTHER ALLERGENS	
	COLD DRY AIR		
		SO_2	SO_2

FIGURE 2. Relative contribution to exercise-induced bronchospasm in an individual who has EIB and ragweed hay fever.

As it is with the three blind men, each describing the elephant only by the part he is touching, so it is with EIB. Recently there has been tremendous refocusing of interest back to mediator release. Histamine and neutrophil chemotactic factor (NCF) release have been studied extensively in EIB and have been shown to play an important role.[42,43,44] Other inflammatory mediators that can be released following vigorous exercise or hyperventilation are presently being studied, including eosinophil chemotactic factor of anaphylaxis (ECF-A), the leukotrienes (LTC_4, LTD_4, LTE_4) and platelet activating factor (PAF).[50,30,45] Many of these mediators may be responsible for late-phase asthma, that is, bronchospasm occurring 4–8 hours after challenge (Fig. 3). Finally, there may be cholinergic influence either centrally mediated or by response to local inflammation. (Table 1).[30,74] Where does this leave us? Dr. Simon Godfrey, a highly respected asthma researcher from Jerusalem, has some practical advice: "What this all means for the asthmatic athlete is probably that he/she should try to avoid exercising in cold, dry conditions and should choose swimming rather than skiing as the preferred sport."[29]

TESTING

Testing for EIB should be considered in any athlete with a prior history of childhood

TABLE 1. MECHANISMS OF EXERCISE-INDUCED BRONCHOSPASM

EARLY REACTIONS

Respiratory Water Loss—resulting in changes in epithelial cell osmolarity
Temperature Change—airway cooling
Cholinergic Response—neurological, inflammation
Mediator Release—histamine

LATE REACTION—MAST CELL DEGRANULATION

Neutrophil chemotactic factor
Eosinophil chemotactic factor
Leukotrienes (LTC_4, LTD_4 and LTE_4)

asthma, chronic cough, present or past history of chest problems or allergies. Prior to testing, PFT's should be within 80% of predicted normal levels before exercise challenge.[21] Medications for treating asthma should be withheld from 8–24 hours, depending on the drug. Beta agonists and theophylline should be withheld for 8 hours (regular acting preparations) or 12 hours (sustained acting preparations), depending on the formulation. Cromolyn sodium should not be used for 24 hours and cholinergic antagonists should not be used for 8 hours. Steroid preparations can be used unless the patient is also being studied for the presence of late phase asthma. Certain antihistamines may have mild anti-asthma properties and are probably best avoided prior to testing.

Equipment necessary for testing depends on the setting and resources available. If a pulmonary function laboratory is available, then a treadmill or cycloergometer is used. Since EIB induces both large and small airway disease, several different pulmonary function parameters may be used including FEF_{25-75}, FEV_1, or peak expiratory flow rate (PEFR). These may be measured on a spirometer or in the case of the PEFR, a peak flow meter. Electrocardiograph monitoring may be advisable for those at risk and a cardiotachometer makes monitoring the heart rate simpler. While not often needed, equipment and drugs necessary to treat the implications of cardiac and pulmonary complications should be readily available.

In the standardized exercise challenge test, the equipment used is somewhat expensive

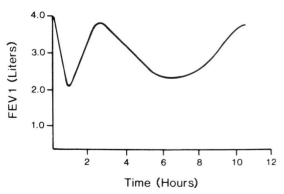

FIGURE 3. Patterns of bronchospasm in early phase. (10 min to 2 hrs) and late phase (4–8 hours) exercise-induced bronchospasm.

and cumbersome. A motor-driven treadmill or a cycloergometer is used. With a treadmill, several criteria are followed. The critical factors are that the workload must be strenuous, continuous and of a duration of 6–8 minutes. A nose clip is provided to induce breathing through the mouth, and the workload is adjusted to between 80–85% of the patient's predicted work capacity[32] or to a heart rate of 90% of predicted maximum values.[21] A formula to predict the maximum heart rate is selected from Table 2. A cycloergometer is much cheaper, less cumbersome and the workload can be adjusted more easily. From a practical standpoint, the subject is coached to achieve a heart rate of between 170–200 per minute (lower in older populations) and to maintain this rate for 6–8 minutes. After baseline pulmonary functions are obtained, strenuous exercise is initiated for 6–8 minutes and then subsequent PFTs are obtained every 5 minutes for 20–30 minutes; generally the greatest fall in PFT is observed at 10 minutes post-exercise. Results are expressed as a percentage decrease:

$$\% \text{ decrease} = \frac{\text{Baseline PFT} - \text{lowest PFT value after exercise} \times 100}{\text{Baseline PFT}}$$

A decrease of 15% or more is considered a positive challenge. Ideally, since EIB is enhanced in cold air with low humidity, testing should not be done in a room with high temperature and humidity. To determine the protective effects of certain drugs, the PFT is measured before the drug is administered and again just before exercise.

In an office setting, elaborate equipment is often neither available nor affordable. Nevertheless, it may be still possible to determine whether exercise provokes bronchospasm. A baseline PFT obtained by an office spirometer or peak flow meter along with a resting heart rate is obtained. The patient is then made to run around the building or up and down flights of stairs in an attempt to sustain a heart rate of 170–200 beats per minute continually for 6–8 minutes. PFT's are then measured every five minutes for 20–30 minutes. While this is certainly not ideal or standardized, it does give some indication of whether bronchospasm is induced and does not cost the typical $200–400 charged by many pulmonary function labs.

An extension of laboratory or office testing is to measure lung function changes on the playing fields. A peak flow meter or portable spirometer may be used to monitor obstructive lung changes under actual sporting conditions, either in practice or actual competition. The advantage of this setting is that it is cheap, it duplicates the actual "field" conditions, and it permits the assessment of drug effectiveness.

Several precautions in performing exercise challenges must be observed. It may be inadvisable to do more than one or two challenges in a day on the same subject, since a period of "refractoriness' may ensue following successive periods of exercise. Also, some patients may *not* experience EIB when challenged under warm, humid conditions and may experience EIB only under cold, dry conditions. Additionally, others may not experience significant problems with EIB unless exposed to air pollutants, allergens or other pulmonary irritants. Testing these individuals under office or laboratory conditions may not provoke bronchospasm, leading to the erroneous conclusion that EIB is not present. Clearly patients at risk for cardiac problems or those who are taking beta blockers should be tested with extreme caution. Fatalities have been reported in these individuals when tested.[61] A final note about

TABLE 2. MAXIMUM PREDICTED HEART RATE ACCORDING TO AGE

AGE	209−0.74x AGE	205 − $\frac{\text{AGE}}{2}$	220−AGE	225−AGE*
8	203	201	212	217
12	200	199	208	213
16	197	197	204	209
20	194	195	200	205
30	187	190	190	195
40	179	185	180	185
50	172	180	170	175
60	164	175	160	165

*Recommend using this formula for predicting maximum heart rate since it is simple to remember and provides appropriate range to achieve during exercise challenge.

testing: elaborate and sophisticated laboratory studies cannot substitute for a careful, thoughtful medical history and examination by an astute physician.

TREATMENT

Many drugs are used in the treatment and prevention of EIB (Table 3). The beta-2 specific agonists are the most effective agents in the treatment of EIB.[52] The beta-2 specific drugs include albuterol, terbutaline and bitolterol. Other beta-2 specific agents available in Europe and other countries but not in the United States, include fenoterol and rimeterol.

Other sympathomimetic agents used in asthma with effectiveness include metaproterenol, isoetharine, isoproterenol, ephedrine and adrenalin. Most of these drugs are familiar and time-honored in the treatment of asthma. However, they are not as beta-2 specific and have been banned by the International Olympic Committee (Table 4).

Albuterol (Ventolin, Proventil), terbutaline (Brethaire, Bricanyl) and bitolterol (Tornalate) are administered by aerosol 10–60 minutes before exercise. Numerous studies have shown that prior administration may effectively inhibit bronchospasm for as long as 3 to 6 hours.[58,51,40,37] Delivery by metered dose inhalers (MDI) or nebulizers results in more rapid onset of action, fewer side effects and greater effectiveness than by oral administration.[67] Usually two puffs by MDI are sufficient, although as many as 4–6 puffs may be

TABLE 3.   LIST OF EFFECTIVE DRUGS IN EXERCISE INDUCED BRONCHOSPASM

MOST EFFECTIVE
- Albuterol
- Terbutaline
- Bitolterol

EFFECTIVE
- Cromolyn
- Metaproterenol
- Theophylline

EFFECTIVE IN PREVENTING LATE-PHASE ASTHMA
- Cromolyn
- Inhaled Steroids

TABLE 4.   SYMPATHOMIMETIC AMINES BANNED OR PERMITTED IN OLYMPIC AND NCAA COMPETITION

BANNED
Adrenaline
Ephedrine
Isoetherine
Isoproterenol
Metaproterenol

PERMITTED (With a letter from team physician)
Albuterol
Bitolterol
Fenoterol*
Rimeterol*
Terbutaline

*Not currently available in the United States

even more effective. When using the oral form, it is advisable to take the drug 1 hour before exercise, since the onset of action is delayed by the slower intestinal absorption.

Cromolyn sodium given a few minutes before exercise protects as many as 70% of patients with EIB, probably by preventing mast cell degranulation and inhibiting mediator release.[39] However, it is not as effective as the beta-2 specific agents and the duration of action is not as long. Further, since it does not cause bronchodilation, baseline PFTs are not improved. However, it is as effective as theophylline and calcium-channel blockers and is more effective than atropine and ketotifen. It has the added advantage of being effective against late reaction asthma and of having virtually no known side effects. It was previously thought that the Spinhaler delivery system with its lactose powder capsule was less effective because of the irritant effect of lactose on the airways; however, several investigators have showed no difference between cromolyn delivered by Spinhaler and cromolyn delivered by MDI (non-lactose containing).[15]

Theophylline, perhaps the most widely used anti-asthmatic drug in the United States, has been shown to be effective in preventing EIB.[73,24,20] Although less effective than inhaled beta-2 specific agonists,[40] sustained use of theophylline may be more effective than taking a single dose before exercise.[24] Chronic use of theophylline appears to exert a potent prophylactic effect[9] and more recent data suggest a possible anti-inflammatory effect as well.[73] Several studies have shown a correlative effect between serum theophylline levels and the degree of bronchodilation;[44] therefore, Weinberger argues for maintaining a serum theophylline level between 10–20 μg/ml.[54] Occasionally, it may be beneficial to combine theophylline with a beta-2 specific agonist.[33,41,72] However, the combination of these two agents may increase side effects or have potentially dangerous cardiotoxicity,[21] particularly under conditions of hypoxia. Therefore, appropriate caution should be exercised. A search for effective, but safer, xanthine drugs is underway.[54,55]

Atropine and ipratropium bromide have been studied with conflicting results in EIB,[57,11,14,71] although they are now generally felt to be moderately effective agents.[74] The use of ipratropium is preferred to atropine since the side effects are less. The onset of action is between 1–2 hours and the duration of protection is about 3–5 hours. At the present time, its use is somewhat limited in EIB since it requires a near-normal baseline pulmonary function test.

Other, newer or experimental drugs are being evaluated (Table 5). The cromolyn-like drugs have been studied extensively but thus far have been disappointing in clincal trials. Anti-inflammatory/antihistamine agents have also been investigated, with ketotifen showing possible promise. Calcium antagonists such as nifedipine taken in doses of 20 mg 30 minutes prior to exercise may afford some protection.[16,15] For a summary of the newer drugs in the treatment of asthma, see the nice review by Dr. Furukawa.[27]

The experience of the U.S. swimmer in the 1972 Olympics was a sad one and, therefore, any athlete competing on an organized level should check carefully with the appropriate governing boards as to which drugs are acceptable in the treatment of asthma. Table 6 lists the drugs approved by the International Olympic Committee and the National Collegiate Athletic Association. Table 4 includes a list of banned anti-asthmatic drugs and Table 7 lists banned drugs that might inadvertently be used by the allergic athlete. Particular care must be focused on anti-allergic agents, since many can be obtained over the counter in ubiquitous "cold" preparations. Table 8 lists other banned drugs that might be prescribed for the asthmatic athlete. Not infrequently, asthmatics have persistent coughing and some widely available cough medications, such as PennTuss or Dimetapp with Codeine, may be used without the athlete knowing they contain drugs that may cause disqualification.

NON-PHARMACOLOGIC MODALITIES THAT MAY MINIMIZE EIB

Conditioning. Although there were documented reports of exercise conditioning prescribed for asthma as far back as the 1500s,[47] most physicians unfortunately do not encourage exercise programs for asthmatics. Certainly, increased physical fitness results in a reduced ventilation rate during exercise as well as reduced heart rate; and older reports suggest that increased physical conditioning causes reductions in the requirements for anti-asthmatic medications, decreases in the frequency and severity of asthma, and a decline in work and school absences.[26,56] In a Norwegian study, bicycling challenge before and after training demonstrated a significant decrease in EIB.[25] More recent studies have shown that even children with chronic, severe asthma can engage in strenuous, long-distance exercise without adverse effects provided they receive the proper medications. However, even with optimal conditioning, highly strenuous exercise can provoke EIB in certain individuals,[66] so the physician needs to use appropriate judgment.

Inducing "Refractoriness" by Short Bursts of Activity. It has been known for quite some time that short bursts of repeated physical activity decrease EIB.[66,53,49] Schnall and Landau reported that seven 30-second periods of running separated by short intervals appeared to protect their small patient sample.[18] Subjects appear to be "protected" from EIB for 1–3 hours.

Other Protective Maneuvers. Long distance running may permit athletes to "run through" their EIB.[70] Whether this is true refractoriness or merely enhances endurance remains unknown.[60] Nevertheless, there are asthmatic athletes who tolerate running long

TABLE 5.   NEW OR EXPERIMENTAL AGENTS

I. CROMOLYN-LIKE AGENTS	
1. Proxicromil	Mildly effective in asthma and exercise-induced bronchospasm: investigation suspended when malignancies occurred in long-term animal studies.
2. Doxantrazole	More active than cromolyn *in vitro,* but ineffective in clincial asthma and exercise-induced bronchospasm.
3. Fenprinest	Investigational dosages indicated drug was ineffective; higher dosage ranges are now being studied.
II. CROMOLYN-LIKE ACTIVITY WITH DIFFERENT CHEMICAL STRUCTURE	
1. Lodoxamide	In aerosol form, somewhat effective. Orally, effective but significant side effects.
2. Bufrolin	300 times more potent than cromolyn *in vitro* but only slightly effective in clincial studies.
3. Nivimedone	25 to 30 times more potent than cromolyn sodium *in vitro;* only slightly effective clinically.
III. ANTI-INFLAMMATORY/ANTIHISTAMINE	
1. Tiaramide	Anti-inflammatory agent with anti-asthmatic properties; clinical studies indicated effectiveness; however studies in the United States were suspended when seizures occurred in several patients.
2. Ketotifen—Oral Antihistamines	5,000 times more potent than cromolyn *in vitro.* In clinical trials, effectiveness appears to be comparable to theophylline and cromolyn. Results with exercise bronchospasm unclear.
3. Azatadine (Trinolan)	Antihistamine and *in vitro* inhibitor of mediator release. However, the high dosages required to prevent exercise-induced bronchospasm are associated with considerable side effects.
IV. CALCIUM CHANNEL BLOCKERS	
1. Verapamil/Nifedipine	Studies suggest some protection against exercise-induced bronchospasm but without bronchodilatory effect.
V. IPRATROPIUM BROMIDE	
	Quaternary derivative of atropine. Effective in asthma, particularly bronchitic asthma; however, results in preventing exercise-induced bronchospasm are controversial.
VI. STEROIDS	
1. Budesonide-Steroid Aerosol	Some protection after prolonged treatment.

distances, and this effect may be due to endogenous catecholamine release during exercise. While it is important for athletes to warm up before engaging in vigorous exercise, this is especially important for asthmatic individuals. Each session should begin with a warm-up period of 10–15 minutes of stretching exercises and calesthenics. Likewise, following vigorous exercise the asthmatic athlete should "warm down" for about 10 minutes.[35,26,46] A well-planned conditioning program of increasing intensity should be devised for each asthmatic. The training program should allow the athlete to exercise different muscle groups, with particular focus on strengthening the upper body musculature. Generally, breathing exercises may be of benefit, and particular attention should be paid to breathing in a slow, deep and rhythmic pattern, allowing for more efficient air flow and relaxation. Hyperventilation should be avoided. The athlete should be encouraged to breathe through the nose whenever possible since the filtering and warming

TABLE 6. SYMPATHOMIMETIC VASOCONSTRICTORS*

BANNED

Ephedrine
Phenylephrine
Phenylpropanolamine
Pseudoephedrine
Tetrahydrozoline

PERMITTED

Topical cromolyn sodium
Topical nasal steroids**

---

*Used for hay fever, etc.
**Permitted with letter from team physician.

TABLE 8. DRUGS THAT MIGHT BE USED BY THE ASTHMATIC ATHLETE THAT ARE BANNED FROM USE DURING COMPETITION

All sympathomimetic amines (except beta$_2$ specific)

  Includes virtually all oral decongestants and many topical decongestants for the eyes

Opiate analgesics and antitussives (non-opiates acceptable—e.g., dextromethorphan, diphenhydramine)

effects of the nasal passage may lower the risk of EIB;[65] however, with increasing workload, mouthbreathing is invariably necessary to meet the metabolic requirements of very strenuous exercise. Additionally, patients with nasal obstruction from allergic rhinitis tend to mouth breathe, thus negating the air-conditioning effects of the nasal passages. Occasionally, wearing a surgical face mask to warm and humidify the air around the mouth may help to prevent EIB.[59] When possible, athletes should try to avoid exercising vigorously in cold, dry, polluted air.

While athletes should be encouraged to choose activities that they enjoy, certain sports such as tennis, swimming, baseball or volleyball, which are associated with short exercise bursts, may be much better tolerated. Activities that require prolonged, vigorous exercise, such as long distance running, competitive bicycling, downhill or

TABLE 7. THERAPEUTIC AGENTS FOR EXERCISE-INDUCED BRONCHOSPASM ACCEPTABLE TO THE INTERNATIONAL OLYMPIC COMMITTEE MEDICAL COMMISSION AND THE NATIONAL COLLEGIATE ATHLETIC ASSOCIATION

Atropine sulfate
Caffeine*
Corticosteroids**
Cromolyn sodium
Methylxanthines—theophylline
Sympathomimetic amines (beta$_2$ specific only)**

---

*Caffeine is a *weak* bronchodilator, which is banned if urinary concentration >15 μg/ml for NCAA and > 12 μg/ml for Olympic competition.
**Requires letter from team physician.

cross-country skiing, ice skating and basketball, are often poorly tolerated. Nonetheless, with proper conditioning, "warm-up" periods, and repetitive short exercise bursts to induce a "refractory" period, along with appropriate pharmacotherapy, the athlete may be able to participate in these vigorous activities on a competitive level. It is important for the physician, coaching staff and affected athletes to work together.

EXERCISE-INDUCED ANAPHYLAXIS

Exercise-induced anaphylaxis, while uncommon, can be a frightening and potentially fatal entity. The first author of this chapter has seen five cases referred to the University of Nebraska for evaluation, including one individual who nearly expired on two occasions but was fortunately given adrenalin by his wife, who happened to be a nurse. Not all cases are as dramatic; however, the following case example demonstrates that this can be a frightening experience.

CASE REPORT. A 16-year-old active teenage girl went out on a tennis date after dinner with a boy whom she wanted to impress. After several minutes of exercise, she began feeling warm, itched, and noticed an erythematous rash with some urticaria. She was too embarrassed to say anything and continued playing. She then began to have facial swelling and a choking sensation. Nevertheless, since she wanted to make a favorable impression, she continued to play. Subsequently, she had difficulty breathing, felt faint, and her face became increasingly swollen. Reason prevailed, and she was taken to the emergency room where the pediatrician on call gave her adrenalin, intravenous steroids and antihistamines. Over the next 24 hours, her symptoms gradually abated. On questioning, she had experienced two less-severe episodes while in gymnastics class during the previous two years. She could not remember whether she had eaten shortly before the exercise periods, and she had engaged in similar activities previously without precipitating these symptoms.

While exercise-induced anaphylaxis was known in the past, it was only recently described as a syndrome by Sheffer and Austen in 1980.[62] It is an unpredictable and potentially life-threatening reaction consisting of erythema, pruritus, urticaria, angioedema, laryngospasm and hypotension (Table 9). In addition, patients may experience gastrointestinal symptoms including cramping, nausea, vomiting and diarrhea. Headaches may also be associated. There appear to be several risk factors, although a major consideration is that symptoms may come on unexpectedly, or conditions that brought on the first attack may not precipitate other attacks. Nevertheless, prior food ingestion before exercise has been associated with exercise-induced anaphylaxis. For reasons that are not clear, celery has been implicated in several of the cases.[38] Whether this represents a cross reactivity with celery antigen and ragweed antigen remains to be shown. Prior ingestion of shellfish and also of aspirin have been reported. The intensity of the exercise also appears to be an important factor, in that the intensity varies directly with the likelihood and severity of symptoms.[63] A positive personal or family history of allergies may be present in some patients and weather conditions may also play a factor. Unlike EIB, exercise-induced anaphylaxis appears to be associated more commonly with hot, humid weather conditions.

It is somewhat difficult to treat an entity when the cause is not clearly defined and the attacks may be sporadic. Nevertheless, in those suffering a previous attack, it may be advisable to avoid eating before exercise and also to avoid exercising on hot, humid days. Since intensity of exertion appears to be related to the severity of symptoms, less intense exercise may be advisable. Clearly, if warmth and itching occur, especially on the palms and soles, the individual should stop exercising immediately. The individual should not exercise alone and should advise his or her companion(s) that an attack might

TABLE 9. EXERCISE-INDUCED ANAPHYLAXIS

I. **SIGNS AND SYMPTOMS**
  Generalized pruritus
  Generalized urticaria
  Angioedema (face, palms of the hands and soles of the feet)
  Upper respiratory symptoms
  Choking and difficulty swallowing
  Gastrointestinal symptoms, cramping, nausea, diarrhea
  Headaches

II. **RISK FACTORS? (Factors are unproven)**
  Positive personal or family history of allergies
  Food ingestion—shellfish, celery, aspirin
  Weather conditions—seem more common with hot, humid weather conditions
  Intensity of exercise—appear to be worse with highly vigorous exercise

III. **PREVENTION/PRECAUTIONS**
  Reduction in intensity of exertion
  Avoidance of exercise on hot, humid days
  Avoid eating before exercise
  Immediate availability of an individual capable of treating anaphylaxis

  Medications:
    Pretreatment with antihistamines partially effective
    Pretreatment with beta adrenergic agents and theophylline compounds of unproven benefit

occur and what first aid measures should be taken. An Epi-pen or Ana-kit should be available, and the individual and/or companion(s) should be taught how to administer these medications.

Pretreatment with antihistamines has been partially effective, however, preadministration of theophylline or beta-adrenergic compounds has not been shown to be beneficial.[69]

Appropriate, rapid treatment of anaphylaxis is mandatory. Subcutaneous adrenalin should be given immediately and antihistamines such as diphenhydramine or hydroxyzine should be given. Steroids and intravenous fluids can also be given if warranted. Distinction must be made from other exercise-associated severe events such as myocardial infarct and arrhythmias, cerebral vascular accidents, "heat stroke" and syncope.

SUMMARY

Exercise-induced bronchospasm is a very common and underdiagnosed problem.

Symptoms encountered may not necessarily relate to those classically associated with asthma, such as wheezing. Awareness and proper recognition by the physician and coach can enable proper treatment of this entity. Appropriate conditioning, warming up, inducing "refractoriness," engaging in sports that are less likely to provoke EIB, and the aggressive and appropriate use of medications will allow athletes to enjoy sports and compete effectively. A second entity, exercise-induced anaphylaxis, is being described more frequently. Appropriate recognition and precautions are necessary.

ACKNOWLEDGEMENTS. The secretarial assistance of Michele Wallace, Kim Schamp, and Mary Heck was greatly appreciated.

REFERENCES

1. Anderson SD: Current concepts of exercise-induced asthma. Allergy 38:289–302, 1983.
2. Anderson SD: Is there a unifying hypothesis for exercise-induced asthma? J Allergy Clin Immunol 73:660–65, 1984.
3. Anderson SD, Schoeffel RE, Follet R: Sensitivity to heat and water loss at rest and during exercise in asthma patients. Eur J Respir Dis 63:459–71, 1982.
4. Anderson SD, Schoeffel RE: Respiratory heat loss and water loss during exercise in patients with asthma. Eur J Respir Dis 63:472–800, 1982.
5. Anderson SD, Silverman M, Konig P, et al: Exercise-induced asthma. Br J Dis Chest 69:1–39, 1975.
6. Bar-Yishay E, Godfrey S: Mechanisms of exercise-induced asthma. Lung 162:195–204, 1984.
7. Ben-Dov I: Refractory period after exercise-induced asthma unexplained by respiratory heat loss. Am Rev Respir Dis 125:530–34, 1982.
8. Ben Dov I, Bar-Yishay E, Godfrey S: Exercise-induced asthma without respiratory heat loss. Thorax 37:730–31, 1982.
9. Bierman CW, Shapiro GG, Pierson WE, et al: Acute and chronic theophylline therapy in exercise-induced bronchospasm. Pediatrics 60:845, 1977.
10. Bierman CW, Spiro SG, Petheram I: Characterization of the late response in exercise-induced asthma. J Allergy Clin Immunol 74:701–06, 1984.
11. Borut TC, Tashkin DP, Fischer TJ, et al: Comparison of aerosolized atropine sulfate and SCH 1000 on exercise-induced bronchospasm in children. J Allergy Clin Immunol 60:127–33, 1977.
12. Cerrina J, Denjean A, Alexandre G, et al: Inhibition of exercise-induced asthma by a calcium antagonist, nifedipine. Am Rev Respir Dis 123:156–60, 1981.
13. Chan Yeung MM, Vyas MN, Grzybowski S: Exercise-induced asthma. Am Rev Respir Dis 104:915–23, 1971.
14. Chan-Yeung M: The effect of ScH 1000 and disodium cromoglycate on exercise-induced asthma. Chest 71:320–23, 1977.
15. Corkey C, Mindorff C, Levison H, Newth, C: Comparison of three different preparations of disodium cromoglycate in the prevention of exercise-induced bronchospasm. Am Rev Respir Dis 125:623–26, 1982.
16. Corris PA, Nariman S, Gibson GH: Nifedipine in the prevention of asthma induced by exercise in histamine. Am Rev Respir Dis 128:991–92, 1983.
17. Deal EC, McFadden ER, Ingram RH, Jaeger JJ: Hyperpnea and heat flux. J Appl Physiol 46:476–82, 1979.
18. Deal EC, McFadden ER, Ingram RH, Jaeger JJ: Esophageal temperature during exercise in asthmatic and non-asthmatic subjects. J Appl Physiol 46:484–90, 1979.
19. DeCotiis BA, Braman SS, Corrao WM: Pulmonary function studies and the prevalence of bronchial hyperreactivity in patients with allergic rhinitis. Am Rev Respir Dis 122:64, 1980 (abstract).
20. Dusdieker L, Green M, Smith G, et al: Comparison of orally administered metaproterenol and theophylline in the control of chronic asthma. J Pediatr 101:281–87, 1982.
21. Eggleston PA, Beasley PP, Kindley RT: The effects of oral doses of theophylline and fenoterol on exercise-induced asthma. Chest 79:399–405, 1981.
22. Eggleston PA: Methods of exercise challenge. J Allergy Clin Immunol 73:666–69, 1984.
23. Ekwo E, Weinberger MM: Evaluation of a program for the pharmacologic management of children with asthma. J Allergy Clin Immunol 61:240, 1978.
24. Ellis EF: Inhibition of exercise-induced asthma by theophylline. J Allergy Clin Immunol 73:690–92, 1984.
25. Fitch TK: Sport, physical activity and the asthmatic. In Oseid S, Edwards AM (eds): The Asthmatic Child in Play and Sport. Pittman Press, London, 1983, p 249.
26. Fitch KD, Morton AR, Blanksby BA: Effects of swimming training on children with asthma. Arch Dis Child 51:190–94, 1976.
27. Furukawa CT: Other pharmacologic agents that may effect bronchial hyperreactivity. J Allergy Clin Immunol 73:693–98, 1984.
28. Godfrey S: Exercise-induced asthma. Allergy 33:299–37, 1978.
29. Godfrey S: Introduction. Symposium on Special Problems in Management of Allergic Athletes. J Allergy Clin Immunol 73:630–33, 1984.
30. Gross NJ, Skorodin MS: Anticholinergic, antimuscarinic bronchodilators. Am Rev Respir Dis 129:856–70, 1984.
31. Hahn AG, Anderson SD, Morton AR, et al: A reinterpretation of the effect of temperature and water content of the inspired air in exercise-induced asthma. Am Rev Respir Dis 130:575–79, 1984.
32. Henriksen JM, Dahl R: Effects of inhaled budesonide alone and in combination with low dose terbutaline in children with exercise-induced asthma. Am Rev Respir Dis 128:993, 1983.
33. Joad JP, Ahrens RC, Lindgren SD, Weinberger MD:

Relative efficacy of maintenance therapy with theophylline, inhaled albuterol and the combination for chronic asthma. J Allergy Clin Immunol 79:78–85, 1987.

34. Johnson WR, Buskirk ER (eds): Science and Medicine of Exercise in Sports, 2nd ed. New York, Harper and Row, Inc., 1980, p 125.

35. Jones RV, Williams H, Zarabbi V, et al: The use of training programs in asthmatic children. *In* Oseid S, Edwards AM, eds: The Asthmatic Child in Sport and Play. Pittman Press, London, 1983, p 312.

36. Katz HR, Stevens RL, Austen KF: Heterogeneity of mammalian mast cells differentiated in vivo and in vitro. J Allergy Clin Immunol 76:250–59, 1985.

37. Kettelhut BV, Kobayashi RH, Kobayashi AD: Pharmacologic management of asthma in infants and young children. Neb Med J 71:295, 1986.

38. Kidd JM, Cohen SH, Sosman AJ, Fink JN: Food-dependent exercise-induced anaphylaxis. J Allergy Clin Immunol 71:407–11, 1983.

39. Konig P: The use of cromolyn in the management of hyperreactive airways and exercise. J Allergy Clin Immunol 73:686–89, 1984.

40. Kraan J, Koeter GH, Mark T, et al: Changes in bronchial hyperreactivity induced by four weeks of treatment with anti-asthmatic drugs in patients with allergic asthma: A comparison between budesonide and terbutaline. J Allergy Clin Immunol 76:628, 1985.

41. Lee HS, Evans HE: Albuterol by aerosol and orally administered theophylline in asthmatic children. J Pediatr 101:632–35, 1982.

42. Lee TH, Nagy L, Nagakura T, et al: Identification and partial characterization of an exercise-induced neutrophil chemotactic factor in bronchial asthma. J Clin Invest 69:889–99, 1982.

43. Lee TH, Nagakura T, Papageorgiou N, et al: Exercise-induced late asthmatic reactions with neutrophil chemotactic activity. N Engl J Med 308:1502–05, 1983.

44. Lee TH, Nagakura T, Papageorgiou N, et al: Mediators in exercise-induced asthma. J Allergy Clin Immunol 73:634–39, 1984.

45. Lewis RA, Robin JL: Arachidonic acid derivatives as mediators of asthma. J Allergy Clin Immunol 76:259–64, 1985.

46. Lilker ES, Manicatide M, O'Hara W, Lasachuk K: Exercise-induced asthma is prevented by warm-down. Am Rev Respir Dis 131:A48, 1985.

47. Major RH: A note of history of asthma. *In* Underwood EA (ed): Science, Medicine and History. London, University Press, 1953, p 522.

48. McFadden ER, Ingram RH: Exercise-induced asthma: Observations on the initiating stimulus. N Engl J Med 301:763–69, 1979.

49. McNeill RS, Nairn JR, Millar JS, et al: Exercise-induced asthma. Quart J Med 35:55–67, 1966.

50. Nadel JA: Inflammation and asthma. J Allergy Clin Immunol 73:651, 1984.

51. Nelson HS: Beta adrenergic agonists. Chest 82:33S, 1982.

52. Newhouse MT, Dolovich MB: Control of asthma by aerosols. N Engl J Med 315:870–74, 1986.

53. Orenstein DM, Reed ME, Grogan FT, Crawford LV:

Exercise conditioning in children with asthma. J Pediatr 106:556–60, 1985.

54. Persson, CG: Overview of effects of theophylline. J Allergy Clin Immunol 78:780–87, 1986.

55. Persson CG: Development of safer xanthine drugs for treatment of obstructive airways. J Allergy Clin Immunol 78:817, 1986.

56. Petersen KH, McElhenney TR: Effects of a physical fitness program upon asthmatic boys. Pediatrics 35:295–99, 1965.

57. Poppius H, Salorinne Y: Comparative trial of salbutamol and an anticholinergic drug, SCH 1000, in prevention of exercise-induced asthma. Scand J Respir Dis 54:142, 1973.

58. Reed CE: Adrenergic bronchodilators: Pharmacology and toxicology. J Allergy Clin Immunol 76:335–41, 1985.

59. Schachter EN, Lach E, Lee M: The protective effect of a cold weather mask on exercise-induced asthma. Ann Allergy 46:12–16, 1981.

60. Schnall RP, Landau R: Protective effects of repeated short sprints in exercise-induced asthma. Thorax 35:828, 1980.

61. Schwartz S, Davies S, Juers JA: Life-threatening cold and exercise-induced asthma potentiated by the administration of propranolol. Chest 73:100–01, 1980.

62. Sheffer AL, Austen KF: Exercise-induced anaphylaxis. J Allergy Clin Immunol 66:106–11, 1980.

63. Sheffer AL, Austen KF: Exercise-induced anaphylaxis. J Allergy Clin Immunol 73:699–703, 1984.

64. Sheppard D, Eschenbacher WL: Respiratory water loss as a stimulus to exercise-induced bronchoconstriction. J Allergy Clin Immunol 73:640–42, 1984.

65. Shturman-Ellstein R, Zeballos RJ, Buckley JM, et al: The beneficial effect of nasal breathing on exercise-induced bronchoconstriction. Am Rev Respir Dis 118:65–73, 1978.

66. Siegel SC: Summary. International Symposium on Special Problems of Allergic Athletes. J Allergy Clin Immunol 73:745–48, 1984.

67. Sly RM: Beta adrenergic drugs in the management of asthma in athletes. J Allergy Clin Immunol 73:680–85, 1984.

68. Smith SB: Exercise-induced asthma: Diagnostic clues with recommendation for treatment. Postgrad Med 77:42–45, 1985.

69. Songsiridej V, Busse WW: Exercise-induced anaphylaxis. Clin Allergy 13:317–21, 1983.

70. Sterns, DR, McFadden ER, Breslin FJ, Ingram RH: Reanalysis of the refractory period in exertional asthma. J Appl Physiol 50:503–08, 1981.

71. Tinkelman DG, Cavanaugh MJ, Cooper DM: Inhibition of exercise-induced bronchospasm by atropine. Am Rev Respir Dis 114:87–94, 1976.

72. Vandewalker ML, Kray KT, Weber RW, et al: Addition of terbutaline to optimal theophylline therapy. Chest 90:198–203, 1986.

73. Weinberger M, Hendeles L: Theophylline use: An overview. J Allergy Clin Immunol 76:277–84, 1985.

74. Yeung R, Nolan GM, Levison H: Comparison of the effects of inhaled SCH 1000 and fenoterol on exercise-induced bronchospasm in children. Pediatrics 66:109–14, 1980.

12 Medical Syndromes Unique to Athletes

MORRIS B. MELLION, M.D.

There are a number of medical syndromes or problems that are rare or even nonexistent in those portions of our population that do not exercise regularly or intensely. Most of these syndromes are at first extremely perplexing to physicians who have only cursory experience working with athletes. These patients are different in that they maintain an extremely active, physically intense lifestyle. This chapter will focus on eight areas that encompass many of the more common athletic syndromes.

OVERTRAINING

There is a well-documented but poorly understood syndrome in which the training program of the athlete exceeds the body's physiological and pyschological limits, and the individual's whole system seems to break down. The result is a major setback in both performance and general well-being, which takes weeks, and sometimes months, of rest to resolve. This problem results from a short- to medium-term, often massive, increase in training volume and/or intensity over a previously substantial baseline. It is not merely the result of a few days of "overdoing it."

Overtraining, or "staleness," is a multisystem problem whose pathophysiology is only partly understood. The athlete feels "run down" and tired, and experiences sleep difficulty and loss of appetitie. Resting heart rate and heart rate recovery time after exercise increase. The athlete loses weight and notes a heavy-legged feeling when exercising. Muscle pain is common, and performance suffers, often dramatically. Illnesses and injuries are common in this setting.[1,2,6] Table 1 is a list of common problems seen in overtrained athletes.

The hallmark of overtraining is an increase in basal resting heart rate. Most highly trained endurance athletes will have an early morning basal heart rate of 50 beats per minute or less. This phenomenon is known as "athletic bradycardia." Those who monitor their resting pulse immediately upon awakening each morning often note the remarkable consistency of this measurement for a given training state. As fitness improves, the basal heart rate decreases, but as the athlete experiences even incipient overtraining, the rate increases. Rises of five to ten beats per minute are considered indicative of overtraining,[1,6] but anecdotal information from some athletes with very consistent basal heart rates indicates that they become concerned with changes as small as two beats per minute. Recent research involving multiday, extreme long-distance runs indicates that the morning heart rate does correlate with marked increases in long-distance running mileage above the established training level, and may be a useful tool for anticipating and preventing overtraining. Cardiac catheterization data before and after a run across the United States averaging 42 miles per day, six days per week, revealed a 15% drop in stroke volume with a compensatory increase in heart rate and arteriovenous oxygen difference.[3] These findings suggest the importance of cardiac muscle fatigue in overtraining.[3,6] Other reports in ultramarathoners suggesting impaired left ventricular performance due to severe endurance running would support this hypothesis.[8,9]

The broad range of symptoms in many overtrained athletes may be due to a widespread response to hypothalamic dysfunction. Barron and colleagues compared the responses of four overtrained athletes with those of six marathoners. The overtrained

129

TABLE 1.   COMMON PROBLEMS IN
OVERTRAINED ATHLETES*

PSYCHOLOGICAL

Fatigue
Apathy (loss of motivation)
Sleep difficulty
Anorexia
Depression
Irritability and restlessness

PHYSIOLOGICAL

Increased basal heart rate
Weight loss (both fluid and body fat)
Chronic muscle soreness
Heavy feeling in legs
Gastrointestinal disturbances
Lymphadenopathy
Frequent illnesses and infections
Frequent overuse injuries
Poor healing of overuse injuries
Increased evening fluid intake
Exaggeration of postural blood pressure drop

PERFORMANCE

Decreased speed
Decreased endurance
Increased heart rate recovery time after exercise
Decreased coordination

*Adapted from Baron JL, Noakes TD, Levy W, Smith C, Millar RP: Hypothalamic dysfunction in overtrained athletes. J Clin Endocrinol Metabol 60:803–806, 1985; Brown RL, Frederick EC, Falsetti HL, Burke ER, Ryan AJ: Overtraining of athletes: a round table. Phys Sportsmed 11:93–110, 1983; and Dressendorfer RH, Wade CE, Scaff JH: Increased morning heart rate in runners: a valid sign of overtraining? Phys Sportsmed 13:77–86, 1985.

athletes exhibited lower cortisol, ACTH, growth hormone, and prolactin responses than the well-trained marathoners. The differences disappeared after four weeks of rest.[1]

A muscle overuse syndrome has been identified in long-distance runners pushing their mileage and themselves to their limits. Serum creatinine kinase is elevated, and thigh muscle circumference is decreased with no accompanying drop in estimated body fatness.[5] Interestingly, the opposite effect can be seen by "tapering" training over a period of two weeks before competition. In this circumstance there are marked gains in muscle power and maximum performance during competition.[4] The sports medicine literature is replete with stories of athletes who had unplanned periods of one to three weeks of rest before a major competition and performed their personal best.[2]

Richard L. Brown, administrator and exercise physiologist at Athletics West, provides five indicators that may warn of incipient overtraining: (1) decreased post-workout weight; (2) increased evening fluid intake; (3) later time to bed; (4) increased morning pulse rate; and (5) decreased hours slept. All five of these indicators suggest "an increased risk of illness or injury in the next two or three days." Brown identifies the morning heart rate and the time to bed as "the two most immediate and critical indicators."[2]

The treatment for incipient overtraining syndrome is to cut back training volume and intensity. There is good evidence that aerobic power may be maintained, once it is established, despite rather dramatic reductions in training frequency.[7] Thus, the strategy of "training holidays" is sound. Once the overtraining syndrome has reached its full dimensions, there may be no choice but for the athlete to break off from serious training for a period of several weeks to months.

REFERENCES

1. Barron JL, Noakes TD, Levy W, et al: Hypothalamic dysfunction in overtrained athletes. J Clin Endocrinol Metab 60:803–806, 1985.
2. Brown RL, Frederick EC, Falsetti HL, et al: Overtraining of athletes: a round table. Phys Sportsmed 11:93–110, 1983.
3. Bruce RA, Kusumi F, Culver BH, Butler J: Cardiac limitation to maximal oxygen transport and changes in components after jogging across the US. J Appl Physiol 39:958–964, 1975.
4. Costill DL, King DS, Thomas R, Hargreaves M: Effects of reduced training on muscular power in swimmers. Phys Sportsmed 13:94–101, 1985.
5. Dressendorfer RH, Wade CE: The muscular overuse syndrome in long-distance runners. Phys Sportsmed 11:116–130, 1983.
6. Dressendorfer RH, Wade CE, Scaff JH: Increased morning heart rate in runners: a valid sign of overtraining? Phys Sportsmed 13:77–86, 1985.
7. Gullmo A, Broome A, Smedberg S: Herniography. Surg Clin N Am 64:229–244, 1984.
8. Hickson RC, Rosenkoetter MA: Reduced training frequencies on maintenance of increased aerobic power. Med Sci Sports Exerc 13:13–16, 1981.
9. McKechnie JK, Leary WP, Noakes TD, et al: Acute pulmonary oedema in two athletes during a 90-km running race. S Afr Med J 56:261–265, 1979.
10. Niemala KO, Palatsi IJ, Ikaheimo MJ, et al: Evidence of impaired left ventricular performance after an uninterrupted competitive 24-hour run. Circulation 70:350–356, 1984.

ANEMIA, "PSEUDOANEMIA," AND IRON DEFICIENCY

As athletes have become increasingly aware that anemia and even iron deficiency alone can affect performance, especially in endurance training and competition, the burden has fallen upon physicians to understand, evaluate, and treat a group of partly understood problems lumped under the heading of "sports anemia." In daily practice there is a hazy area in the decision-making process about whether a borderline hemoglobin or hematocrit warrants an anemia work-up and treatment. The situation is made more difficult in athletes because what appears to be a true anemia may not be an anemia at all but a "pseudoanemia," and what appears to be normal hematologic status may be masking an iron deficiency of rather significant proportions.

This section will (1) discuss the "pseudoanemia" of sports; (2) identify the common mechanisms causing true anemia in the athlete; (3) clarify the role of iron deficiency, with or without anemia, in athletic performance; and (4) suggest a therapeutic plan for these problems.

Athletic Pseudoanemia. Intensive endurance exercise conditioning causes major increases in plasma volume[1,3,9,27] as well as in total red blood cell mass and total body hemoglobin.[1,3,9] Because the increase in plasma volume exceeds the increments of red blood cell and hemoglobin production, the standard hematologic measures of red blood cell count, serum hemoglobin and packed red blood cell volume (hematocrit) may appear depressed.[3,15,19] Plasma volume in well-conditioned runners has been shown to exceed that in non-runners by as much as 31%, while total red blood cell mass and total body hemoglobin have been documented to be 18% and 20% higher in runners than controls, respectively.[1,3]

Some authors have called this phenomenon "sports anemia;"[4,15,19,36] but since others have used the same term to describe a broader range of anemias in athletes, it may be clearer to call it "athletic pseudoanemia." In a study of 12 male runners in a 20-day, 312-mile road race, hemoglobin fell from 16.0 to 13.4 gm/dl, RBC from 5.17 to 4.36

million/cu mm, and hematocrit from 47.7% to 40.7%, with no concurrent drop in running performance.[15] Another study demonstrated that when a group of cross-country runners decreased their running mileage, their hemoglobin and hematocrit readings rose back toward preseason levels.[19]

Is the dilution effect of plasma volume expansion in the blood a functional adaptation to exercise training that improves performance? The answer to this question is not clear. Crowell and Smith suggested that most efficient oxygen delivery to tissue takes place when the hematocrit is 40%; at this level there would be a compromise between the oxygen-carrying capacity of the blood and the vascular resistance to increasing blood viscosity.[11] Recent studies on blood doping (blood boosting), however, demonstrate increased performance in response to red blood cell transfusions, which raise the hematocrit well above the 40% level.[2,34]

Athletic "pseudoanemia" is a benign condition requiring no medical management. Iron, B_{12}, and folate supplementation have no effect on it. The problem for the physician is to differentiate it from true anemia, which does require therapy and monitoring.

Iron Deficiency in the Athlete. Although athletes are subject to all of the anemias that afflict other populations, the specific anemia problem related to exercise is iron deficiency. In a study of 52 elite Canadian distance runners, 29% of the men and 82% of the women were iron-deficient.[5] Numerous other studies demonstrate deficient iron stores in both male and female endurance athletes and ballet dancers.[16,25,28,35]

Research has shown that iron deficiency in athletes results from a combination of (1) insufficient iron intake, (2) inadequate iron absorption, and (3) accelerated iron loss. The Recommended Dietary Allowance (RDA) of iron is 10 mg/day for men and 18 mg/day for women.[18] The average iron content of Western diets is 5–6 mg/1000 Kcal; hence, assuming normal rates of iron absorption and loss, the average man requires a 2000 Kcal diet and the average woman, a 3000 Kcal diet to obtain adequate iron intake without supplementation. Endurance athletes, especially women, often fall below these dietary levels.[4,5,7] Additionally, there is evidence of an iron absorption defect as well. The rate of radioactive iron absorption in a study of iron-depleted runners is only half that seen in a control group of iron depleted blood donors.[16]

Endurance athletes lose more iron than their sedentary counterparts. Basal iron loss in urine, stool, sweat, skin, and hair is estimated at 0.5–1.0 mg/day with an additional 0.5 mg/day average additional loss due to menstruation. Measured loss in a cohort of eight long distance runners followed for 2 years with radioactive iron studies averaged 2 mg/day.[16] This increase is multifactorial. Intense exercise can waste iron by microscopic or gross hematuria, hemoglobinuria, and myoglobinuria.[13,23,31] Profuse sweating can cause up to 1 mg/day iron loss.[22,33,29] Microscopic or frank gastrointestinal bleeding, common in runners, can produce additional iron loss.[24,32] The result is a significantly elevated iron requirement for athletes to maintain an equilibrium.

Diagnosis of Iron Deficiency and Iron Deficiency Anemia. A staging system is commonly employed to elucidate the relationship of iron deficiency to the development of clinical anemia (Table 2).[4,10,28] Stage 1, "prelatent" iron deficiency is characterized by markedly diminished or absent bone marrow iron stores. The diagnosis is generally made by measuring serum ferritin, which correlates with the body's iron stores. Levels below 20 ng/ml suggest absent bone marrow iron, but higher levels may also correspond to significant depletion in athletes, since heavy training may elevate serum ferritin levels spuriously.[4] Erythropoiesis occurs in Stage 1, but the red cells may be iron-deficient. Since the literature in this area is confusing and often contradictory, the clinician must make an arbitrary decision about what ferritin level warrants therapy. Until there is a generally accepted consensus, it seems reasonable to use replacement iron in athletes with ferritin levels below 20 or 25 ng/ml and to be suspicious at levels between 20 and 50 ng/ml.

Stage 2 is "latent" iron deficiency. The serum iron stores are depleted, and hemoglobin and other red blood cell parameters may be reduced but within the normal range. As serum iron levels drop, total iron binding capacity increases reactively; and transferrin satuation is decreased as well. Transferrin saturation below 16% indicates too low an iron store available to the developing red blood cell for normal erythropoiesis.[10] Erythropoiesis continues or is slowed in Stage 2, and the red cells are iron-deficient.

Stage 3 is "manifest" iron deficiency characterized by anemia. Hemoglobin drops below 12 gm/100 ml in women and 14 gm/100 ml in men.[8] In black athletes the diagnosis of anemia is slightly more difficult, because the normal hemoglobin level in black children and adults is 1 gm/100 ml lower than in their white counterparts, and this difference is not accounted for by dietary or socioeconomic considerations.[20,21] Red blood cell count, hematocrit, and red blood cell indices as well may reflect the severity of the anemia.

Effects of Iron Deficiency With and Without Anemia on Performance. Hemoglobin is the freight car of the body's oxygen transport system. A major reduction in hemoglobin will produce an obvious diminution of muscle function, particularly when the athlete is attempting to exercise at a maximal level. The body can compensate for mild anemia at submaximal loads by increasing ventilation and cardiac output, and by increasing RBC levels of 2,3-diphosphoglycerate, which, in turn, enhances oxygen release from hemoglobin to the tissues. A point is reached where the anemia is so severe or the work demand is so high that the compensating mechanisms are no longer adequate and performance is diminished.

In the absence of clinical anemia iron deficiency can also affect maximum performance levels. Iron is a basic component of myoglobin, which transports and stores oxygen in muscle, and of cytochrome C, which is necessary for oxidative metabolism. Both have been found to be depleted in iron-deficient rats,[17] and treatment with iron is therapeutic.[12,14] Iron deficiency without anemia has been shown to diminish oxidative metabolism in humans, necessitating more energy production by less efficient muscle anaerobic metabolism and causing accumulation of lactate in the blood.[26,30] Similarly, in laboratory animals it dramatically reduces exercise time to exhaustion.[17]

Treatment. In most situations of estab-

TABLE 2. STAGES OF IRON DEFICIENCY*

STAGE	CHARACTERISTIC	SERUM FERRITIN	SERUM IRON	TOTAL IRON BINDING CAPACITY	TRANSFERRIN SATURATION	HEMOGLOBIN	BONE MARROW IRON STORES
1. Prelatent	Marrow iron depletion	↓	N	N	N	N	0–trace
2. Latent	Serum Iron depletion with iron-deficient erythropoiesis	↓	↓	↑	↓	N–low N	0
3. Manifest	Iron deficiency anemia	↓	↓	↑	↓	↓	0

*Adapted from: Clement DB, Sawchuk LL: Iron status and sports performance. Sports Med 1:65–74, 1984; Cook J: Clinical evaluation of iron deficiency. Semin Hematol 19:6–18, 1982; Parr RB, Bachman LA, Moss RA: Iron deficiency in female athletes. Phys Sportsmed 12:81–86, 1984.

lished iron deficiency in athletes, dietary iron is unlikely to provide adequate replacement. This source of iron should not be overlooked, because heme-iron contained in red meat, poultry and fish is much more readily absorbed than the non-heme iron found in non-meat foods and iron supplements. Indeed, a small amount of meat in the diet appears to enhance the absorption of non-heme iron from other sources. Ascorbic acid supplementation is also well known to enhance non-heme iron absorption.[6]

Oral iron supplementation should be given in the form of a ferrous salt yielding approximately 65 mg of elemental iron one to three times daily, depending on the severity of the deficiency. Typically, one to two doses daily are adequate for the anemia and iron deficiency seen in athletes. The most commonly used preparations are ferrous sulphate, fumarate, and gluconate. Absorption is better on an empty stomach. Gastrointestinal side effects are less common with the fumarate and gluconate and less frequent when the dose is started small and gradually increased. Ascorbic acid in 250 mg doses may be given concurrently with the iron, and commercial preparations are available that combine this absorption enhancer with iron in a single dose.

This discussion is not complete without mention of overtreatment with iron. As athletes, coaches and trainers have become increasingly aware of the importance of iron for performance, many athletes have started taking large and often excessive doses of iron without physician supervision. Hemochromatosis from iron supplementation is a rare but real complication. Athletes of Mediterranean heritage should be screened for thalassemia, and black athletes should be evaluated for sickle cell disease before iron therapy is instituted.

REFERENCES

1. Brotherhood J, Brozovic B, Pugh LGC: Haematological status of middle- and long-distance runners. Clin Sci Mol Med 48:139–145, 1975.
2. Buick FJ, Gledhill N, Froese AB, Spriet L, Meyers EC: Effect of induced erythrocythemia on aerobic work capacity. J Appl Physiol 48:636–642, 1980.
3. Bunch TW: Blood test abnormalities in runners. Mayo Clin Proc 55:113–117, 1980.
4. Clement DB, Sawchuk LL: Iron status and sports performance. Sports Med 1:65–74, 1984.
5. Clement, DB, Asmundson, RC: Nutritional intake and hematological parameters in endurance runners. Phys Sports med 10:37–43, March 1982.
6. Clydesdale FM: Physiochemical determinants of iron bioavailability. Food Technol 37:133–138, 1983.
7. Cohen JL, Potosnak L, Frank C, Baker H: A nutritional and hematologic assessment of elite ballet dancers. Phys Sportsmed 12:81–86, 1984.
8. Committee on Iron Deficiency: Iron deficiency in the United States. JAMA 203:119–124, 1968.
9. Convertino VA, Brock PJ, Keil LC, et al: Exercise training-induced hypervolemia: role of plasma albumin, renin, and vasopressin. J Appl Physiol 48:665–669, 1980.
10. Cook J: Clinical Evaluation of iron deficiency. Semin Hematol 19:6–18, 1982.
11. Crowell JW, Smith EE: Determination of the optimal hematocrit. J Appl Physiol 22:501–504, 1967.
12. Dallman PR, Schwartz HC: Myoglobin and cytochrome response during repair of iron deficiency in the rat. J Clin Invest 44:1631–1638, 1965.
13. Davidson RJL: March or exertional haemoglobinuria. Semin Hematol 6:150–161, 1969.
14. Davies KJA, Maguire JJ, Brooks GA, et al: Muscle mitochondrial bioenergetics, oxygen supply, and work capacity during dietary iron deficiency and repletion. Am J Physiol 242:E418–E427, 1982.
15. Dressendorfer RH, Wade CE, Amsterdam EA: Development of pseudoanemia in marathon runners during a 20-day road race. JAMA 246:1215–1218, 1981.
16. Ehn L, Carlmark B, Hoglund S: Iron status in athletes involved in intense physical activity. Med Sci Sports Exerc 12:61–64, 1980.
17. Finch CA, Miller LR, Inamdar AR, et al: Iron deficiency in the rat: physiological and biomechanical studies of muscle dysfunction. J Clin Invest 58:447–453, 1976.
18. Food and Nutrition Board Committee on Dietary Allowances, National Research Council: Recommended Dietary Allowances. Washington, D.C.: National Academy of Sciences, 1980.
19. Frederickson LA, Puhl J, Runyan WS: Effects of training on indices of iron status of young female cross country runners. Med Sci Sports Exerc 15:271–276, 1983.
20. Garn SM, Ryan AS, Owen GM: Iron matched black-white hemoglobin differences after correction for low transferrin saturations. Am J Clin Nutr 34:1645–1647, 1981.
21. Garn SM, Smith NJ, Clark DC: Lifelong differences in hemoglobin levels between blacks and whites. J Nat Med Assoc 67:91–96, March 1975.
22. Green R, Charlton R, Seftel H, et al: Body iron excretion in man: a collaborative study. Am J Med 45:336–353, 1968.
23. Knochel JP, Schlein EM: On the mechanism of rhabdomyolysis in potassium depletion. J Clin Invest 51:1750–1758, 1972.
24. McMahon LF, Ryan MJ, Larson D, Fisher RL: Occult gastrointestinal blood loss in marathon runners. Ann Intern Med 100:846–847, 1984.

25. Nickerson HJ, Tripp AD: Iron deficiency in adolescent cross-country runners. Phys Sportsmed 11:60–66, 1983.
26. Ohira Y, Edgerton VR, Gardner GW, et al: Work capacity, heart rate, and blood lactate responses to iron treatment. Br J Haematol 41:365–372, 1979.
27. Oscai LB, Williams BT, Hertig BA: Effect of exercise on blood volume. J Applied Physiol 24:622–624, 1968.
28. Parr RB, Bachman LA, Moss RA: Iron deficiency in female athletes. Phys Sportsmed 12:81–86, 1984.
29. Paulev P-E, Jordal R, Pedersen NS: Dermal excretion of iron in intensely training athletes. Clin Chimica Acta 127:19–27, 1983.
30. Schoene RB, Escourrou P, Robertson HT, et al: Iron repletion decreases maximum exercise lactate concentrations in female athletes with minimal iron-deficiency anemia. J Lab Clin Med 102:306–312, 1983.
31. Siegel AJ, Hennekens CH, Solomon HS, Van Boeckel B: Exercise-related hematuria: findings in a group of marathon runners. JAMA 241:391–392, 1979.
32. Stewart JG, Ahlquist DA, McGill DB, et al: Gastrointestinal blood loss and anemia in runners. Ann Intern Med 100:843–845, 1984.
33. Vellar OD: Studies on sweat losses of nutrients: iron content of whole body sweat and its association with other sweat constituents, serum iron levels, hematological indices, body surface area and sweat rate. Scand J Clin Lab Invest 21:157–167, 1968.
34. Williams MH, Wesseldine S, Somma T, Schuster R: The effect of induced erythrocythemia upon 5-mile treadmill run time. Med Sci Sports Exerc 13:169–175, 1981.
35. Wishnitzer R, Vorst E, Berrebi A: Bone marrow iron depression in competitive distance runners. Int J Sports Med 4:27–30, 1983.
36. Yoshimura H: Anemia during physical training (sports anemia). Nutr Rev 28:251–253, 1970.

PROTEINURIA, HEMATURIA, AND "ATHLETIC PSEUDONEPHRITIS"

Over one hundred years ago, Leube reported finding protein in the urine of soldiers who had just undergone strenuous exercise, whereas there was no protein in the early morning specimens from the same men.[6] In 1910, Barach found protein, red blood cells, and hyaline and granular casts in the urine of marathon runners.[2] In 1956, Gardner identified protein, red blood cells, and a wide variety of cellular and granular casts in the urine of a group of 47 football players and correlated the incidence of these findings with the increasing intensity of physical activity. Noting that the urine in healthy athletes would clear of these findings after "a few days of less strenuous activity," he proposed the term "athletic pseudonephritis" to distinguish this transient phenomenon in the athlete from the urinary findings of glomerulonephritis.[10]

Effects of Exercise on Renal Function. Exercise may cause a reduction in renal blood flow, and the extent of this reduction varies with the intensity of exercise. Research has shown that moderate exercise (50% of the individual's maximum aerobic capacity) may cause renal blood flow to drop nearly 30%, while strenuous exercise may cause it to fall as much as 75%. These changes appear within the first ten minutes of exercise. Both the afferent and efferent arterioles of the renal glomeruli constrict in response to sympathetic nervous system stimuli and the increased circulating levels of epinephrine and norepinephrine related to the exercise load. Secondly, the glomerular filtration rate decreases during exertion as well, but not to the same extent. An intense exercise load may reduce the glomerular filtration rate by up to 50% of the resting value. Hydration level is also an important determinant of glomerular filtration rate, and intense exercise increases circulating levels of plasma anti-diuretic hormone, thus decreasing urine flow and conserving plasma volume.[15]

"Athletic Pseudonephritis". It is now well established that strenuous exercise produces increased excretion of protein, red and white blood cells, and both cellular and non-cellular renal tubular casts in a variety of contact and non-contact sports.[1,2,4,5,7,10,15,17] These findings are transient and will disappear if the athlete rests for one to several days.[1,5,10,14,15,17] Recents studies have demonstrated that the majority of urinary sediment findings in "athletic pseudonephritis" are renal in origin.[5,7,14,15,19] It appears that the kidney responds to the reduced renal blood flow during exercise with increased glomerular permeability and decreased renal tubular reabsorption of protein.[13,15] One hypothesis is that the renal vasoconstriction in response to the exercise load causes many glomeruli to stop functioning. After exercise, when these glomeruli resume function, they may leak protein and, presumably, blood cells.[15,19] The urinary sediment findings correlate with the intensity of the exercise,[1,10,15,19] and the state of hydration[15,16] and the interaction between these.[12]

Gross Hematuria. A separate syndrome of gross hematuria in runners has been well documented. It consists of grossly bloody urination, occasionally without warning symptoms, but sometimes preceded by urinary frequency and tenesmus. Painless blood clots as large as 0.5×1.0 cm have been reported. Evaluation with excretory urograms has been consistently negative. Cystoscopic examinations have varied with the interval between symptoms and examination. Early cystoscopies have revealed localized bladder contusions with loss of bladder epithelium and the presence of fibrinous exudates. The syndrome has been identified in both male and female runners. Early urinalysis will show RBC's. This syndrome is also benign, and all urinary findings disappear within a few days.[3,8,9]

Urinary Screening. Traditionally, preparticipation athletic screening has included urine testing by dipstick for protein, blood, and glucose. A recent study demonstrated that of 701 high school students undergoing athletic screening, 40 had proteinuria and one had glycosuria. Repeat testing with first-voided morning specimens revealed normal urine in all students, and a glucose tolerance test was normal in the student with glycosuria.[11] Consequently, routine urinary screening is no longer recommended.[18]

If a urinalysis is obtained for other reasons, and an athlete has abnormal sediment, it may be necessary that the athlete rest completely for several days before the urinary findings revert to normal. In some individuals, even a small amount of exercise may produce an abnormal urine.

REFERENCES

1. Alyea EP, Parish HH: Renal response to exercise—urinary findings. JAMA 67:807–813, 1968.
2. Barach, JH: Physiological and pathological effects of severe exertion (marathon race) on the circulatory and renal systems. Arch Intern Med 5:382–405, 1910.
3. Blacklock, NJ: Bladder trauma in the long-distance runner: "10,000 metres haematuria." Br J Urol 49:129–132, 1977.
4. Boileau M, Fuchs E, Barry JM, Hodges CV: Stress

5. Campanacci L, Faccini L, Englaro E, et al: Exercise-induced proteinuria. Contrib Nephrol 26:31–41, 1981.
6. Castenfors J: Renal function during prolonged exercise. Ann N Y Acad Sci 301:151–159, 1977.
7. Fassett RG, Owen JE, Fairly J, et al: Urinary red-cell morphology during exercise. Br Med J 285:1455–1457, 1982.
8. Fred HL: More on grossly bloody urine of runners. Arch Intern Med 138:1610–1611, 1978.
9. Fred HL, Natelson EA: Grossly bloody urine of runners. South Med J 70:1394–1396, 1977.
10. Gardner KD: "Athletic pseudonephritis"—alteration of urine sediment by athletic competition. JAMA 161:1613–1617, 1956.
11. Goldberg B, Saraniti A, Witman P, et al: Pre-participation sports assessment—an objective lesson. Pediatrics, 66:736–745, 1980.
12. Helzer MJ, Latin RW, Mellion MB, et al: The effect of exercise intensity and hydration on athletic pseudonephritis. Med Sci Sports Exerc 18(Suppl): S76, 1986.
13. Javitt NB, Miller AT: Mechanism of exercise proteinuria. J Appl Physiol 4:834–839, 1952.
14. Kincaid-Smith P: Haematuria and exercise-related haematuria. Br Med J 285:1595–1597, 1982.
15. Poortmans JR: Exercise and renal function. Sports Med 1:125–153, 1984.
16. Riess RW: Athletic hematuria and related phenomena. J Sports Med Phys Fitness 19:381–388, 1979.
17. Siegel AJ, Hennekens CH, Solomon HS, van Boeckel B: Exercise-related hematuria: findings in a group of marathon runners. JAMA 241:391–392, 1979.
18. Smith NJ (ed): Sports Medicine: Health Care for Young Athletes. Evanston, Illinois, American Academy of Pediatrics, 1983.
19. White HL, Rolf D: Effects of exercise and of some other influences on the renal circulation in man. Am J Physiol 152:505–516, 1948.

"RUNNER'S HIGH" AND EXERCISE ADDICTION

"Then, some time into the second hour comes the spooky time. Colors are bright and beautiful. Water sparkles, clouds breathe, and my body, swimming, detaches from the earth. A loving contentment invades the basement of my mind, and thoughts bubble up without trials. I find the place I need to live if I am going to live."[6]

Mandell's description of "the second second wind" is a literary example of what many call "the runner's high." Runner's high is a euphoria often experienced late in a long, slow distance run, and sometimes after the run, by well-conditioned athletes who typically run more than twenty miles weekly. In one survey, 69% of 424 runners have experienced a "high period," and this group reported that an average of 44% of their runs elicited a "high."[2]

Although there are no well-proven explanations for runner's high at present, there are several hypotheses, foremost of which is that it is a response to endogenously produced opiates, termed endorphins. In 1974, Hughes discovered two pentapeptides, each of which functioned "as an endogenous mediator at central morphine receptor sites."[5] Two years later, a larger peptide called beta-endorphin was shown to have the same type of activity on naturally occurring opiate receptors in the brain.[4] These three compounds and several others with similar effects have become collectively known as endorphins. In 1980, Appenzeller and associates demonstrated a relationship between intense endurance exercise and serum beta-endorphin levels.[1] This finding initiated speculation about whether the increased beta-endorphin production might cause "behavioral alterations" such as the runner's high.

Exercise Addiction. Exercise addiction has become a well-recognized syndrome in runners and other endurance athletes. One way to define an addiction is to withdraw the alleged stimulant. In the case of exercise addiction, runners and other athletes who stop experience a broad range of symptoms, including anxiety, restlessness, irritability, nervousness, guilt, muscle twitching, a bloated feeling, and sleep disturbance.[7] Just as endorphins have been implicated as the biological mediator of euphoria in the runner's high, it has also been suggested that they are the etiologic substance in exercise addiction.

Glasser was the first to associate the concept of addiction with exercise. He identified running and meditation as forms of an attainable "positive addiction" that may "strengthen us and make our lives more satisfying."[3] Unfortunately, not all people with exercise addiction have such a positive experience. Glasser envisioned the addiction process as being an extension of normal behavior. The exercise and/or meditation would replace other dysfunctional or self-defeating behaviors in the individual's life.

Morgan, on the other hand, has identified a syndrome of "negative addiction" in which the compulsion to exercise becomes a distortion of normal behavior. He noted a progression that occurs as a formerly sedentary individual becomes a runner and enjoys many of the positive psychological changes that take place. "At this time, daily exercise can become as much a part of the jogger's life as cigarettes for the pack-a-day smoker, alcohol for the alcoholic, and heroin for the mainliner."[7] He pointed out three signals that indicate that the addictive process is developing negatively: less attention to family and other close personal relationships, less concern with external issues such as achievements at work, and a pattern in which "feeling good becomes more important than anything else." The ultimate test of whether someone has an exercise addiction is how he or she responds when told to stop exercising because of a medical condition.[7] Physicians who see large numbers of athletes all have many patients who fail this test simply because they can't stop exercising. Intervention with these patients may be as difficult as it is with any other form of addiction.

REFERENCES

1. Appenzeller D, Standefer J, Appenzeller J, Atkinson R: Neurology of endurance training: V. endorphins. (Abstract) Neurology 30:418–419, 1980.
2. Callen KE: Mental and emotional aspects of long-distance running. Psychosomatics 24:133–141, 1983.
3. Glasser W. Positive Addiction. New York, Harper and Row, 1976.
4. Goldstein A. Opioid peptides (endorphins) in pituitary and brain. Science 193:1081–1086, 1976.
5. Hughes J: Isolation of an endogenous compound from the brain with pharmacological properties similar to morphine. Brain Res 88:295–308, 1975.
6. Mandell AJ: The second second wind. *In* Sachs MH, Sachs ML (eds): Psychology of Running. Champaign, Il, Human Kinetics, 1981, 211–223.
7. Morgan WP: Negative addiction in runners. Phys Sportsmed 7:56–70, Feb, 1979.

INGUINAL HERNIAS IN ATHLETES

Groin pain is a common athletic syndrome that physicians are seeing even more frequently now that heavy-weight training programs have become part of the conditioning regimens for so many sports. It is not uncommon for even high school athletes to be lifting many hundreds of pounds routinely in squats, hipsled, dead lift, and bench press exercises. Many of these athletes will appear with severe, insidious-onset groin pain and a normal musculoskeletal examination. Often a trial of musculoskeletal rehabilitation for suspected "groin pull" will already have failed. In the male athletes, inguinal hernia examination may be normal or at most there may be an increased impulse in the inguinal ring. In both male and female there will be no appreciable bulge over the inguinal ligament during Valsalva maneuver. Often these athletes have seen several physicians and are frustrated by a lack of adequate diagnosis and treatment.

Since the early 1970's the technique of herniography has been clinically available. A non-irritant, radiopaque contrast medium is injected into the peritoneum under fluoroscopy and the patient is then examined radiographically on a tilting x-ray table. Valsalva maneuver generally causes the dye to flow into the hernia sac.[1]

Smedberg and colleagues evaluated 78 athletes with groin pain including 23 athletes with bilateral symptoms. Only 8 of these 101 symptomatic sides demonstrated a palpable hernia on examination. Herniography revealed hernias in 85 of the 101 symptomatic sides and 27 of the 55 asymptomatic sides. Fifty-three athletes went on to surgery, including 10 who underwent bilateral herniorrhaphy. Operative findings correlated well with herniography. The surprising finding in these athletes was that 55% of the hernias in athletes under 30 years of age were direct, as contrasted with previous reports in the 4–10% range in this age group. Surgery resulted in a 69.8% cure rate and 28.6% improvement. The authors followed the patients with the 19 groin sides that did not respond to therapy. Later diagnoses revealed chronic tenoperiostitis of the adductor muscle group in 13, prostatitis in 2, hip joint arthrosis in 1, and no clear diagnosis in 3.[2]

In summary, groin pain in the athlete is often difficult to diagnose. Herniography may be a useful tool for demonstrating occult inguinal hernias. Other diagnoses, particularly tendonitis or tenoperiostitis of the adductor muscles, may accompany the hernia in spite of normal musculoskeletal and hernia examination. Although most performance athletes will opt for surgery after the diagnosis of an inguinal hernia is made, it is prudent to be cautious in advising them about the surgical outcome.

REFERENCES

1. Gullmo A, Broome A, Smedberg S: Herniography. Surg Clin N Am 64:229–244, 1984.
2. Smedberg SGG, Broome AEA, Gullmo A, Roos H: Herniography in athletes with groin pain. Am J Surg 149:378–382, 1985.

DIARRHEA AND GASTROINTESTINAL BLEEDING IN RUNNERS

Few groups of athletes spend more time discussing their bowel function than serious runners. This phenomenon is not the result of some bizarre psychological fixation. On the contrary, it is due to a rather common problem known affectionately as "runner's trots." One study demonstrated that 30% of runners have experienced this difficulty, and 12% of these have noted frank rectal bleeding.[5] For some runners, this diarrhea may be so severe as to be incapacitating. Of those in whom rectal bleeding is a component of the problem, many report a significant, potentially frightening amount of blood loss with these episodes.

In planning strategies for treatment and prevention, it would be extremely helpful to understand the etiology of the problems. Unfortunately, there are several theories, often in conflict with each other.

Runner's Diarrhea.   Many authors believe that runner's diarrhea results from increased gut motility, while others suggest that it is caused by ischemia during intense exercise. When analyzing the data, it appears that there may not be a single unifying hypothesis and that both of these explanations may hold in some cases.

Priebe and Priebe surveyed 425 runners in a 10-kilometer race. Thirty per cent had experienced runner's diarrhea and two-thirds of these provided data that formed the clinical description of their syndrome. Of this group 85% passed semi-formed or watery stools, 67% had low abdominal pain, 63% experienced rectal urgency, 51% had multiple stools and 13% experienced large volume stools. The problem either began after or continued after completion of the run in 54%, and 33% were incontinent. This description is consistent with a disorder of gut motility such as functional bowel syndrome. Indeed, 15% of Priebe and Priebe's subjects had irritable bowel syndrome when not running. Additionally, 13% had known lactose intolerance, and 33% were on a high-fiber diet, which is common in runners. The symptoms of abdominal pain and rectal urgency were relieved by defecation in 72%. Runners who used prophylactic anti-diarrheal medication generally found these agents to be successful in preventing or reducing the diarrhea. The authors concluded in their study that the diarrhea was the result of intestinal motility problems stimulated by intensive running.[5] Additional support for this explanation is provided by evidence that concentrations of motilin and other gastrointestinal regulatory peptides rise during prolonged running.[7]

Gastrointestinal Bleeding. In some runners an intense performance stimulates severe abdominal pain accompanied by grossly bloody diarrhea, often containing large quantities of red, maroon, or clotted blood. Two studies of runners indicate significant levels of fecal blood loss. One study demonstrated increased fecal hemoglobin levels, from a mean of 0.99 mg/gm pre-race to 3.96 mg/gm post-race, with elevations noted in 20 of 24 runners after races of 10 to 42.2 kilometers.[6] The other study showed that 7 out of 36 runners tested after the Boston Marathon had guaiac positive stools, and that these 7 individuals tended to be younger and faster.[4] Indeed, several reports suggest that bleeding may be associated with more strenuous or competitive running.[1,2,3,4]

The pathophysiology of gastrointestinal bleeding in runners is poorly understood. Increased bowel motility may explain runner's diarrhea but not bleeding. The current theory is that during intense efforts, endurance runners may experience relative bowel ischemia. During maximal exercise blood flow is shunted away from the gut and may be reduced by as much as 80%, to a level comparable to that seen in hypovolemic shock. It is hypothesized that the severe reduction in bowel circulation, with perhaps the additional stress of hyperthermic levels of core temperature elevation, produces local areas of ischemic bowel necrosis.[2,3] The resulting discomfort may mimic Crohn's disease or acute appendicitis.[2]

Prevention and Therapy. Management of runner's diarrhea and gastrointestinal bleeding may be difficult because the pathophysiology is not yet clear and because many dedicated runners are not willing to reduce their exercise intensity or to switch sports. The diagnosis of functional bowel syndrome should be entertained where it is consistent with the history. In these cases, dietary manipulations may be helpful, and antidiarrheal agents, which are useful in functional bowel syndrome, may be tried.

Many high-performance runners eat high-fiber or vegetarian diets. These diets tend to decrease the bowel transit time and thereby decrease the intraluminal weight that the athlete carries while performing. Runners like these diets because they may carry five or six pounds less bowel contents through a race. If a high-fiber diet stimulates marked increases in bowel motility, then it may be a problem itself. If, on the other hand, a runner is on a low-fiber diet and has significant "runner's trots," then considering adding fiber to solidify the gut is reasonable.

In patients who are bleeding with their diarrhea, the problem may be more alarming. For them, it is extremely important that they be well hydrated before they run. Since fluid intake itself may be a trigger for the diarrhea in some, these runners may be reluctant to drink immediately before running. For them, it is necessary to build up the plasma fluid volume with aggressive hydration between runs. Additionally, these athletes should also be encouraged to take fluids in smaller quantities but more frequently during the run.

A maneuver that has been shown to have some success is to be cut back the training and competition level 20% to 40% in both mileage and intensity and then to build back up very slowly.

Surprisingly, there are relatively few reports of this phenomenon in other endurance sports such as bicycling, swimming, and cross-country skiing. These other sports may provide alternative outlets for the recreational runner in whom these solutions all fail.

REFERENCES

1. Buckman MT: Gastrointestinal bleeding in long-distance runners. Ann Intern Med 101:127–128, 1984.
2. Cantwell JD: Gastrointestinal disorders in runners. JAMA 246:1404–1405, 1981.
3. Fogoros RN: "Runner's trots:" gastrointestinal disturbances in runners. JAMA, 243:1743–1744, 1980.
4. McMahon LF, Ryan MJ, Larson D, Fisher RL: Occult gastrointestinal blood loss in marathon runners. Ann Intern Med 100:846–847, 1984.
5. Priebe WM, Priebe J-A: Runner's diarrhea—prevalence and clincial symptomatology. Am J Gastroenterol 79:827–828, 1984.
6. Stewart JG, Ahlquist DA, McGill DB, et al: Gastrointestinal blood loss and anemia in runners. Ann Intern Med 100:846–847, 1984.
7. Sullivan SN, Champion MC, Christofides ND, et al: Gastrointestinal regulatory peptide responses in long-distance runners. Phys Sportsmed 12:77–82, 1984.

EXERCISE-INDUCED HEADACHES

There is little data to indicate that athletes are more or less prone to having headaches than others. There are, however, headache syndromes brought on by exercise that may be perplexing to physicians diagnostically as well as frightening to patients. Most of these headache syndromes are benign, but it is often difficult to sort them out from more severe underlying organic problems. In a landmark study, Rooke followed 103 patients diagnosed as having "benign exertional headache" for three or more years after the diagnosis was made. In 10 of these patients, significant intracranial lesions were found, including three Arnold-Chiari deformities, two cases of platybasia, one basilar impression, one chronic and one acute subdural hematoma, and two brain tumors. Sixteen of the patients had hypertension (150/100 or greater), but their blood pressure elevation was not considered to be the etiology of their headaches.[14] The finding that 10% of this group of benign exertional headache patients had significant pathology appears alarming. However, these patients were seen at a nationally famous tertiary referral center, and it is likely that the incidence of underlying organic disease is lower in the general population. Nonetheless, it is obvious that patients presenting with these syndromes need a careful history and physical examination, and an individual assessment and decision about the appropriateness of a CAT scan or neurological consultation.

Acute-Effort Migraine. Acute-effort migraine means a unilateral throbbing retroorbital headache that occurs a few minutes after extremely intense exercise. It is generally preceded by an aura consisting of scintillating scotomata and occasional lateral visual field cuts. It is usually accompanied by nausea and frequently by vomiting and photophobia. Hemiplegic variants are common. The duration is generally a few minutes to an hour, but many of these syndromes will persist for several hours. These headaches are less common in highly conditioned athletes, but many of them were seen in internationally competitive athletes at the Mexico City Olympics, held at an altitude of 5,000 feet.[1,3,10] Treatment is generally not necessary, but standard therapies for classical migraine have been tried in cases of more prolonged or frequent headaches. Prevention techniques include increasing the athlete's conditioning level and avoiding intense exercise when poorly acclimated at high altitude. One detailed case report demonstrates that a long, gradual warm-up in a highly competitive swimmer prevented her headaches.[8]

Vascular Headaches with Prolonged Exercise. A second common syndrome is a vascular headache that comes on more gradually after prolonged low-intensity exercise. It is characterized by intense throbbing pain, unilateral or bilateral and variable in location. It is generally not preceded by a scotoma or focal neurologic signs. Accompanying nausea is common, but vomiting is rare. This type of headache may last from one to many hours. It is commonly seen in the poorly conditioned athlete, and it is often associated with exercise in the heat, dehydration, hypoglycemia, exercise by the poorly acclimated athlete at high altitude, and antecedent alcohol consumption. Treatment consists of analgesics, especially the non-steroidal anti-inflammatory drugs, and treatment of associated conditions. Preventive measures include increasing the level of conditioning and avoiding the associated situations that make the athlete susceptible.[1,3]

Benign Exertional Headache. Benign exertional headache is precipitated by any level of physical activity, including brief or mild episodes. It is generally a throbbing headache but does not exhibit a clearly vascular pattern. Location is variable, but the headache pattern is generally consistent for each patient. Many patients find that increased physical effort or neck movement may intensify the headache. These headaches may last for a few minutes to many hours. These patients may also have headaches associated with other maneuvers that involve increased intrathoracic pressure, such as coughing, sneezing, bending, defecating, and sexual orgasm.[1,3,6] Indomethacin has been shown to be an effective treatment and prophylaxis for this problem.[6] It is likely that a much broader range of nonsteroidal anti-inflammatory drugs would also be effective.

Migraine Precipitated by Minor Head Trauma. There is a migraine syndrome, known as "footballer's migraine," which comes on a few minutes after minor head trauma following which the athlete does not become unconscious. It is a unilateral, throbbing, retro-orbital headache, preceded or accompanied by scintillating scotomata and other visual disturbances. Paresthesias and hemiplegic symptoms are common, as well as nausea, vomiting, and photophobia. These headaches may last from a few hours to two days.[2,3,5,7,11] These headaches should not be confused with the migraine syndrome, which develops following more severe trauma and which appears weeks to months after blunt head trauma.[4] Migraine precipitated by minor head trauma may be managed with standard treatments for classical or hemiplegic migraine. There are not enough data available about whether various forms of migraine prophylaxis will work for athletes with these headaches.

Weightlifter's Headache. There is a syndrome of headache in weightlifters and other people doing resistance forms of exercise that comes on suddenly while straining to lift. The headache is typically occipital and upper cervical, but may extend to the parietal areas. It is a severe, steady burning or "boring" headache. It lasts for days to many weeks and subsides gradually. The etiology is unclear, but it is possibly a form of cervical ligament strain. The treatment is rest; and although there is no mention of physical therapy in the literature, it seems appropriate to start the athlete on a neck rehabilitation program. This type of headache may be recurrent and may necessitate stopping of lifting altogether or stopping the specific exercise which exacerbates it.[12,13]

Exertional Headache in Pheochromocytoma. Episodic headache is a symptom of pheochromocytoma that may be brought on by exertion. The characteristic headache is bilateral, throbbing, and often indistinguishable from classic migraine. It is commonly accompanied by nausea and vomiting. Duration is variable, from a few minutes to a rather prolonged headache. Diagnosis is aided by the fact that these patients are frequently hypertensive without their headache. Their blood pressure during the headache is dramatically elevated, with a series of case reports demonstrating pressure 200-300/ 120-210. These headaches should be managed by treating the underlying pheochromocytoma.[9]

Summary. The exercise-induced headache syndromes are summarized in Table 3. Guides to the evaluation and management of the individual syndromes have been presented, but a repeat word of caution is necessary. Although the incidence of underlying severe organic underlying pathology is likely to be less than the 10% in Rooke's study, these exercise-induced headaches will mask a significant amount of underlying pathology. They should not be treated as trivial and benign until they are carefully evaluated and the potential severe organic etiologies have been ruled out.

REFERENCES

1. Appenzeller O: Cerebrovascular aspects of headache. Med Clin N Am 62:467–480, 1978.

TABLE 3.   EXERCISE-INDUCED HEADACHES

TYPE OF HEADACHE	ONSET	SYMPTOMS	DURATION	OTHER CHARACTERISTICS	PREVENTION	TREATMENT
Acute effort migraine	Few minutes after extremely intense exercise	Scintillating scotomata Unilateral throbbing retro-orbital headache Nausea & vomiting Photophobia Occasional lateral visual field cuts or hemiplegic variants	Generally few minutes to an hour Occasionally several hours	Less common in highly conditioned athletes	Increase conditioning level Long gradual warm-up Avoid intense exercise when poorly acclimated	Generally not necessary If headache prolonged, treat as classic migraine
Vascular headache with prolonged exercise	After prolonged low-intensity exertion	More gradual onset after exercise Intense throbbing pain Variable location Unilateral or bi-lateral No scotoma or focal neurological signs Nausea	One to many hours	Common in poorly conditioned athletes Often associated with: dehydration exercise in heat hypoglycemia exercise at high altitude alcohol consumption	Increase conditioning level Avoid: dehydration excessive heat loss hypoglycemia alcohol exercise at high altitude when poorly acclimated	Analgesics, especially non-steroidals Treat associated conditions
Benign exertional headache	Precipitated by any level of physical activity including brief or mild	Generally a throbbing headache, but not clearly a vascular pattern Variable location but generally consistent for each patient Increased effort or neck movement may intensify headache	Few minutes to many hours	May have headaches associated with other maneuvers which involve increased intrathoracic pressure	Prophylactic indomethacin or other non-steroidal anti-inflammatory drugs	Indomethacin and other nonsteroidal anti-inflammatory drugs—acutely

Syndrome	Onset	Symptoms	Duration	Comments		Treatment
Migraine precipitated by minor head trauma ("Footballer's Migraine")	Few minutes after minor head trauma without unconsciousness	Scintillating scotomata & other visual disturbances. Paresthesias & hemiplegic symptoms common. Unilateral throbbing retro-orbital headache. Photophobia. Nausea & vomiting	Few hours to 2 days	Not to be confused with migraine which develops following severe head trauma & which appears weeks to months after the trauma	Not enough data available for prophylaxis	Treat as classic or hemiplegic migraine
Weightlifter's headache	Sudden onset while straining to lift weights	Occipital, upper cervical. Steady, severe. Burning or "boring"	Days to weeks. Subsides gradually	Possibly a form of cervical ligament strain	May require stopping lifting	Rest. Possible benefit from physical therapy (?)
Exertional headache in pheochromocytoma	Spontaneous or exertion-related	Bilateral throbbing headache often indistinguishable classic migraine. Nausea & vomiting	Variable	Frequent baseline hypertension BP during headache frequently 200-300/120-210		Treat underlying pheochromocytoma
Exertional headache related to organic head and neck lesions	Within a few minutes of exertion	Variable	Generally brief —seconds to minutes	Underlying lesions: Arnold-Chiari deformity platybasia basilar impression subdural hematoma brain tumor		Treat organic lesion

2. Ashworth B: Migraine, head trauma and sport. Scott Med J 30:240–242, 1985.
3. Atkinson R, Appenzeller O: Headaches in sports. Semin Neurol 1:334–344, 1981.
4. Behrman S: Migraine as a sequelae of blunt head trauma. Injury 9:74–76, 1974.
5. Bennett DR, Fuenning SI, Sullivan G, Weber J: Migraine precipitated by head trauma in athletes. Am J Sports Med 8:202–205, 1980.
6. Diamond S, Medina JL: Prolonged benign exertional headache: clinical characteristics and response to indomethacin. Adv Neurol 33:145–149, 1982.
7. Haas DC, Pineda GS, Lourie H: Juvenile head trauma syndromes and their relationship to migraine. Arch Neurol 32:727–730, 1975.
8. Lambert RW, Burnett DL: Prevention of exercise induced migraine by quantitative warm-up. Headache 25:317–319, 1985.
9. Lance JW, Hinterberger H: Symptoms of pheochromocytoma, with particular reference to headache, correlated with catecholamine production. Arch Neurol 33:281–288, 1976.
10. Massey EW: Effort headache in runners. Headache 22:99–100, 1982.
11. Matthews WB: Footballer's migraine. Br Med J 2:326–327, 1972.
12. Paulson GW: Weightlifter's headache. Headache 23:193–194, 1983.
13. Perry WJ: Exertional headache. Phys Sportsmed 13:95–99, 1985.
14. Rooke ED: Benign exertional headache. Med Clin N Am 52:801–808, 1968.

THORACIC OUTLET SYNDROME AND EFFORT THROMBOSIS

Thoracic outlet syndrome and its sequela, effort thrombosis, can occur in athletes in relation to the exertion of their sport, as a result of weight training, or as a response to trauma. It is important to recognize these syndromes because both can impair or stop athletic performance, and because the latter can result in long-term disability if not properly diagnosed and treated.

Thoracic Outlet Syndrome. The thoracic outlet is the space through which the subclavian artery and the brachial plexus pass en route to the axilla. Its bony boundaries are the clavicle, scapula, and first rib. The pectoralis minor and the scalenus anticus and scalenus medius muscles further define this space. Typically, the neurovascular bundle passes between the scalenus anticus and medius. Numerous motions of the shoulder, particularly those involving depression of the shoulder or hyperabduction of the arm,

will exert pressure on the neurovascular bundle. Anatomical variants, including a cervical rib, an abnormal first rib, or congenital hypertrophy of the scalenus muscles may cause severe pressure on the nerves and artery passing through the thoracic outlet. Additionally, exercise may induce scalenus anticus hypertrophy which will result in the same problem. Thoracic outlet syndrome occurs when the compression is great enough to produce symptoms.

The patient generally experiences burning, numbness, and tingling in a variable distribution in the upper extremity. Pain in the upper extremity may imitate a variety of athletic overuse syndromes. Weakness and sensory deficits may occur. Adson's maneuver and the hyperflexion-abduction test may be positive. It is beyond the scope of this discussion to go into the variety of physical examination, laboratory, and x-ray procedures which may be used to diagnose thoracic outlet syndrome.

Thoracic outlet syndrome has been reported in relationship to swimming, the throwing sports, rowing, and weight training.[6,12] Interestingly, it has also been documented in the left arm of concert string players.[9] Personal experience indicates that minor levels of thoracic outlet syndrome are not uncommon. While definitive treatment for these problems is surgical, a trial of physical therapy is generally warranted first.[2,10,11]

Effort Thrombosis. Effort thrombosis is a common variant of thoracic outlet syndrome in which the subclavian or axillary vein becomes acutely thrombosed. It typically occurs in physically active males between the ages of 15 and 40; but with the increasing participation of young women in competitive exercise, it is possible that it may be seen increasingly in young women as well. The right arm is much more commonly involved than the left. Onset is generally abrupt and may follow either a bout of heavy exercise or trauma within 24 hours.

The syndrome initially presents as pain and swelling of the involved extremity. A prominent pattern of venous distension and dilated superficial collateral veins develops over the upper arm, shoulder, neck, and thorax. The extremity may take on a blue or a mottled violaceous discoloration. Both the venous pattern and the discoloration are more prominent when the individual attempts to exercise the extremity. A tender "cord" is often palpable along the course of the axillary vein. Accompanying neurologic and arterial insufficiency symptoms related to thoracic outlet syndrome have been reported as well. The diagnosis is clinical, but confirmation is made by venogram.[1,4,5,8,13]

The traditional treatment of effort thrombosis, rest and anti-coagulation resulted in 68% to 75% chronic problems, consisting of residual pain, swelling, and weakness.[1,3,4,5,13] In many patients, the residual symptoms have been shown to be the result of persistent occlusion of the subclavian and axillary veins, where recanalization has not taken place.[5] Consequently, in the past, several surgeons have advocated early thrombectomy, often with simultaneous relief of the anatomic cause of the venous compression.[1,5] Others have shown some success in correcting the etiologic anatomic problem later on in those patients with persistent disability.[3,7] With the advent of fibrinolytic therapy for the lysis of intravascular clots, early diagnosis of effort thrombosis is even more important. Using this technique, the thrombus may be lysed percutaneously. Because of the high rate of recurrence and sequelae of effort thrombosis, definitive treatment of the underlying thoracic outlet syndrome should then be seriously considered.[13]

REFERENCES

1. Adams JT, De Weese JA: "Effort" thrombosis of the axillary and subclavian veins. J Trauma 11:923–930, 1971.

2. Britt LP: Nonoperative treatment of the thoracic outlet syndrome symptoms. Clin Orthop 51:45–48, 1967.

3. Campbell CB, Chandler JG, Tegtmeyer CJ, Bernstein EF: Axillary, subclavian, and brachiocephalic vein obstruction. Surgery 82:816–826, 1977.

4. Crowell DL: Effort thrombosis of the subclavian and axillary veins: review of the literature and case report with two-year follow-up with venography. Ann Intern Med 52:1337–1343, 1960.

5. Drapanas T, Curran WL: Thrombectomy in the treatment of "effort" thrombosis of the axillary and subclavian veins. J Trauma 6:107–119, 1966.

6. Frankel SA, Hirata I: The scalenus anticus syndrome and competitive swimming: report of two cases. JAMA 215:1796–1798, 1971.

7. Glass BA: The relationship of axillary venous thrombosis to the thoracic outlet compression syndrome. Ann Thorac Surg 19:613–621, 1975.

8. Matas R: Primary thrombosis of the axillary vein caused by strain: report of a case with comments on diagnosis, pathology, and treatment of this lesion in its medico-legal relations. Am J Surg 24:642–666, 1934.

9. Roos DB: Thoracic outlet syndromes: symptoms, diagnosis, anatomy and surgical treatment. Med Prob Perform Art 1:90–93, 1986.

10. Roy S, Irvin R: Sports Medicine: Prevention, Evaluation, Management, and Rehabilitation. Englewood Cliffs, N.J., Prentice-Hall, 1983, pp 189–191.

11. Smith KF: The thoracic outlet syndrome: A protocol for treatment. J Orthop Sports Physical Ther 1:89–99, 1979.

12. Strukel RJ, Garrick JG: Thoracic outlet compression in athletes: a report of four cases. Am J Sports Med 6:35–39, 1978.

13. Vogel CM, Jensen JE: "Effort" thrombosis of the subclavian vein in a competitive swimmer. Am J Sports Med 13:269–272, 1985.

13 Common Skin Problems in Athletes

LOREN H. AMUNDSON, M.D.
MORRIS B. MELLION, M.D.

Every physician dealing with athletes should be aware of the effect of skin problems upon participation and performance. Skin problems are common in athletes; given their frequency, it is important that the sports-oriented physician possess skill in diagnosis and treatment of these problems. Important also is an understanding of the many functions the skin performs, including protection against abrasion and mechanical injury, regulation of the body temperature within close limits, keeping out chemicals and pathogens while protecting the body's fluid content, and filtering out harmful ultraviolet radiation.[1] It is also necessary for the physician to understand skin structure, so as to know how the above tasks are accomplished, and the reader is referred for review to one of several excellent dermatologic texts (see list of recommended texts following references).

The physician should likewise be aware of the many environmental factors that affect the skin and in addition the damage that can be caused by inappropriate care. The importance of skin care should be stressed in health classes.[2] Daily skin care should include fresh clean underclothing and socks, and clean clothing and equipment for practice and competition. Equipment is involved in many sports-related skin problems, as the skin is invariably exposed to trauma during athletic training and competition.[3] Preventive techniques are often not adhered to by athletes, especially student athletes.

Effective management of skin problems in athletes, as with problems of other body systems, follows accurate diagnosis. Fitzpatrick emphasizes that "the trained eye of the physician is the most important single factor in dermatologic diagnosis."[4] Inquiry into the type of sport and level of involvement of the patient is necessary to develop a framework for diagnosis; examples of information required include spatial relationships between a skin eruption and the sport activity, environmental factors such as sunlight, utilization of self-care medication or other therapy, and other aggravating factors.

To be an effective dermatotherapist for the athlete, it is necessary to understand principles of skin care, to be familiar with the pharmacology of topical and systemic agents, and to be acquainted with various physical modes of therapy such as cryotherapy. Glucocorticoids represent the most commonly used topical agents, and it is incumbent upon the sports physician to understand fully the indications and complications of corticosteroid therapy, when used topically, intralesionally or parenterally.[5]

Athletes with bacterial skin infections, viral lesions of herpes simplex and molluscum contagiosum, and infestations should be temporarily disqualified from competition.[6]

INJURY TO THE SKIN

Sun Damage. Sunlight produces both short-term reactions and more serious long-term damage. The athlete and sports physician are usually familiar with short-term conditions, including sunburn and miliaria (sweat gland occlusion). However, the long-term effects of sunlight, including solar elastosis, actinic keratoses and skin cancer are usually far from the mind of the competitive athlete; the sports physician must be able to counsel the student athlete on the need to prevent prolonged sun damage to the skin.

Sunburn (UV-B) is usually not a diagnostic problem, nor is the therapy difficult, although it sometimes interferes with competition. First and second degree sunburn responds well to analgesics and cool compresses whereas systemic steroids can be used to combat acute distress of burns that are more extensive. Aspirin taken 1–2 hours prior to sun exposure may reduce sunburn significantly.[3] Taken in high doses for 24 hours, and started immediately after a significant sun exposure, it may reduce the severity of the burn and provide adequate analgesia.[7] Tanning booths (UV-A) are currently popular, and athletes frequently use them to prevent or control the amount of sunburn obtained through sports participation. However, the long-range effects of UV-A are suspected to cause skin damage, and the use of tanning booths can only be decried.

Protective sun agents provide an appropriate preventive option for the athlete. Sun-blocking agents such as zinc oxide are useful for lips, earlobes, and the nose, especially in swimmers and lifeguards. Sunscreens, especially those with a sun protection factor (SPF) of 15 and above, are effective but must be applied before exposure to the sun and reapplied every few hours after heavy sweating or swimming. Good ones include Creamy Pre-Sun, Sundown, and Supershade.[3] Oily sunscreens may cause folliculitis.[8] Suntan lotions are widely used to speed up the sun's tanning of the skin; although chemicals that react with the skin may produce an artificial tan that lasts a few days, these lotions offer little or no protection against sunburn, especially in swimmers.

Excessive sun exposure frequently leads to a herpes labialis flare-up, necessitating 10 to 14 days for complete resolution. Similarly distressing for the active athlete are a variety of photosensitive and photoallergic reactions, especially in athletes taking a variety of systemic medications[7] (Table 1). "Sun-poisoning" may also occur, especially in those people with type 1 and type 2 skin (light complexion, blue eyes, blonde or red hair). If the exposure is extreme, the patient may present with a toxic clinical picture characterized by fever, chills, nausea and prostration, necessitating aggressive supportive care including

intravenous fluids.[3] Those with sensitive skin should wear a sunscreen whenever significant sun exposure is anticipated, a lifetime preventive activity.

Hypothermia. The skin is likewise susceptible to the effects of cold. Frostnip and frostbite (numb, white patches, especially of the nose, earlobes, digits and male genitalia) are more common in the distance runner, although any sport with skin exposure to a cold environment (e.g., cross-country skiing, winter hiking, ice skating) may be causal. Therapy includes rapid rewarming and protection from trauma; further damage may be prevented by the generous use of friction reducing emollients. Some resultant numbness and superficial erythema, even blistering, may be noted for a few days. Localized skin damage from inappropriate therapy with dry ice and liquid nitrogen does occur, whereas ice massage only rarely causes frostbite.[9]

Localized Conditions

ABRASIONS. Abrasions probably constitute the most common dermatologic lesion seen in athletes. A variety of terms apply: turf burn, mat burn, cinder burn, road rash, raspberry and others. Whatever the cause or location, therapeutic measures must be followed by preventive techniques. Therapy can include initial cleansing with water or hydrogen peroxide, the application of an antibiotic ointment and dry gauze.

Another more recent approach uses Duo-Derm, an occlusive hydrophilic dressing that provides an optimal healing environment for the epithelium, which spreads both from the margins of the abrasion and from the remaining central islands of epithelium in the skin.[10] These dressings are designed to prevent infection, protect the wound and reduce pain. After washing the wound with soap and water, a DuoDerm dressing is applied to the wound and surrounding area with at least an overlapping ¾ inch margin (Fig. 1). As there is usually an accumulation of the tissue fluid that wells up under the dressing initially, it is recommended that the dressing be changed at 24 hours and again if fluid recollects and extends to within ¼ inch of the edge of the

TABLE 1. PHOTOSENSITIVE/PHOTOALLERGIC SUBSTANCES

TOPICAL	SYSTEMIC
Acne medications, vitamin A acid (Retin-A)	Antihistamines, diphenhydramine (Benadryl)
Antifungals	Dyes
Coal tar derivatives	eosin
acridine	fluorescein
anthracene	trypaflavine
phenanthrene	Rose Bengal
pyridine	methylene blue
Cosmetics	Food additives
indelible lipsticks	saccharin
perfumes and aftershave	cyclamates
lotions having essential oils	Miscellaneous
Pigments and dyes	birth control agents
yellow cadmium sulfide	chlordiazepoxide HCI (Librium)
proflavine, acriflavine	furosemide (Lasix)
eosin	Psoralens
anthraquinone	methoxypsoralens
Plants (furocoumarins)	Sulfa drugs and analogues
Soap deodorants (photoallergic)	sulfonamides
halogenated salicylanilides	hypoglycemics:
(tri- and tetrachlor-; brominated)	sulfonylurea (Dymelor)
bithionol	tolbutamide (Orinase)
hexachlorophene	chlorpropamide (Diabinese)
dichlorophene	diuretics:
carbanilides	thiazides (HydroDIURIL)
Sunscreens	phenothiazines:
para-aminobenzoic acid (PABA)	chlorpromazine (Thorazine)
digalloyl trioleate (Sunstick)	promethazine (Phenergan)
	prochlorperazine (Compazine)
	Other antibiotics
	tetracycline
	doxcycline (Vibramycin)
	nalidixic acid (NegGram)
	griseofulvin

dressing. At this time the fluid often has a slightly foul smell, which does *not* indicate infection. If removed, the wound and any dressing materials adhering to it are lavaged gently with water and another piece of Duo-Derm is reapplied. It is left in place until healing is complete, for most abrasions a week or less. One of the advantages of Duo-Derm is that once the dressing is in place there is little or no pain. This process seems to work for all abrasions except the very deepest, which are essentially third degree burns, in which case initial treatment with Silvadene is indicated. Other occlusive dressings include Tegaderm, OP-Site, and Bioclusive, which are polyethylene membranes. They are less effective in large abrasions because they lose their adhesive quality when damp and are less absorbent. Duo-

Derm has a "wet tack" property which provides adherence to wet as well as dry skin.

CHAFING. Intertrigo results from mechanical irritation, regardless of location, and is aggravated by sweating and protective equipment (pads, cups, etc.).[11] Chafing is frequent in runners and bikers, and the nipples, axillae and groin bear the brunt of insult, even to the point of bleeding. Prevention includes cleanliness, loose clothing, talc or Zeosorb to keep the area dry, and/or lubricating creams such as Cramer's Skin Lube and Eucerin. A sports bra may be indicated. Therapy includes air, cool compresses, heat lamps and mild steroid creams.

BLISTERS. Intraepidermal blisters abound in athletes who wear shoes and are also seen in other body areas where friction occurs. Frictional forces are greater if the skin is

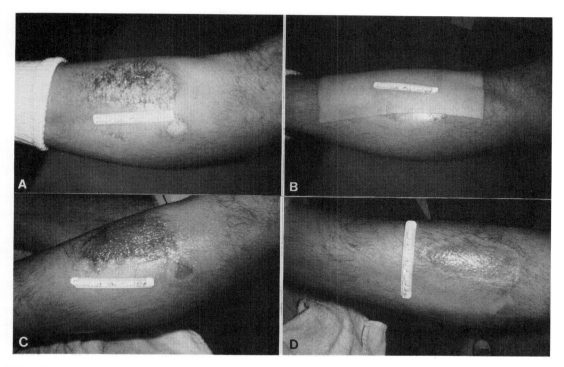

FIGURE 1. *A,* Turf burn, calf, 4.5 by 7.5 centimeters, day of injury. *B,* DuoDerm dressing applied. *C,* Turf burn, calf, 2 days post-injury; reepithialization under way. *D,* Turf burn, calf, 5 days post-injury; wound clean, dry, and well-healed.

moist, less if the skin is dry, greasy or very wet. Some may be prevented by hardening the skin with 10% tannic acid soaks.[6] Other preventive measures include proper shoes and socks, the application of Vaseline to skin or sites of friction in the shoes, the use of talc to reduce moisture, and the use of adhesive tape or moleskin over potential or previous blister sites.[7]

Once a blister has formed there are management options. Some advocate needle aspiration and adhesive taping, using the epidermal layers as an occlusive dressing.[6] Others prefer to remove the blistered layers of skin and expose the base, feeling that this prevents repeat blisters during healing and makes the lesion easier to keep clean and non-infected. Following the removal of the blister roof, a tape adherent such as Tuf-Skin is sprayed on, causing some initial discomfort due to its alcohol content. Following this application, a circular or oval piece of mole-

skin large enough to cover the blister and a ¾ inch border is applied and left in place until healing is complete. Most failures occur from initial neglect of the lesion, then allowing infection to dictate care.

CALLUSES AND CORNS. These lesions, most common on the feet, represent physiological responses to friction or pressure that the skin was not designed to sustain. They are not exclusively confined to the feet, gymnasts and golfers having their share of calluses on the hands and bicyclists occasionally over the ischial rami. Effective therapy depends upon the modification of causative factors, such as changing hand grips or a cycle seat, adjustment of footwear or the use of metatarsal inserts. If additional or ongoing therapy is warranted, it is best provided by intermittent paring and trimming, sanding with a pumice stone, and occasionally by the use of salicylic acid plasters. Such physical or chemical debridement can keep the patient comfortable while removing excessive keratinous accumulation. The less surgical the eradication, the better.

HEMORRHAGE. Several types of soft tissue hemorrhage are seen in the athlete. Subcutaneous ecchymoses occur frequently in the tips of the great and second toes, most often seen in tennis and basketball players and caused by frequent fast starts and stops, in addition to more chronic trauma from long-distant running. Likewise, black heel (talon noir) may be seen on the plantar surface of the heel even in the seasoned athlete (Fig. 2). Prevention rests with thicker socks, moleskin, and emollient creams prior to practice and competition.[12] Diagnosis is sufficient therapy.

Hematomas, seen as blood blisters or contusions in the more superficial intradermal and subcutaneous tissues, and deeper in the muscle with collision/contact sports, may require only limited therapy such as rest, ice, compression and elevation (RICE). More aggressive therapy, especially of deep muscle hematomas, may be indicated to prevent long-term disabilities and complications such as myositis ossificans, more familiar to the athletic trainer and physical therapist than to many physicians.

NAIL HEMORRHAGE. Injuries to the nail may cause it to separate from its underlying bed (onycholysis) or give rise to acute subungual hemorrhage, a more painful condition. Treatment for the former is supportive, whereas evacuating the blood with a hot wire, twirling a needle, or a #11 blade, or yet other methods, will offer instantaneous relief for the latter. Loss of the nail will depend upon the extent of the injury.

LACERATIONS. A variety of lacerations occur in the competitive athlete. Assurance of an immune tetanus status is comforting. Appropriate wound care, including surgical repair, insures the best protection against infection and promotes early healing.

BITES AND STINGS. For those athletes sensitive to a variety of insect bites, common mosquito repellents containing diethyltoluamide deter most would-be invaders.[7] Unattended insect bites frequently lead to infection and must be monitored by those responsible for the athlete, especially in those environments combining sweat, dirt and occlusion. For those athletes demonstrating systemic sensitivity to stinging insects (bees, wasps, and others) the physician must instruct the athlete as to risks and make injectable adrenalin available to those responsible for on-field evaluation and care. Several self-contained "bee sting kits" are available commercially, and one belongs in the field athletic bag.

INGROWN NAIL. Ingrown nails occur fre-

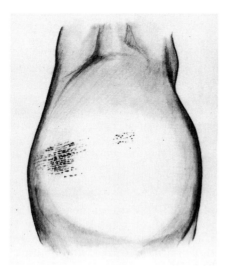

FIGURE 2. Black heel ("talon noir"), a form of ecchymosis.

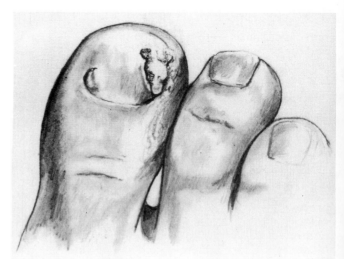

FIGURE 3. Ingrown toenail with excessive granulation tissue (pyogenic granuloma).

quently, usually when the configuration of the nail approaches a semi-circle in cross-section. Other causes include trimming the nails too deeply at the corners and the use of tight-fitting footwear, especially in tennis, basketball and in long distance running. Neglected nails can produce an extreme amount of periungual inflammation, sometimes leading to the development of excessive granulation tissue (pyogenic granuloma), usually next to a great nail, which is also more commonly ingrown (Fig. 3).

The treatment of an ingrown nail necessitates appropriate care of the inflammatory periungual tissue, including nail removal, and sometimes of accompanying systemic infection, plus the need for appropriate footwear. Cutting the great toe nail straight across without snipping off the protruding corners is the best preventive measure. A pyogenic granuloma, usually presenting as "proud flesh" with a moist glistening top, may arise anywhere on the skin, usually following trauma, but most often arises in conjunction with an ingrown nail. This lesion can be handled simply by applying silver nitrate, freezing with liquid nitrogen, shaving off the lesion with curettement of the base, snipping across the base with scissors, or tying off a pedunculated lesion with suture material. Hemostatics are usually indicated to deal with a vigorous ooze created by cutting into the growth.

DERMATOFIBROMA. Dermatofibroma results from microtrauma to the skin, common in the athlete, along with the residuals of localized infections such as folliculitis. Most are seen where repeat shaving of hair and taping occur, commonly on the legs. This small, slightly elevated, firm papule, often brownish to purple in color, usually measures less than 1 cm across (Fig. 4). The lesion is benign and no therapy is indicated.

STRIAE. Striae result from the loss of dermal collagen and elastic supporting fibers that allow the dermis to pull apart.[6] The lesions are initially red to dusky blue and later change to permanent, pale atrophic fracture lines.[7] Seen most frequently in athletes who gain considerable weight and/or muscle, weight lifters and gymnasts, these permanent skin changes are also seen in some growing teenagers, females having a higher incidence.[8] Topical and systemic steroids can also cause striae, especially in intertriginous areas following the use of topical fluorinated steroids.[13] Striae are most common over the anterior shoulder, breasts, lower back, abdomen, buttocks, and thighs, running perpendicular to the direction of skin tension.

GREEN HAIR. Cosmetic discoloration of the hair, most often greenish in tint, may be seen in blonde swimmers. Chlorine additives are often considered responsible and may create bleaching effects with blonding of hair; however copper deposition in the hair matrix is the reason for the green tint.[3] Shampooing after swimming usually prevents this problem. Therapy with 3% peroxide bleach in a 2 to 3 hour session is helpful, as is local application of a commercially available chelating agent (Metalex).

OTHER PHYSICAL FACTORS

Heat. Erythema ab igne, revealing characteristic hyperpigmentation and reticulated erythema, is sometimes seen after prolonged use of local heat for treatment of persistent painful joints or muscles.[14] Prevention is the key.

Cold. Erythema pernio sometimes follows exposure to a cold, wet environment, skin lesions developing 12–24 hours after the injury. Edematous red to blue plaques are seen, most commonly on the anterior shins, and usually disappear in one to two weeks.[14] Therapy is rarely indicated.

Dry skin may occur during prolonged cold exposure in winter sports, secondary to loss of hydration in the keratin layer. The skin appears dry and roughened, may crack, chap and lead to eczema; hence the names dry skin eczema, winter itch, asteatotic eczema, or eczema craquele. Therapy includes moisture (bathing) followed by lubricants (Alpha Keri, Domol), plus bland emollients applied several times daily (Tables 2, 3). Humidification of the home environment and improved general skin care are preventive.

Moisture. Hyperhidrosis is common in many high energy athletes and may adversely affect manual dexterity and aggravate several pedal skin problems.[15] Twenty per-

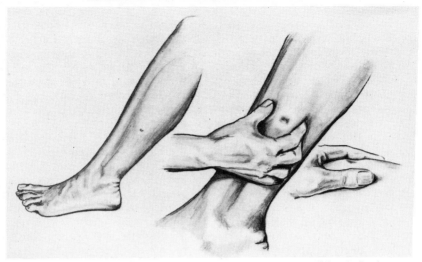

FIGURE 4. Dermatofibroma. This is a benign lesion that "dimples" when pinched.

cent aluminum chloride in anhydrous ethyl alcohol (Drysol) applied to completely dried palms and soles at bedtime may be helpful. Strict attention to product directions is important.

PHYSICAL URTICARIA

The interesting but distressing group of induced urticarias have a common pathogenesis in histamine. IgE is involved in some, but complement does not appear to play a role.[16] Physical exertion, pressure, cold, heat, solar, aquagenic and cholinergic factors may lead to exercise-related forms of urticaria, aided by rapid changes in body temperature and by emotional stress—all factors common to sports activities.

Prevention is difficult, short of total avoidance of inciting factors.[3] Gradual exercise may be used to "desensitize" athletes to this form of urticaria, while pharmacologic intervention is often not successful. Therapy used in selected cases includes antihistamines such as diphenhydramine (Benadryl), cyproheptadine (Periactin) and hydroxyzine (Atarax, Vistaril), corticosteroids and sunscreens.[16] Occasionally, two of the above H_1 antihistamines must be used in combination to obtain an adequate result. Another approach is to use an H_1 antihistamine plus the

H_2 antihistamine cimetidine (Tagamet) in combination (Table 4).

Exercise-induced anaphylaxis may be seen in these athletes, symptoms occurring within five minutes of exercise or delayed until exercise is completed.[16] The patient typically experiences pruritus, usually generalized, fol-

TABLE 2. LUBRICANTS AND EMOLLIENTS FOR DRY SKIN

Ointments/Creams (water-in-oil, oil-in-water emulsions)
Lanolin based
  Aquaphor
  Nivea
  Eucerin
  Keri
Petroleum based
  Lanolor
  Keri Creme
  Cold Cream USP
  Hydrophilic ointment USP
  Vaseline Dermatology Formula
Lotions (suspensions of powder in water)
  Lubriderm
  Cetaphil
  Wondra
  Aloe Vera
  Esoterica Dry Skin
  Eucerin
  Vaseline Intensive Care
  Wibi
  Alpha Keri
  Lacthydrim
  Ultra-Mide

TABLE 3. AMOUNT OF OINTMENT OR CREAM NEEDED
FOR TOPICAL USE

AREA COVERED	ONE APPLICATION (Gm)	ONE APPLICATION THREE TIMES DAILY FOR ONE WEEK (Gm)
Hand, face, head or anogenital region	2	45
One arm, or anterior, or posterior trunk	3	60
One leg	4	90
Entire body	30–60	1000

lowed by urticaria. The severity varies, and may progress to include bronchospasm, hypotension, arrhythmias and GI symptoms—true anaphylaxis, which must be treated as such. This exercise-induced syndrome is more common in those with a family history, including similar problems such as atopic eczema and asthma. The topic is covered more fully in another chapter.

CONTACT DERMATITIS

Allergic Dermatitis. Dermatitis is an inflammatory process of the epidermis and upper dermis. Common symptoms and findings include itching that leads to scratching, reddening of the skin, along with the development of papules and even blisters when the process is acute; more chronic cases reveal thickening and lichenification. Allergic contact dermatitis, the prototype being poison ivy, is common in susceptible athletes, especially those exposed to weedy areas during training or competition; these individuals develop specific T cell antibodies against the allergen.

TABLE 4. PHYSICAL URTICARIAS

INCITING FACTOR	SUGGESTED THERAPY*
Solar	Sunscreens
Cold	Cyproheptadine
Heat	H$_1$ Antihistamines
	Cyproheptadine
Cholinergic	Cyproheptadine
Exertion, pressure	H$_1$ Antihistamines
	H$_2$ Antihistamines
	Hydroxyzine

*Combinations of medications sometimes indicated.

Other common allergic causes include paraphenylenediamine (blue and black) clothing dyes, nickel-containing metal, all "caine" containing medicaments and benzoin preparations (Tincture of benzoin, Tuf-Skin)[17]. Other potent skin sensitizers such as ethylenediamine and neomycin also put the athlete at risk for dermatitis and are best not used at any time. Clear finger nail polish applied to the metal may prevent nickel dermatitis from buttons, shoulder pads and other equipment.

Irritant Dermatitis. Assessment of irritant contact dermatitis is often not difficult; it is usually due to physical and mechanical agents, and the history and location of the lesions are diagnostic. Common irritants include adhesive tape, lime, dry ice, astroturf, poorly fitting gear, cold-pack chemicals from a leak in "liquid ice," a variety of clothing fibers, rubber-containing straps, pads, leather gloves, shoes and chin straps, and a variety of skin products. The hallmark of therapy is to eliminate the continued exposure to the irritant. Often one need suggest only symptomatic relief such as cool, wet compresses or the use of antipruritic lotions and creams (no "caines"), including topical steroids, for less active dermatitis. At times systemic antihistamines are indicated, which may interfere with athletic performance. Rarely, a short course of systemic steroids may be necessary.

INFECTIONS

Bacterial Infections. Temporary cessation of athletic activities is often indicated for common pyoderms, including impetigo and furunculosis (boil).[17] Diagnosis is usually easy; impetigo represents a superficial infection of the skin caused by the Staphylococcus or Streptococcus or a combination of the two, whereas furunculosis, most commonly a staphylococcal sebaceous gland abscess, forms as an infection deep in the hair follicle. Both commonly occur in athletes and are aggravated by sweat, dirt and occlusion. Those athletes wearing heavy protective padding, as in hockey and football, are susceptible to a type of bacterial folliculitis called "acne mechanica." Seventy percent of boils develop after a bruise or break in the skin, most being located on the extremities. Associated causative factors include skin lubricants, elbow and forearm pads, whirlpool baths and athletic tape.[18] Prevention is important but difficult—finishing the season is curative.

Impetigo can often be cleared by using warm wet compresses, a 5–10% benzoyl peroxide solution, or a topical antibacterial ointment such as Bacitracin. An oral course of penicillin or erythromycin is indicated, since untreated streptococcal skin infections may lead to acute glomerulonephritis. Furuncles may develop deeper pockets and become fluctuant, necessitating incision to facilitate rapid drainage. A single stab wound is sufficient (without a wick).[15] Antibiotics are not ordinarily necessary in the treatment of a furuncle; however widespread, recurrent, or resistant furunculosis may best be aided by culture and appropriate systemic therapy. Adhesive tape used to secure a gauze dressing can produce enough injury in the adjacent stratum corneum to foster new lesions in the same area; therefore circumferential dressing is preferred if at all possible. Some sports physicians find that Bacitracin or triple antibiotic ointment applied to an area of furunculosis reduces the development of satellite lesions.

A recent addition to the folliculitis field is hot tub folliculitis, caused by the pseudomonas organism. The papulovesiculopustular lesions, occasionally heralded by mild systemic symptomatology and located in areas where the skin has been covered by swimwear or other clothing, are usually diagnostic and may be accompanied by an external Pseudomonas otitis.[19] The course is benign and self-limited, rarely necessitating diagnostic testing or therapeutic measures. Other Pseudomonas infections seen in athletes include "green" lesions of the nails and interdigital webs; the latter are best treated with gentamicin (Garamycin) ointment.

One to 3 mm discrete craters are frequently seen on the soles of tennis and basketball players. This condition, pitted keratolysis, is precipitated by hyperhidrosis (external or essential), aggravated by occlusive footwear, and caused by the Corynebacterium species.[14] Therapies include 5% formalin soaks and oral erythromycin. A less common bacterial infection in the crural area is erythrasma, also caused by Corynebacterium species. Seen most frequently in long distance runners in temperate climates, this infection may be characterized by a foul odor; it responds to systemic erythromycin.

External otitis (swimmer's ear) is the bane of aquatic participants.[20] Effective therapy includes otic wicks saturated with an acetic acid (VōSoL HC) or antibacterial ear drop (Colymycin S Otic), followed by measures that promote a more aerobic environment for the external ear, including removal of excess cerumen. Prevention of recurrent otic dermatitis externa in susceptible individuals may include the use of VōSoL or Burow's solution (Domeboro), used after swimming and post-competition showers. A hair dryer may also be helpful.

Fungal Infections.   Fungal infections, prototypes being dermatophytic tinea pedis ("athletes foot") and tinea cruris ("jock itch"), also include moniliasis and tinea versicolor. Diagnosis of most fungal infections can be made from clinical features, those often altered by self-treatment using a variety of OTC preparations.

Fungal infections commonly result from the macerating effects of chronic perspiration reducing the natural barrier effects of the stratum corneum. Tinea pedis is a common infection of the lateral intertoe spaces, especially in post-pubertal males. Tinea cruris is common in men and rarely seen in women. *Candida albicans,* an opportunistic yeast, can cause much trouble in warm moist parts of the body. Classic involvement of intertriginous areas and the easily identifiable 1–2 mm satellite lesions just beyond the main area of dermatitis make the diagnosis easily apparent. Tinea versicolor, seen commonly in swimmers and divers, creates more cosmetic than medical concerns for the student athlete; it usually fluoresces gold to orange under Wood's light.[7]

Preventive measures include daily changes of socks and shorts, absorbing foot powder and leather shoes, and daily cleansing of athletic shower and dressing facilities. Therapy may involve modification of the athlete's conditioning or training, allowing a more optimal environment to exist for a period of time. The availability of Monistat-Derm makes therapy for dermatophytic and monilial infections very effective, ably backed up by a variety of other topical antifungal agents. Three percent selenium sulfide shampoo, applied and left on for 3–5 min after a shower, and repeated daily for 5 days, constitutes a satisfactory course of treatment for tinea versicolor.

Viral Infections.   Common warts are usually easy to recognize because of the resemblance to a cauliflower sprig, the surface often including crypts or invaginations, irregular and rough, and accompanied by black dots representing thrombosed capillary tips. Warts rarely interfere with athletic competition and have a low rate of infectivity. While the plantar wart is caused by the same virus, it often looks different due to the weight-bearing surface. Warts tend to be self-limited and the athlete that has no symptoms and is willing to wait may be justly rewarded, as most warts resolve spontaneously within a few months, presumably a response to immunologic activity. These common lesions can be effectively treated by a variety of methods including liquid nitrogen, carbon dioxide stick, intermittent application of strong acids, home therapy with weak acids such as 10% salicylic acid and 10% lactic acid in flexible collodion (Duofilm), by gentle electrodesiccation, curettage under local anesthesia, and other less common methods such as 0.025% Retin A gel and 2-5% 5 FU. A greater confluence of warts, called a mosaic, often several centimeters in width, is best handled by the application of a commercial 40% salicylic acid plaster, cut to the shape of the warts and held in place with adhesive tape for 2-3 days. Following removal and foot soaks or a bath, including gentle clear-

ing of the remaining debris, a new plaster can be reapplied for another several days. Continued therapy for one to two months will often cause the wart to regress. Elliptical excision of warts should be avoided, especially on the plantar surface, and strong acids, liquid nitrogen and cautery should not be used during the athletic season. For therapy of troublesome, painful plantar warts during the athletic season, weekly injection of 1% xylocaine into the base of the wart until it shells out can be recommended (Fig. 5). The wart usually responds to therapy in one to three weeks, occasionally requiring more prolonged therapy.[21]

Another viral infection, molluscum contagiosum, produces small translucent papules (2–4 mm) that may be single, grouped or inoculated along a scratch (Koebner's lines). While lesions may occur most anywhere on the body, the hands and face are common locations, including the face and upper body of boxers and wrestlers. The translucent quality and umbilication of this small papule simplifies the diagnosis. A variety of therapies that evacuate the papular "molluscum body" include a tiny stab of the papule with a knife blade, light spark from an electric needle, application of liquid nitrogen, or the continued diligent application of salicylic and lactic acid preparations.

Herpes simplex virus can affect any cutaneous location or adjacent mucosa in the athlete; however, the most frequent locations are the face and hands, often following sun exposure or trauma, respectively. Common in wrestlers, along with impetigo, it is known as "herpes gladiatorum." The most effective preventive measure is daily scrubbing of the mats after practice and competition, often done by the wrestlers themselves, who know the competitive price of an acute episode. If a trigger factor can be reasonably assumed, the athlete may be able to avoid it, usually a significant saving to conditioning and competition. The lesions are initially small, 1–2 mm vesicles grouped together on an erythematous base. An initial attack may be dramatic, with considerable pain, adenopathy and fever. As to care for the acute eruption, therapies abound, including old fashioned maneuvers such as wet compresses, rubbing alcohol, ethyl ether, tincture ben-

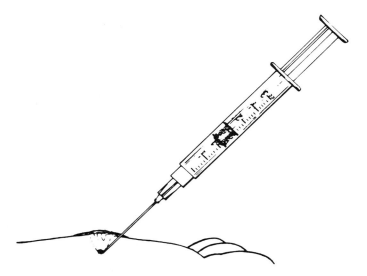

FIGURE 5.   Technique for injecting 1-2 cc of Lidocaine into the base of a plantar wart.

zoin or 4% zinc solution. Five to ten percent benzoyl peroxide and other drying agents are also used in the acute blistering phase, to be followed by a variety of bland creams or ointments when the lesions begin crusting.[17] Acyclovir (Zovirax) is an antiviral agent now available for topical, oral and systemic use. Its best indication in the athlete may be prophylaxis in situations where recurrent attacks produce an unusual degree of distress or frequent extended periods away from competition.

INFESTATIONS

Pediculosis.   Lice, more the bane of the younger classroom student (head lice) than the student athlete (pubic lice), most commonly occur under circumstances of inadequate hygiene. However, the camaraderie of athletes often puts them in close physical contact, as do athletic endeavors. Pubic lice (crabs) are therefore not uncommon and affect mature adults of both sexes and all socioeconomic strata. Head and pubic lice spread by this close personal contact are easily eradicated by a single application of gamma benzene hexachloride (Kwell) products. Nits on eyelashes, sometimes a secondary area for pubic lice to inhabit (similar hairshaft diameter), can be removed by

nightly application of generous amounts of petrolatum to the eyelids at bedtime, until cleared.[22] Head lice, less common in the athlete, may be also treated with a newer product, permethrin cream rinse (Nix), also used as a single application.

Scabies.   Still at epidemic levels in this country, one may suspect scabies in athletes complaining of generalized itching, worse at night and seen especially in those participating in sports leading to close body contact. Because the female mite can survive one to three days off the body, scabies can be spread by fomites such as towels, uniforms and equipment.[13] While proof of infestation is gratifying (recovering the mite from a burrow), a high index of suspicion and environmental factors often lead to appropriate assumptions and therapy. Itchy papules of the breast areolae or penis are nearly pathognomonic. Therapy is effective with a single application (neck to toes) of Kwell lotion in the evening after a bath. Rebathing the next day completes one treatment cycle, which is usually sufficient. Therapy for scabies is not complete without provision of systemic antipruritics as it may take 3–4 weeks for the itching to subside, this being completed when the inflammatory skin changes have been replaced with normal epithelium. Judicious use of topical corticosteroids may be helpful, however widespread skin involvement often makes this therapy impractical and expensive. If multiple cases are seen in the same athletic environment, it behooves the physician to personally supervise the application of a scabicide to all close contacts.

EXACERBATION OF PRE-EXISTING DERMATOSES

Athletes appear in the training room, on the practice field, and in competition with a variety of skin problems common to their age groups. As stated earlier, prevention is a key to skin problems, which can affect participation and performance; this applies equally to exacerbation of pre-existing skin problems seen in the athlete. Environmental factors play a significant role—the combination of sweat, dirt, and occlusive protective equipment combine to aggravate several pre-existing skin conditions including acne, atopic dermatitis, dyshidrosis and seborrheic dermatitis. These will be discussed further.

Acne. Acne is rarely a diagnostic problem. Much more difficult is the control of this distressingly common skin affliction of youngsters, especially during competitive athletic seasons in many sports. Control of acne is attainable however, and the objectives are twofold; short-term cosmetic results and long-term prevention of scarring. Preventive and therapeutic measures include the wearing of loose-fitting, dry, clean, absorbent cotton clothing, and avoidance of abrasive skin cleansers and constant picking at acne lesions.[23] Diet is not a factor. In spite of athletic lifestyles and environment, much can be done to improve the lot of the athlete with acne by employing the judicious use of benzoyl peroxide, retinoic acid derivatives and broad-spectrum antibiotics, both topical and systemic. Most athletes find sunshine to be helpful, noticing improvement in acne during the summer with worsening during the winter. A special problem is the athlete with frequent cystic acne, who may perform at less than full capacity while the cysts, most common on the face, neck and upper trunk, develop, mature, and either drain or resorb, this being psychologically distressing to the athlete for as long as 3 or 4 weeks. Once a cyst

has developed, hot compresses and a small incision to drain its contents when fluctuant are helpful. A more recent innovation, the early intralesional injection of 0.1 to 0.3 ml of ¼% triamcinolone acetonide suspension usually leads to rapid disappearance of the cyst with no surgical trauma to the skin surface.[1] This procedure also lessens the likelihood of secondary infection compared to a wound drained by surgical means. An athlete with severe acne may benefit from dermatologic consultation, especially if Accutane, a derivative of vitamin A, is considered for "curative" systemic use.

Atopic Dermatitis. Athletes with an atopic background are at risk to develop this condition, or for aggravation of their lifelong "curse," especially if elements have been present since infancy or childhood. The chronic thickening and excoriation of flexural areas at the elbows and knees often flare during athletic competition. These athletes are also at increased risk to develop exercise-related urticaria and anaphylaxis, exercise-induced bronchospasm (EIB, asthma), and allergic rhinitis (even progressing to nasal polyps). They likewise may develop aspirin sensitivity.

The treatment for a flare-up of atopic eczema is both rewarding and frustrating. Appropriate avoidance of excessive soap during bathing will be helpful, along with frequent use of bland emollients such as Vaseline or Eucerin, sometimes used in conjunction with topical corticosteroids. A short course of systemic corticosteroids may offer considerable relief for a flare-up that threatens to interfere with athletic competition but should be used judiciously if at all. Other measures useful during flareups include adequate rest, generous oral hydration, relief from emotional tension and the use of systemic antipruritic agents. Fall and winter sports participants are at greater risk for flare-up of atopic eczema, and many do not learn the need for continuing gentle topical care; for this reason the sports physician must frequently provide a "pep talk" to ensure the compliance with measures allowing them to be available for optimal participation.

Dyshidrosis. A common dermatitic condition affecting both the younger and more mature athlete is dyshidrosis (Fig. 6). Deep seated vesicles affecting the hands and feet,

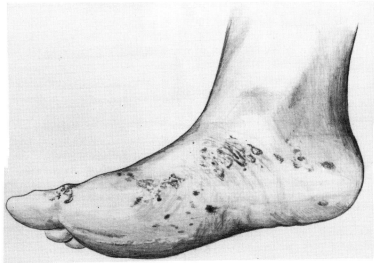

FIGURE 6.   Deep seated vesicles of dyshidrosis.

or both, constitute common locations, lying along sides of the digits and on the palms or soles. Bullae are occasionally produced, and when they do occur secondary infection is common, especially in the active athlete. Differential diagnosis includes fungal dermatophytosis, a variety of contact dermatitides and atopic dermatitis. These athletes, uncomfortable during significant flare-ups, usually display ongoing hyperhidrosis. Wet compresses in the acute stage (Domeboro), often followed by topical therapy (even steroids) plus more lubricating emollients (Eucerin) for chronic cases, are mainstays of therapy. Continuing therapy also is important as an acute flare-up can cause distressing interference with athletic competition— the hands of a golfer or gymnast, the feet of a runner, basketball or football player.

Seborrheic Dermatitis. All athletes are acquainted with the attention to grooming in the media, the ever-expanding variety of dandruff-fighting shampoos and conditioners. When itching is added to dandruff one can assume an inflammatory process is present, or seborrheic dermatitis. In some cases the scaliness becomes heavy and the process even exudative. Additional areas of involvement, besides the scalp, may include the central forehead, ear canals, central face, mid-chest, axillae, umbilicus, groin, and intergluteal cleft. Treatment of seborrheic der-

matitis, regardless of location, requires frequent scalp shampooing. This therapy alone will often make the dermatitis located elsewhere easier to control. Topical steroid solutions are also used as an adjuvant to scalp care. If other areas of the body require therapy, mild hydrocortisone creams or Cetacort lotion is usually helpful. Flare-ups may be seen during a particularly tense athletic season, and the physician must be ready to intercede.

CONCLUSION

The sports physician can effectively diagnose and treat most skin disorders seen in the athlete. Many are preventable and most respond to therapy without significant side effects. Encouraging the athlete's compliance to the treatment regimen of course augments the chance of successful outcome, and one can relate compliance to the athlete's dedication to success. Noncompliance is less likely to be a factor if the physician and athlete have a sound doctor-patient relationship, and the physician dedicated to sports is more likely to cultivate this type of contact. Another member of the sports medicine team, the certified athletic trainer, is most helpful in prevention, early diagnosis and supervision of therapy.

ACKNOWLEDGMENT: The authors wish to thank certified athletic trainers Margaret Schmidt Amundson and Mark Loren Amundson for sharing their clinical experiences during the preparation of this chapter.

1. Amundson LH, Caplan RM: The skin and subcutaneous tissues, in Taylor RB (ed): Family Medicine: Principles and Practice, 2nd ed. New York, Springer Verlag, 1983, pp 1069-1144.
2. American Academy of Pediatrics Committee on Sports Medicine: The athlete and the skin, in Smith NJ (ed): Sports Medicine: Health Care for Young Athletes. Evanston, Il, American Academy of Pediatrics, 1983, pp 130-141.
3. Basler RSW: Skin lesions related to sports activity. Primary Care 10:479-494, 1983.
4. Fitzpatrick TB, Eise AZ, Wollf K, et al: Dermatology in General Medicine, 2nd ed. New York, McGraw Hill, 1979.
5. Louis DS, Honkin FM, Eckenrode JF: Cutaneous atrophy after corticosteroid injection. Am Fam Physician 33:183-186, 1986.
6. Bergfeld WF: The diagnosis and treatment of dermatologic problems in athletes, in Schneider RC, (ed): Sports Injuries: Mechanisms, Prevention, and Treatment. Baltimore, Williams and Wilkins, 1985, pp 636-651.
7. Liteplo MG: Sports-related skin problems, in Vinger PF, Hoerner EF, (eds): Sports Injuries: The Unthwarted Epidemic. John Wright, Boston, 1982, pp 188-202.
8. Bergfeld WF, Taylor JS: Trauma, sports and the skin. Am J Ind Med 8:403-413, 1985.
9. McMaster WC: Cryotherapy. Phys Sportsmed 10:112-119, 1982.
10. Mertz PM, Marshall DA, Eaglstein WH: Occlusive dressings to prevent bacterial invasion and wound infection. J Am Acad Derm 12:662-668, 1985.
11. Webster SB: How I manage jock itch. Phys sportsmed 12:109-113, 1984.
12. Bodine KG: Black heel. J Am Podiatry Assoc 70:201, 1980.
13. Birrer RB: Common skin problems of athletes, in Birrer RB (ed): Sports Medicine for the Primary Care Physician. Norwalk, CT, Appleton-Century-Crofts, 1984, pp. 239-248.
14. Houston SD, Knox JM: Skin problems related to sports and recreational activities. Cutis 19:487-491, 1977.
15. Stauffer LW: Skin disorders in athletes: Identification and management. Phys Sportsmed 11:101-121, 1983.
16. Eisenstadt WS, Nicholas SS, Velick G, Enright T: Allergic reactions to exercise. Phys Sportsmed 12:95-104, 1984.
17. Bergfield WF: Dermatologic problems in athletes. Primary Care 10:151-160, 1984.
18. Bartlett PC, Martin RJ, Cahill BR: Furunculosis in a high school football team. Am J Sports Med 10:371-374, 1982.
19. Randt GA: Hot tub folliculitis. Phys Sportsmed 11:74-80, 1983.
20. Levine N: Dermatologic aspects of sports medicine. J Am Acad Derm 3:415-424, 1980.
21. Drez Jr D: Forefoot problems in runners, in Mock RP (ed): Symposium on the Foot and Leg in Running Sports, Am Acad Ortho Surg. St. Louis, The C.V. Mosby Co., 1982, pp 73-75.
22. Schamberg IL: Dermatoses of the groin. J Fam Pract 8:825-833, 1979.
23. Hudson A: How I manage acne in athletes. Phys Sportsmed 11:117-120, 1983.

RECOMMENDED DERMATOLOGY TEXTS

Behrman H, Labow T, Rozen J: Common Skin Diseases, 3rd ed. New York, Grune & Stratton, 1978.

Burnett J, Robinson H: Clinical Dermatology for Students and Practitioners. New York, Yorke Medical Books, 1978.

Callen J, Stawiski M, Voorhees J: Manual of Dermatology. Chicago, Year Book, 1980.

Fitzpatrick T, Eisen A, et al: Dermatology in General Medicine, 3rd ed. New York, McGraw-Hill, 1987.

Mark R, Samman P: Dermatology. New York, Appleton-Century-Crofts, 1977.

Moschella S, Pillsbury D, Hurley H: Dermatology. Philadelphia, W.B. Saunders, 1985.

Pillsbury D, Heaton C: A Manual of Dermatology, 2nd ed. Philadelphia, W.B. Saunders, 1979.

Sauer G: Manual of Skin Diseases, 4th ed. Philadelphia, J.B. Lippincott, 1980.

Stewart W, Danto J, Maddin S: Dermatology: Diagnosis and Treatment of Cutaneous Disorders. St. Louis, C.V. Mosby, 1978.

14 Principles of Musculoskeletal Rehabilitation

GUY L. SHELTON, R.P.T., A.T.C.

Adequate rehabilitation of the musculoskeletal system is essential for the early, safe return of the athlete to participation. Since every athlete is different in goals, level of skill, level of participation, and degree of competitiveness, the specific rehabilitation program must be customized for that athlete. The "cookbook" approach, where each athlete with a specific problem is handed the same sheet of exercises for that given problem, is not suitable. Most athletes will follow an exercise program better if they feel knowledgeable about the program and confident that it is designed for them.

The primary care physician's role is to arrive at an accurate diagnosis, initiate a definitive treatment program, and follow up appropriately to insure that healing, treatment and rehabilitation goals are being met. Orthopaedic or other referral is warranted when a specific diagnosis cannot be made, when the definitive treatment might include surgery or specialized immobilization, or when a seemingly minor problem fails to respond to appropriate measures. Physical therapy should be considered a basic component of the treatment program.

The physical therapist or athletic trainer performs a musculoskeletal evaluation to establish a baseline from which progress is measured, and a customized treatment and rehabilitation program is initiated. The therapist teaches the athlete the components of the program, its rationale, proper exercise techniques, and guidelines for progressing or limiting activities. Appropriate motivation of the athlete should be provided along with the exercise instruction. If an athlete has problems with the rehabilitation program, then the therapist can re-evaluate and modify the athlete's program. In short, the therapist serves as the athlete's teacher and coach for the rehabilitation program.

GOALS OF THE REHABILITATION PROGRAM

The overall goal of the treatment and rehabilitation program is to return the athlete to his or her desired level of participation as soon as safely possible. Consideration must be given to the amount of healing time required for the specific injury, length of time away from participation, the athlete's compliance with the treatment and rehabilitation program, and the athlete's motivation to return to play. With many injuries, the athlete may face deadlines to get well and resume participation. These deadlines often conflict with the time required for adequate healing and rehabilitation. While these participation considerations must occasionally be addressed, they should be carefully thought through so as not to jeopardize the long-term ability of the athlete to participate.

In order to decrease recovery time and promote healing, swelling and tissue congestion in the injured area must be controlled and reduced. Furthermore, nutrient supply for rebuilding injured tissue must be facilitated. Morbidity is decreased by minimizing deconditioning through early initiation of the reconditioning program. It is also important to prevent further injury by allowing adequate healing and providing appropriate protection during recovery.

STEPS IN TREATMENT AND REHABILITATION

Prevention. The initial step in treatment of athletic injuries is prevention. The old adage that "an ounce of prevention is worth a pound of cure" is certainly true when dealing with injuries. There are four aspects of prevention: the physical condition of the athlete, proper equipment, a safe playing environment, and the preparticipation physical examination. Even the recreational athlete must be aware of his or her level of fitness and skill. Enhanced flexibility and strength as well as athletes' recognition of their own skill level and physical limitations help to prevent injuries. Appropriate use of both standard and special protective equipment, clothing, and footwear decreases the risk of injury. The playing surface, surrounding environment, and the atmospheric conditions are factors in certain injuries. A preparticipation screening examination, particularly in interscholastic athletes, those with previous injuries, and those over 35 years old or with cardiac risk factors present, may help identify certain pre-existing conditions that either need further work-up or definitive treatment. This approach may prevent the underlying conditions from causing a new injury or a re-injury in a previously injured area.

Triage and Initial Management. Once an injury occurs the triage process must begin. An evaluation on the field must be done to rule out any life-threatening problem. This must be done within the examiner's skill level. An "on the field diagnosis" or working assessment must be made until a more specific diagnosis can be determined. The initial management of the injury must also be determined. This might include basic first aid measures and simple treatment, stabilization of the more seriously injured patient, rapid transportation to an emergency facility for definitive care, or a combination of the three. Initial management could also mean referral to an orthopedic surgeon or other specialist for further evaluation. It is important to stress that any decision made at this point be a conservative one.

Basic Athletic First Aid. Early implementation of basic athletic first aid helps minimize pain and swelling, protects the athlete from further injury, and facilitates an early start with the rehabilitation activities. The steps in basic athletic first aid are best remembered by the acronym PRICES: *P*rotection, *R*est, *I*ce, *C*ompression, *E*levation, and *S*upport.

Protection means protecting the injured area from further injury. In cases of lower extremity injuries, crutches (Fig. 1) should be used if ambulation causes *any* pain, swelling,

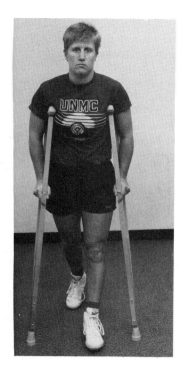

FIGURE 1. Partial weightbearing with axillary crutches protects an injured lower extremity.

limping, or buckling of the extremity. This should be continued until these symptoms are not present and more serious injury is ruled out. Sometimes the use of an immobilizer or splint is warranted, especially if the athlete is in significant pain or if a fracture is suspected. In upper extremity injuries, a sling may be used to provide protection for the injured part. Protective positioning instructions to the athlete help the athlete avoid inadvertent positions that could cause additional stress to the injury. In any situation when the severity of the injury is in question, the use of a stretcher to transport the athlete provides maximum protection and decreases the likelihood of further injury.

Rest from use of the injured part also helps prevent further injury. The need for rest in more severe injuries is apparent, but absolute rest in minor injuries is usually too strict. If one can be sure that an injury is not serious in nature, then relative rest may be employed. Relative rest means providing enough protection to keep the athlete asymptomatic. Some lower extremity injuries, for example, may not require crutches but may require abstaining from running or cutting even if the athlete can walk without symptoms.

Ice causes vasoconstriction and thus limits the blood flow to the injured area.[31,42] It further decreases tissue metabolism and thus reduces tissue damage.[31,42] Ice also decreases firing of pain nerve receptors,[31,42] which helps reduce muscle spasm. Many methods of cooling tissue have been used. Chipped ice packs and reusable frozen gel packs have been shown to provide better deep cooling than chemical cold packs and circulating freon gas.[43] Immersion of the injured part in iced water is also effective. Ice massage with a block of ice directly on the skin is useful over a small area. Treatment duration varies with the intensity of the cold and the patient's tolerance. A maximum of 30 minutes of cold followed by at least 30 minutes without cold packs is a general rule to use. Shorter treatment durations must be used if patient tolerance dictates.

Compression is used in conjunction with ice to provide a physical limitation to the space that swelling may occupy. This also helps the edema dissipate so that it can be more readily reabsorbed by the circulatory system. Generally, elastic or double-knit compression bandages are wrapped distally to proximally, overlapping about one half the width of the bandage. Pneumatic and hydraulic compression devices are also helpful but are somewhat costly.

Elevation is a simple matter of using gravity to assist fluid to run downhill. By elevating the injured part above the level of the heart, venous return is enhanced and extravascular fluid is drained away from the injured area. This is especially effective when combined with ice and compression.

Support is a form of protection but implies a more functional type of protection. This would be appropriate for minor injuries without any significant symptoms, when the athlete is going to return to play right away. An example of this would be supportive taping of the ankle for a minor ankle sprain.

Definitive Diagnosis and Treatment. Since a problem must be adequately defined before it can be properly solved, one must reach a specific, definitive diagnosis. Often this is the point where the primary care physician first encounters an athlete. A detailed history and physical examination will provide sufficient information to make the diagnosis in many cases. Sometimes x-rays or other tests will be necessary. Referral to orthopedic, sports medicine, or another consultant is appropriate whenever the diagnosis or treatment approach is not clear.

The treatment program generally takes one of three forms. Treatment with immobilization should be used with some fractures and certain types of severe sprains. However, immobilization can have detrimental effects on muscle function, fitness and articular cartilage nutrition. While immobilization may be the only proper way to treat certain injuries, a functional or rehabilitative treatment program must also be included following immobilization to help the athlete return to participation as soon as safely possible.

Second, surgical treatment should be undertaken in unstable fractures, certain severe sprains and strains, and as final definitive treatment for some problems for which more conservative treatment has failed. As with immobilization treatment, functional or rehabilitative treatment should always be included in the follow up care postoperatively. In many surgical cases, some form of gentle rehabilitative exercises and other treatments may be initiated immediately after surgery.

Third, functional treatment involves progressive exercise and activity. It should be initiated as soon as possible following injury, immobilization or surgery. This minimizes the deconditioning, the detrimental effects of immobilization, and the recovery time. The remainder of this chapter will be devoted to various aspects of the functional or rehabilitative treatment program.

Treatment with Physical Modalities

Cold, heat, water, sound, electricity and air have long been utilized in treating musculoskeletal injuries. However, treatment with these various physical agents does not constitute the primary, long-term treatment in any situation. They may be used to control acute symptoms or those occurring during rehabilitation. This may allow certain therapeutic exercises to be initiated sooner and progressed more rapidly. Diathermy, electrical stimulation, infrared light and ultrasound should only be applied by individuals licensed or certified to do so, due to the possible dangers inherent with these modalities.

The use of cold in the acute management of injuries has already been discussed. Ice can also be used to control flare-ups of inflammation during the rehabilitation period. Ice massage can provide local analgesia to painful areas prior to exercise or deep friction massage.

Therapeutic heat is used to facilitate circulation in an injured area. Warmer tissues are also easier to stretch.[47] Heat can be applied through moist heat packs, hot water bottles, electric heating pads, warm compresses, short wave and microwave diathermies, infrared light, ultrasound, and whirlpool baths.

A good compromise sometimes used is contrast treatment. The injured part is warmed for 1–4 minutes and then cooled for 1–2 minutes. The ratio of heat time to cool time is adjusted based on the likelihood of creating swelling. Shorter heat times and longer cool times are used in more acute situations.

Swelling should always be monitored when using any form of heat. Any increase in swelling or other signs of inflammation as a result of any heating modality indicates a need to stop the heating and apply cold immediately.

Electrical stimulation has several potentially useful benefits. It can be used to facilitate muscle contraction as the initial part of a strengthening or re-education program.[3] Transcutaneous electrical nerve stimulation (TENS) may be used to assist with pain control in acute injuries.[34] Iontophoresis, the use of a continuous direct current to infiltrate therapeutic medications into tissues, can be helpful in treating local areas of inflammation and scar tissue.[9,23]

Ultrasound has several useful therapeutic effects.[23] It can be used to create heating deep in tissues. Phonophoresis uses the mechanical effects of ultrasound to drive medications, mixed in creams and applied topically, into tissues. This is most commonly used with hydrocortisone for anti-inflammatory

effect. The mechanical effects of ultrasound help decrease tightness in collagen tissue.

EMG biofeedback displays a measure of the muscle contraction being performed and allows the athlete to monitor muscle activity during contraction. Additional feedback to the athlete helps maximize muscle contraction during rehabilitation. This is especially useful in conjunction with electrical stimulation to facilitate and re-educate muscles following immobilization or surgery.

Again, these physical agents are used only as an adjunct to therapeutic exercise in the rehabilitation program. With the exception of basic heat and cold, the application of the above modalities should only be done by professionals trained in such application.

Therapeutic Exercise

The most important physical modality used in the rehabilitation of the athlete is therapeutic exercise. No matter what the athlete's level—recreational, fitness, or competitive—anyone trying to resume an active, vigorous activity must, at some point, undergo some active, vigorous retraining. Several points must be considered in designing and implementing a program of therapeutic exercise.

First, and probably most important, the program must be accomplished without persistent symptoms.[27] Increased pain, swelling, limping, instability, or alteration of mechanics signal that the injured part is not able to handle the stresses being applied to it. Using symptoms and functional milestones rather than a timetable as a barometer for progress allows the athlete to be advanced when ready and held back when not ready for more stressful activities. Table 1 illustrates a functional "timetable" for ankle-sprain rehabilitation.

Second, no "cookbook" program is going to work well for each athlete.[53] While general treatment goals may be similar for a given injury type, the specific program is based on the goals of the individual athlete. The healing constraints, level of irritation, progress to date, and the athlete's tolerance of the exercise program determine the currently appropriate exercise program and readiness of the athlete to progress. Knowledge of existing ex-

TABLE 1.   SAMPLE REHABILITATION PROGRAM FOR ANKLE SPRAINS BASED ON SYMPTOMS AND FUNCTIONAL MILESTONES

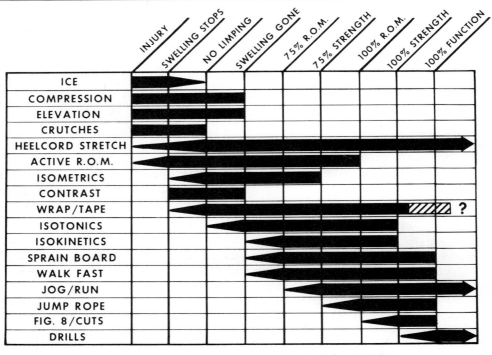

ANKLE SPRAIN REHABILITATION

Adapted from Garrick JG: A practical approach to rehabilitation. AM J Sports Med 9:67, 1981.

ercise techniques, creativity in modifying old exercises and developing new exercise techniques, and knowledge of injury pathology, biomechanics, and kinesiology help the practitioner create a customized exercise program for the athlete.

Third, the exercise program must be realistic but adequate. Other than the seriously competitive athlete very few will devote several hours a day to the rehabilitation program. However, all phases of rehabilitation must be addressed or the program will be incomplete and less effective.

Fourth, all components of the exercise program must be goal-oriented. Each activity should have a specific reason for inclusion in the program. Extraneous exercises add to the time required to complete the daily program and thus increase the rate of noncompliance.

Fifth, time must be spent maintaining and improving conditioning in the uninjured areas and the fitness of the athlete. A prolonged period of relative inactivity during healing and rehabilitation can cause a significant decline in the athlete's physical condition. Neglecting these components will only increase the time needed to get back to performance levels once healing and injury rehabilitation are complete.

Finally, the athlete must be educated about the various rehabilitation activities. He or she must not only understand the exercise techniques and protocols, but the rationale for doing the program a certain way. The athlete must be an active participant in the rehabilitation process. If the athlete knows how to monitor progress and problems, then he or she can make some modifications in the program without total dependence on the supervising medical or allied health professional.[40]

Strengthening   Exercises.   Strengthening

exercises include isometric, isotonic, and isokinetic techniques. Isometric exercises are muscle contractions against resistance so that there is no effective joint movement. Resistance can be readily adjusted by altering the effort of the muscle being contracted. Therefore these exercises are suitable for strengthening in acute and subacute stages of recovery, since additional stress to the injured tissues can be adjusted by the athlete according to comfort. Gentle, repetitive isometric contractions around the joint also facilitate the hemodynamic circulation around the injury and thus decreases swelling. Isometric strengthening extends about 20° around the specific joint position.[29] A technique known as "multiple angle isometrics," where isometric exercises are done at about every 20° through the available range of motion, can be used to work on isometric strength through the range while minimizing irritation.[15]

Isotonic exercises[22] are muscle contractions performed against a constant resistance. Resistance is applied via ankle weights, weight machines, free weights, elastic bands, or the athlete's body weight. The speed of the contraction can be varied by the athlete. Variable resistance isotonic exercise is a hybrid of isotonic exercise using exercise machines such as Eagle (Cybex, Ronkonkoma, NY), Nautilus (Nautilus, DeLand, FL), and Universal (Universal Gym Equipment, Cedar Rapids, IA) equipment. The speed of contraction is still varied by the patient, the machine resistance is fixed, but the load experienced by the limb is varied by the use of cams or variable length lever arms. In all modes of isotonic exercise, there is a concentric, or shortening contraction, phase and an eccentric, or lengthening contraction phase. Eccentric contractions require more muscle energy expenditure, put more stress on the muscle,[19] and are the most important contraction mode for many athletic activities. Various strategies for weight training have been used.[16,30,55]

Isokinetic exercises[22] are muscle contractions against a fixed speed of movement in which the resistance not only varies but accommodates through the range of motion according to the input ability of the musculoskeletal lever system. Examples include Cybex and Orthotron machines (Cybex, Ronkonkoma, NY), the Kin/Com machine (Chattecx, Chattanooga, TN), and the Lido system (Loredan Biomedical, Davis, CA). Isokinetics have several advantages over isotonic and isometrics. Isokinetics load the musculoskeletal lever system maximally through the range of motion. Isokinetic resistance also accommodates to pain, fatigue, and other factors that affect muscle force output and is therefore relatively safe to use in injury situations. The controlled, faster speeds of movement allow individual muscle training at more functional limb speeds. Equipment cost and availability are two drawbacks to isokinetic exercise.

In any strengthening mode, the muscle must be overloaded in order to strengthen. Overload can be accomplished by increasing the intensity or resistance, increasing the number of repetitions, increasing the frequency of the workouts, increasing the speed of movement, changing the mode of exercise, or a combination of the above.[46] However, with a healing injury, the intensity of the exercise is probably the most critical parameter to control. Too much intensity (resistance) too soon in the healing process is more likely to cause increased symptoms.[33] Therefore, a high repetition, low resistance approach is generally used initially.[33,53] Progression to a more traditional low-repetition, high-resistance program is done as symptoms allow.

Additionally, the mode and technique of the exercise may create inappropriate stresses on the healing injury. Modified standard exercise techniques must be made with certain injuries to avoid these stresses or provide appropriate stimulus.[2,18,24,26,53] Careful consideration to and understanding of the specific injury and the associated biomechanics is essential for a safe and tolerable strengthening program. Selected strengthening exercises are illustrated in Figures 2 through 26 (following text of chapter).

Flexibility Exercises. Flexibility exercises are essential to any rehabilitation program. Adequate joint range of motion allows normal kinesiological relationships to occur between limb segments during activity. Good tissue extensibility, especially after surgery, is essential for pain-free tissue excursion during movement. Appropriate musculotendinous flexibility allows more efficient muscle action at extremes, decreases joint compression forces, and decreases musculotendinous overstress.[1,51]

Joint range of motion decreases when injury causes inflammation. Pain causes inhibition of normal muscle function. Swelling increases the pressure within the joint and decreases the ability of the joint to move. Prolonged limitation of motion causes the joint capsule, muscle and tendon to adaptively shorten and further restrict motion. Gentle active range of motion exercises can be started as soon as swelling is under control.[21] Assisted or passive range of motion exercises are helpful to increase range of motion beyond active limits or where active exercises are too uncomfortable. In situations where adaptive shortening has occurred, passive joint mobilization exercises performed by the physical therapist can be helpful.[48] Some of these exercises can be taught to the athlete. In all situations, emphasis must be placed on increasing range of motion gradually without increasing symptoms. In cases of severely restricted range of motion due to adaptive shortening, more vigorous assisted and passive exercises can be done by the physical therapist with appropriate modalities to control symptoms.

Inadequate musculotendinous flexibility is a contributing or causative factor in many types of injuries[1,12,19,38,51,53] Inflexibility increases the force against which antagonistic muscles must contract, thus increasing fatigue and decreasing efficiency of these muscles.[49] Forces in joints, tendons, and other associated structures are also increased by inflexibility, increasing risk of overstress and injury.

Following injury, musculotendinous flexibility decreases due to spasm of muscles around the injury in an effort to protect and guard the injured area. When inflammation or immobilization limits joint range of motion, normal extensibility of the musculotendinous unit cannot be maintained. Gentle stretching exercises are begun as soon as comfortable following an injury. Emphasis is placed on smooth, static stretching technique.[1,4,47] Ballistic or bouncing stretches stimulate the stretch reflex,[19] and the resulting muscle contraction prevents the muscle

from elongating. Ballistic stretching may also create undue force on the injured area and increase inflammation. As range of motion increases and inflammation decreases, additional stretching techniques are included for associated and uninjured areas.

The athlete must be taught to stretch properly. Adequate time must be allowed so that the repetitions can be held long enough for the muscles to adapt to a more flexible, elongated position. The tension must be felt in the intended area but pain should not be experienced. Repetitions must be performed frequently enough to allow lengthening adaptations to summate over time and thus improve flexibility. The specific exercise prescription must be tailored to the individual athlete's own initial level of tightness, specific injury, and tolerance. Anderson[1] illustrates many stretching techniques from which techniques for the exercise prescription can be created. This book is an excellent reference for physicians, therapists, and the athlete. Figures 27 through 45, at the end of this chapter, illustrate selected flexibility exercises.

Endurance. Endurance activities should be included in the rehabilitation program as soon as possible following injury.[27] The relative inactivity that occurs during healing and recovery time creates significant detraining effects that can decrease performance.[19] Any activity designed to maintain or increase cardiovascular endurance following injury must also avoid any undue stress that might cause re-injury. Bike riding (Fig. 46, see end of chapter), single-leg stationary bike riding, upper extremity ergometer training (Fig. 47, see end of chapter), swimming, non-weight-bearing running in a pool, or cross country skiing may all provide adequate cardiovascular stimulus while altering stresses on a lower extremity injury. Running or riding a stationary bike can provide a similar effect for upper extremity injuries. Again, no symptoms should be created.

Individual muscle endurance also deteriorates following injury. Certain muscle enzymes decrease with detraining.[19] This inhibits the muscle's ability to utilize oxygen and sustain force of contraction. Rehabilitation programs that include a larger number of repetitions at appropriate intensity levels help maintain and regain muscular endurance.

Coordination and Agility. Coordination and agility training is necessary for the athlete to transform the strength, flexibility and endurance gained into full-speed performance skills. Magill[32] states that practice is essential for one to learn skills. Practice variability helps the athlete learn a variety of motor patterns necessary to match the variety of responses a given performance may require.[32] A similar process of skill acquisition is required during rehabilitation as the athlete relearns the skill following injury and detraining.

Additionally, tissues that have not been subjected to performance-level stresses for a period of time will be unable to adapt to a sudden resumption of such stresses without risking further injury. Magill[32] states that tasks high in complexity should be practiced in parts rather than as a whole. A gradual progression through increasingly more complex functional activities is advocated by most authors.[6,7,10,11,17,22,25,28,33,37,39,45,54] Emphasis is placed on proper performance of the skill, no increase in symptoms, and demonstration of confidence with the skill.

Proprioception activities form the basis of coordination and agility activities.[20,36] For lower extremity injuries, bicycling,[41] weight shifting, single-leg standing, uniaxial and multiaxial (Fig. 48, see end of chapter) balance board activities,[20,27,39] and mini-trampoline drills[53] facilitate proprioceptive responses in the rehabilitating limb. For upper-extremity injuries, weight bearing through the arms in various positions (sitting push-ups, wall push-ups) and weighted-ball or weighted-implement activities are used.[50]

All progressive functional exercise sessions are begun with a thorough warm-up program. Warming up consists of getting the blood flowing and stretching all key areas for the activity being done. Exercise sessions are always concluded with a cool-down session, consisting of stretching as above and applying ice to the recovering area to minimize symptoms. The athlete begins with the most basic step in the program, works until he achieves the performance criteria, and progresses to the next step *only* in the absence of symptoms. Tables 2 and 3 provide suggested steps of progression for lower and upper extremity injuries respectively.

Protective Equipment

Protective equipment has long been used to prevent injury. Protective equipment is also essential to help prevent re-injury. Standard protective equipment for a given sport must be adjusted for proper fit. For many recreational sports, the main item of protective equipment is appropriate footwear.

Modified protective equipment may be needed for certain injuries. Additional padding secured inside standard football shoulder pads may provide additional protection for a contusion or acromioclavicular sprain. An oversize football thigh pad may be taped to the thigh to protect a thigh contusion from re-injury in any contact sport.

Special protective equipment includes special padding, taping and bracing (see Chapter 21). Virtually any area of the body may be protected from direct contact with either prefabricated or custom made padding. Taping and bracing are sometimes helpful in limiting the extreme motion in an unstable joint. *However, taping and bracing should complement the rehabilitation program not substitute for it.*[33,52] There should be a specific need for the supporting device. The specific taping procedure or brace applied should provide the desired support and not be just a placebo.[33] However, even the simplest wrap or sleeve may provide cutaneous proprioceptive feedback and thus facilitate dynamic stability of the joint.[27]

EVALUATION FOR RETURN TO PARTICIPATION

At some point during the rehabilitation process a decision must be made as to whether the athlete may return to participation. In the circumstance of a team athlete, various individuals have specific roles in this decision-making process. The physician who provided definitive treatment must make the judgment that adequate healing has taken place. There should be no swelling, pain, or limping.

The team physician, athletic trainer, coach

TABLE 2. PROGRESSIVE RUNNING PROGRAM

STEP	*Progression Criteria*
Bicycle	30–45 minutes.
Walk	2 miles in 30 minutes or less.
Jog	Jog 50 yards, walk 50 yards up to 1/4 mile, increase total distance to 1 mile, then increase jogging and decrease walking until jogging 1 mile straight through.
Run	Increase jogging to 2–4 miles, then increase pace to pre-injury level.
Sprint	Take 10–15 yards to build up to 1/2 speed, sprint at 1/2 speed for 40 yards, take 15-20 yards to slow down and stop. Gradually work from 1/2 to 2/3 to 3/4 to full speed. Do 10–20 sprints per session.
Figure 8	Gently jog a large (20–30 yard) figure 8. Gradually run the 8 faster. Then decrease the size of the 8 by 2–3 yards at a time so that the cutting is progressively sharper. Work down to a 4–5 yard 8. Do 10–20 figure eights at a session.
Basic drills	Work into jumping rope, power jumping activities, stairs, backward running, side step running, side crossover running, quick starts and stops, cutting and other basic drill activities important to the athlete's specific sport.
Sports drills	Target these fine tuning drills to the specific activity the athlete wants to resume.

TABLE 3. PROGRESSIVE PITCHING PROGRAM

STEP	*Progression Criteria*
Short toss	Toss ball 10–15 feet for accuracy using good throwing mechanics.
Long toss	Stand in short center field. Throw ball so that it rolls to second base. Then throw so that ball reaches second base in four bounces, then three bounces, then two and finally one. Use good mechanics and throw for accuracy.
Mound toss	From the mound throw at 1/2 speed toward the plate. Emphasize accuracy and mechanics.
Straight throws	Throw straight pitches progressively faster up to 3/4 speed.
Breaking throws	Throw curve and slider pitches progressively faster up to 3/4 speed.
Speed	Increase speed on all pitches toward full speed while maintaining good mechanics and accuracy.
Special pitches	Add any specialty pitches to program.
Fielding	Work on fielding ground balls and throwing to various bases from gradually more awkward positions.

or a combination of the three must be sure that the athlete is functionally ready to return. Full rehabilitation is the main criterion. Strength is documented through manual[14,35] or isokinetic[15] muscle testing. Flexibility testing and goniometry reveal recovery of mobility. Return of endurance, coordination and agility is documented by comparing functional and agility tests to pre-injury levels. The athlete must then demonstrate full-speed performance[17,39] of his specific sports skills under the watchful eye of these individuals.

The coach's responsibility is to support the athlete as he works through the rehabilitation process. At no time should the coach try to have the athlete force himself to do an activity beyond what the injury permits.

Finally, the athlete himself must take an active role in the decision to return to play. The athlete is best aware of how the injured area feels. He must be encouraged to be honest in judging whether the injury is ready. There must not be any lack of confidence on the athlete's part in the performance of his skills nor any increase in symptoms after the performance.

This team of individuals may not be available to provide guidance to the recreational athlete in deciding when to return to participation. The primary physician and the physical therapist must educate the athlete in the parameters to monitor and guidelines to follow. The recreational athlete should heed this advice and strive to be both aware of any symptoms that occur and honest with himself in dealing with these symptoms.

If there is ever a doubt as to whether the athlete is ready for participation, then clearance to resume must be withheld until all doubt is cleared.

GENERAL REHABILITATION PRINCIPLES FOR SPECIFIC INJURY TYPES

Fractures. Early rehabilitation of fractures should always be designed with respect to the type of fracture and method of immobilization or protection. Muscles near the fracture may be exercised only if the risk of disrupting healing is minimal. Fitness of the uninjured limbs and the cardiovascular system should be maintained as much as safely possible. Once healing has occurred and immobilization and protection discontinued, then specific rehabilitation of the injured limb may be initiated, with emphasis on regaining full range of motion and strength lost during healing.

Sprains. Ligament injuries present a challenge to those involved with their rehabilitation. If surgery or immobilization is required, early rehabilitation guidelines used for fractures should be followed. The range of motion and strengthening program should be designed to avoid undue stress on the healing static stabilizers and to not create symptoms. Strengthening should be maximized in muscles responsible for providing dynamic stability. Coordination and agility activities should focus on helping the entire limb regain synergistic function, with the dynamic stabilizers being retrained to help support the joint. Taping or bracing may at times provide additional support but thorough rehabilitation provides the quickest and safest return to activity.

Strains and Contusions. Muscle injuries also require thorough rehabilitation for return to play with the least risk of re-injury. Stretching exercises should be started gently as soon as possible following injury. Full flexibility must be eventually regained so that the muscle is able to adapt to the extremes of activity. Injuries to the muscle cause some loss of strength. Decreased function during healing also decreases strength. Therefore rehabilitation of the muscle to full strength is essential for full return to activity. With deep contusions, the risk of developing myositis ossificans is always present. Strict adherence to the PRICES principle, cautious use of passive stretching, and conservative progression are the keys to preventing this disabling complication of deep muscle contusions.

Overuse Injuries. Repetitive tissue stress can lead to chronic inflammation and inability to participate in sports. Treatment and rehabilitation seems most effective when multifaceted. Relative rest is essential to control the inflammation. Alternate activities provide partial participation to help maintain fitness while decreasing irritating stress. Deep friction massage mechanically increases circulation locally and breaks up scar tissue.[13] Ice helps decrease inflammation. It also provides some analgesia prior to deep friction massage. Anti-inflammatory medication may also be helpful. Injections are rarely used and never into major load-bearing tendons.

Inflexibility can contribute to musculoskeletal overstress. Therefore a well-rounded stretching program is an essential part of rehabilitation. Appropriate strengthening helps recondition the total limb and sometimes helps correct contributing mechanical faults. Eccentric loading has been reported to be useful in treating tendinitis.[12]

Errors in training and mechanical faults with performance can contribute to additional stress.[27] These can be magnified with the high repetition of competitive endurance activities and thus must be identified and corrected. Often a coach or other individual knowledgeable in a particular sports skill is employed to help identify and correct these faults.

SUMMARY

Musculoskeletal injuries are serious in that they can keep the competitive, recreational or fitness athlete from normal participation. This can have detrimental effects on the athlete's physical and emotional well-being. Therefore timely and complete rehabilitation is necessary to minimize these detrimental effects.

The PRICES principle is used as first aid in all musculoskeletal injuries. Once a definitive diagnosis is made, a specific course of treatment is initiated. In all forms of treatment, rehabilitative exercises should be started as soon as feasible. As the athlete progresses, presence or absence of symptoms determines the athlete's rate of progress and readiness to return to participation.

ACKNOWLEDGEMENTS. The author would like to thank Laura Peter for serving as model for the photographs in this chapter.

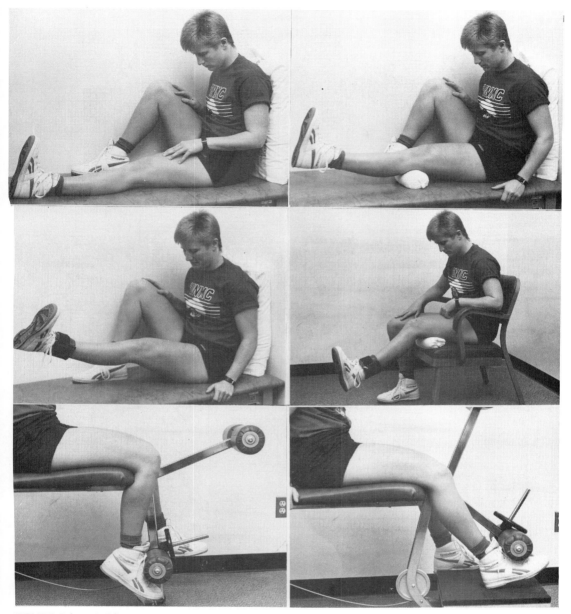

FIGURE 2 (top left).   Isometric quadriceps setting. Used in the early stage after injury to decrease swelling.

FIGURE 3 (top right).   Terminal knee extension. Used in regaining full active extension and in early quadriceps strengthening. May be done as the initial phase of leg raise.

FIGURE 4 (center left).   Straight leg raise with external rotation. Used for quadriceps strengthening. External rotation component used in athletes with patellofemoral problems biases strength toward vastus medialis obliquus (VMO).[53]

FIGURE 5 (center right).   Knee extension with ankle weights. Relatively low intensity exercise but still can cause irritation with patellofemoral problems or acute injuries. Used mostly during intermediate rehabilitation.

FIGURE 6 (bottom left).   Knee extensions on a weight machine. Used in advanced rehabilitation. Not a physiologic method of quadriceps strengthening.

FIGURE 7 (bottom right).   Knee extensions, −45° starting position. Used for quadriceps strengthening. Less pressure on patellofemoral joint than full knee extension techniques in Figures 5 and 6.

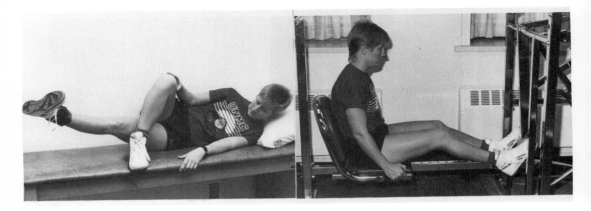

FIGURE 8 (left).   Hip adduction sidelying. With quadriceps set at onset, this can provide additional stimulus to the VMO to improve patellofemoral stability.

FIGURE 9 (right).   Leg press. Closed kinetic chain strengthening for quadriceps and hip extensors. More physiologic method than knee extensions.

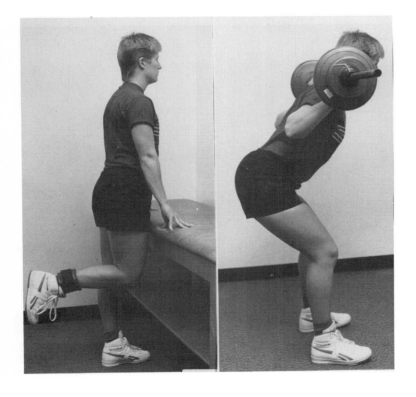

FIGURE 10 (left). Knee curls standing for hamstring strengthening. May also be done prone on knee curl machine.

FIGURE 11 (right). Mini-squat. Partial depth is preferred over the traditional parallel squat. Keeping shins vertical lessens shear forces at knee. Used in intermediate and advanced phases.[44]

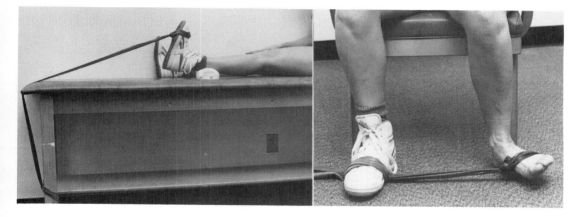

FIGURE 12 (left).   Ankle dorsiflexion. Used for ankle rehabilitation. Also helpful for patellar tendinitis when eccentric phase is emphasized.[5]

FIGURE 13 (right).   Ankle eversion. Used to strengthen dynamic stabilizers with inversion ankle injuries.

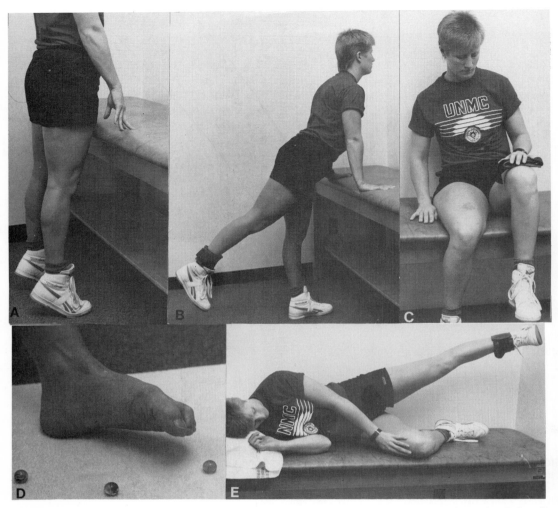

FIGURE 14. (above). *A,* Toe raises. Used to strengthen calf. Start on both legs, progress to only one leg. *B,* Standing hip extension. *C,* Sitting hip flexion. *D,* Toe curls. Marbles or small, smooth stones are grasped by the toes. Used to strengthen foot intrinsic muscles. *E,* Sidelying hip abduction.

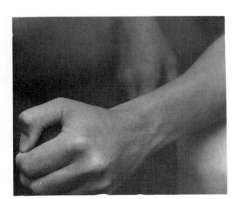

FIGURE 15 (left). Grip strengthening. Used for generalized forearm and hand strengthening. Also helps circulation in upper extremity following injury.

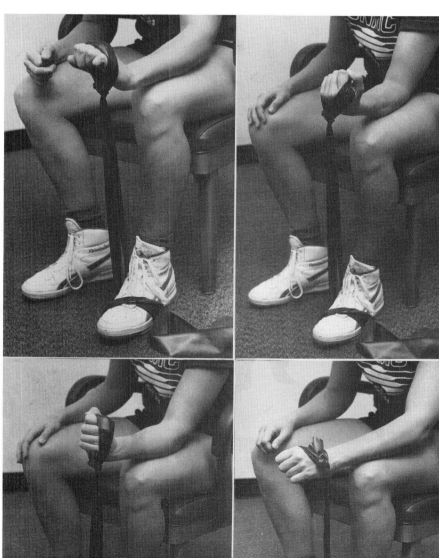

FIGURE 16. Wrist extension **(top left)** and flexion **(top right)** using elastic band.

FIGURE 17 (bottom left). Wrist radial deviation using elastic band.

FIGURE 18 (bottom right). Forearm pronation using elastic band.

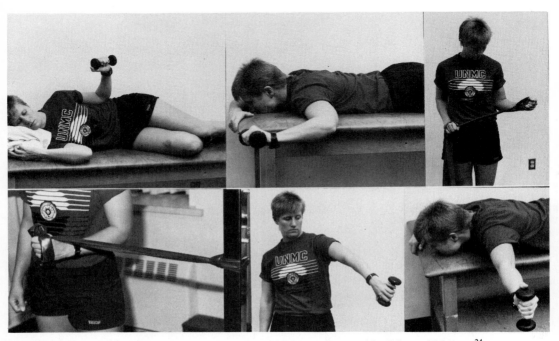

FIGURE 19 (top left).   Shoulder external rotation sidelying as suggested by Jobe and Moynes.[24]

FIGURE 20 (top center).   Shoulder external rotation prone   as suggested by Jobe and Moynes.[24]

FIGURE 21 (top right).   Standing external rotation using elastic band.

FIGURE 22 (bottom left).   Standing internal rotation using elastic band.

FIGURE 23 (bottom center).   Isolated strengthening for the supraspinatus as suggested by Jobe and Moynes.[24]

FIGURE 24 (bottom right).   Horizontal abduction prone with arm externally rotated for rotator cuff strengthening as suggested by Blackburn.[8]

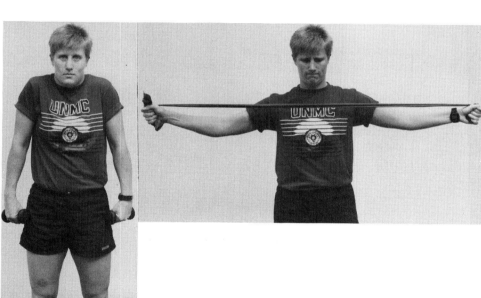

FIGURE 25 (left).   Shoulder shrug/scapular adduction for scapulothoracic stability.

FIGURE 26 (right).   Scapular adduction with elastic band for scapulothoracic stability.

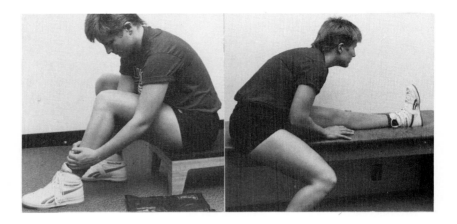

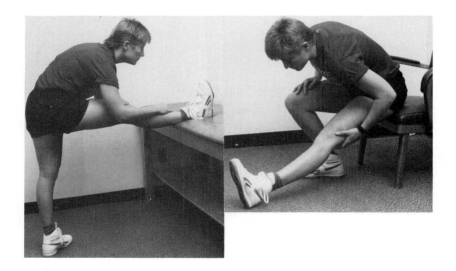

FIGURE 27 (top left). Assisted knee flexion from a low seat. Low seat keeps hip lower than knee and minimizes substitute movement of lifting hip instead of flexing knee.

FIGURE 28 (top right). Hamstring stretching—long sitting at edge of table or couch.

FIGURE 29 (bottom left). Hamstring stretching standing.

FIGURE 30 (bottom right). Hamstring stretching from chair with foot on floor.

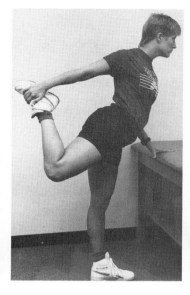

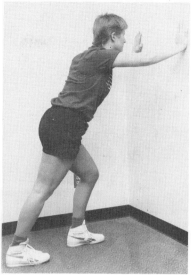

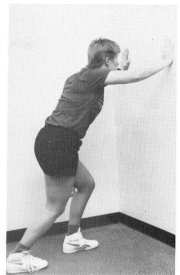

FIGURE 31. Quadriceps stretching. Care should be taken not to acutely flex the knee in athletes with patellofemoral problems.

FIGURE 32. Heelcord stretching—knee straight. Used to stretch the gastrocnemius muscle.

FIGURE 33. Heelcord stretching—knee bent. Used to stretch the soleus muscle and Achilles tendon.

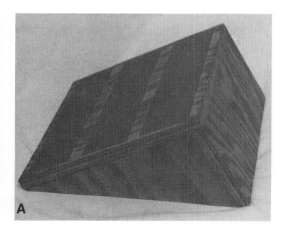

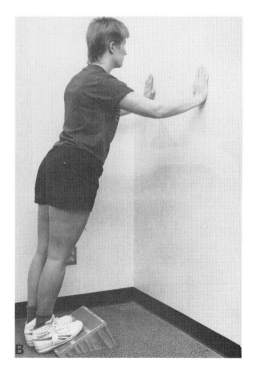

FIGURE 34. *A,* Slant board (12″x12″x6″ high) to increase stretch on calf.[38,39] *B,* Heelcord stretching using slant board.

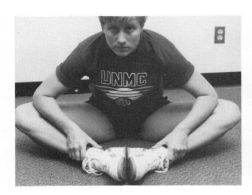

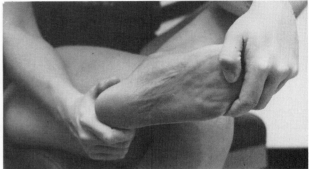

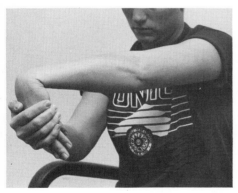

FIGURE 35 (top left).   Adductor stretch.

FIGURE 36 (top right).   Plantar fascia stretch. Done manually to increase flexibility as a treatment for plantar fasciitis.

FIGURE 37 (bottom left).   Wrist extensor stretch. Used for lateral epicondylitis.

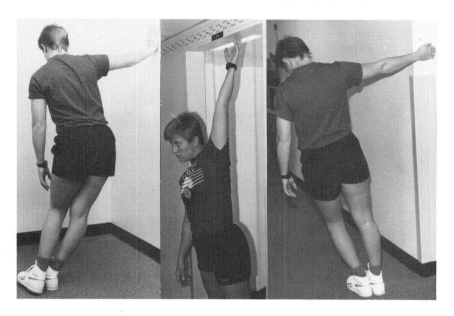

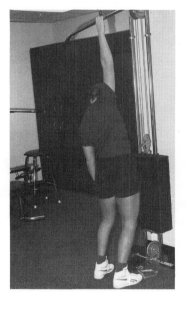

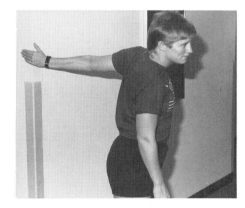

FIGURE 38 (top left). Iliotibial band stretch. Used for iliotibial band friction syndrome.

FIGURE 39 (top center). Shoulder flexion stretch using doorway to anchor hand.

FIGURE 40 (top right). Distraction stretch for glenohumeral joint. Useful as early stretching exercise in impingement syndrome and rotator cuff problems.

FIGURE 41 (bottom left). Overhead version of exercise in Figure 40. This is more advanced technique and should be achieved gradually.

FIGURE 42 (bottom right). Horizontal abduction stretch.

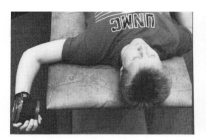
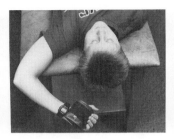
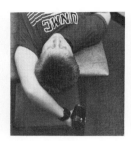

FIGURE 43 (left).   Supine external rotation stretch in 90° abduction as suggested by Jobe.[24]

FIGURE 44 (center).   Supine external rotation stretch in 135° abduction as suggested by Jobe.[24] Progression of stretch in Figure 43.

FIGURE 45 (right).   Supine external rotation stretch in 180° abduction as suggested by Jobe.[24] Progression of stretch in Figure 44. Very helpful with shoulder problems in throwing athletes.

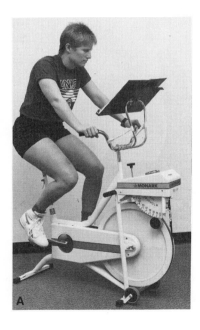

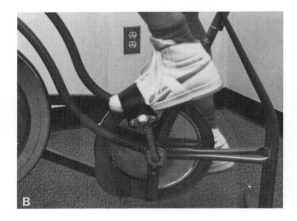

FIGURE 46. *A,* Stationary bicycle riding. Seat height, pedalling resistance, pedalling speed and pedalling phase effort can be adjusted for treatment of various injuries. *B,* Use of toe straps on stationary bicycle to stabilize foot on pedal and facilitate upward pull during the upstroke phase.

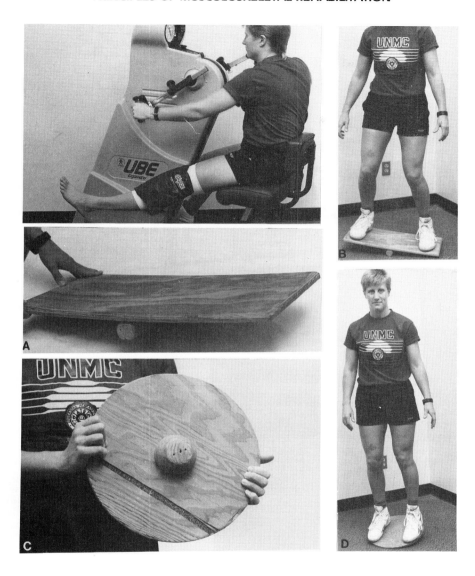

FIGURE 47 (top left).   Upper Body Exercise (UBE) Ergometer (Cybex, Ronkonkoma, NY). Used for maintenance of aerobic capacity during rehabilitation and upper extremity endurance training.

FIGURE 48.   *A,* Uniaxial balance board (12″x24″ with 2″ tall pivot on bottom). *B,* Uniaxial balance board in use. Foot position can be varied to balance side to side or front to back. *C,* Multiaxial balance board (15″ diameter with 2″ semi-sphere on bottom). *D,* Multiaxial balance board in use. As balance ability is achieved, the athlete's attention is diverted by playing catch in order to make the reactions more automatic.

REFERENCES

1. Anderson B: Stretching, Bolinas, California, Shelter Publications, 1980.
2. Antich TJ, Brewster CE: Modifications of quadriceps femoris muscle exercises during knee rehabilitation. Physical Therapy 66:1246, 1986.
3. Baker LL: Neuromuscular electrical stimulation in the restoration of purposeful limb movements. *In* Wolf SL: Electrotherapy. New York, Churchill Livingstone, 1981.
4. Beaulieu JE: Developing a stretching program. Phys Sportsmed 9:59, 1981.
5. Black JE Alten SR: How I manage infrapatellar tendinitis. Phys Sportsmed 12:86, 1984.
6. Blackburn TA: Rehabilitation of anterior cruciate ligament injuries Orthop Clin North Am 16:241, 1985.
7. Blackburn TA: The off-season program for the throwing arm. *In* Zarins B, Andrews JA, Carson WG: Injuries to the Throwing Arm. Philadelphia, W.B. Saunders, 1985.
8. Blackburn TA: Treatment of throwing injuries. Presented at the Cybex Isokinetic Seminar, Las Vegas, NV, October, 1985.
9. Boone DC: Applications of iontophoresis. *In* Wolf SL: Electrotherapy. New York, Churchill Livingstone, 1981.
10. Brewster CE, Moynes DR, Jobe FW: Rehabilitation for anterior cruciate reconstruction. Ortho Sporte Phys Ther 5:121, 1983.
11. Curl WW, Markey KL, Mitchell WA: Clinical Orthopaedics and Related Research 172:133, 1983.
12. Curwin S, Stanish WD: Tendinitis: Its Etiology and Treatment, Lexington, Massachusetts, D.C. Heath, 1984.
13. Cyriax J: Textbook of Orthopaedic Medicine, Vol. 1, 8th ed. London, Bailliere Tindall, 1982.
14. Daniels L, Worthingham C: Muscle Testing: Techniques of Manual Examination. Saunders, Philadelphia, 1972.
15. Davies, GJ: A Compendium of Isokinetics in Clinical Usage, 2nd ed. La Cross, Wisconsin, S & S Publishers, 1984.
16. DeLorme TL: Restoration of muscle power by heavy resistance exercise. J Bone Joint Surg, 27A:645, 1945.
17. Donley PB: Standards of fitness to return to activities for knee injuries. Bulletin of the Sports Medicine Section American Physical Therapy Association 4:9, 1974.
18. Einhorn AR: Shoulder rehabilitation: equipment modifications, J Orthop Sports Phys Ther 6:247, 1985.
19. Fox EL, Mathews DK: The Physiologic Basis of Physical Education and Athletics. Philadelphia, Saunders College Publishing, 1981.
20. Freeman MAR, Dean MRE, Hanham IWF: The etiology and prevention of functional instability of the foot. J Bone Joint Surg 47B:678, 1965.
21. Garrick JG: A practical approach to rehabilitation. Am J Sports Med 9:67, 1981.
22. Gould JA, Davies GJ: Orthopaedic and sports rehabilitation concepts. *In* Gould JA, Davies GJ: Orthopaedic and Sports Physical Therapy. St. Louis, C.V. Mosby, 1985.
23. Griffen JE, Karselis TC: Physical Agents for Physical Therapists. Springfield, Illinois, Charles C. Thomas, 1982.
24. Jobe FW, Moynes DR: Delineation of diagnostic criteria and a rehabilitation program for rotator cuff injuries. Am J Sports Med. 10:336, 1982.
25. Jones AL: Rehabilitation for anterior instability of the knee: Preliminary report. J Orthop Sports Phys Ther. 3:121, 1982.
26. Jurist KA, Otis JC: Anterioposterior tibiofemoral displacements during isometric extension efforts, Am J Sports Med. 13:254, 1985.
27. Kellett J: Acute soft tissue injuries—a review of the literature. Med Sci Sports Exer. 18:489, 1986.
28. Kerlan R: My bag of tricks for treatment of common throwing shoulder problems. Presented at Injuries to the Throwing meeting, Atlanta, Georgia, February 11, 1983.
29. Knapik JJ, Ramos MV, Wright JE: Non-specific effects of isometric and isokinetic strength training at a particular joint angle. Med Sci Sports Exer, 12:120, 1980.
30. Knight KL: Knee rehabilitation by the daily adjustable progressive resistive exercise technique. Am J Sports Med. 7:336, 1980.
31. Lehmann JF, DeLateur BJ: Cryotherapy. *In* Lehmann JF: Therapeutic Heat and Cold, Baltimore, Williams and Wilkins, 1982.
32. Magill RA: Motor Learning: Concepts & Applications, Dubuque, Iowa, W. C. Brown, 1980.
33. Malone T, Blackburn TA, Wallace LA: Knee rehabilitation. Phys Ther, 60:54, 1980.
34. Mannheimer JS, Lampe GN: Clinical Transcutaneous Electrical Nerve Stimulation, Philadelphia, F. A. Davis, 1984.
35. Marino M, Nicholas JA, Gleim GW, et al: The efficacy of manual assessment of muscle strength using a new device. Am J Sports Med 10:360, 1982.
36. Marino M: Current concepts on rehabilitation in sports medicine: research and clinical interrelationships. *In* Nicholas JA, Hershman EB: The Lower Extremity and Spine in Sports Medicine, Vol. 1. St. Louis, C. V. Mosby, 1986.
37. Markey KL: Rehabilitation of the anterior cruciate deficient knee. Clin Sports Med 4:513, 1985.
38. McCluskey GM, Blackburn TA, Lewis T: Prevention of ankle sprains. Am J Sports Med 4:151, 1976.
39. McCluskey GM, Blackburn TA, Lewis T: A treatment for ankle sprains. Am J Sports Med, 4:158, 1976.
40. McKenzie RA: The Lumbar Spine: Mechanical Diagnosis and Therapy. Waikanae, New Zealand, Spinal Publications, 1981.
41. McLeod WD, Blackburn TA: Biomechanics of knee rehabilitation with cycling. Am J Sports Med, 8:175, 1980.
42. McMaster WC: A literary review on ice therapy in injuries. Am J Sports Med, 5:124, 1977.
43. McMaster WC, Liddle S, Waugh TR: Laboratory evaluation of various cold therapy modalities. Am J Sports Med 6:291, 1978.

44. Miller BG: Prophylactic care of the knee. Presented at the Total Care of the Knee Before and After Injury meeting, Overland Park, Kansas, May 17, 1985.

45. Paulos L, Noyes FR, Grood E, Butler DL: Knee rehabilitation after anterior cruciate ligament reconstruction and repair. Am J Sports Med 9:140, 1981.

46. Sanders M, Sanders B: Mobility: active-resistive training. *In* Gould JA, Davies GJ: Orthopaedic and Sports Physical Therapy. St. Louis, C. V. Mosby, 1985.

47. Sapega AA, Quedenfeld TC, Moyer RA, Butler RA: Biophysical factors in range-of-motion exercise. Phys and Sportsmed 9:57, 1981.

48. Saunders HD: Orthopaedic Physical Therapy: Evaluation and Treatment of Musculoskeletal Disorders, 1982.

49. Sealey DG: Practical considerations in flexibility exercises for knee and lower extremity. *In* Hunter LY, Funk FJ: Rehabilitation of the Injured Knee. St. Louis, C. V. Mosby, 1984.

50. Shelton GL: Rehabilitation of selected shoulder injuries. Presented at the Cybex Isokinetic Seminar, Las Vegas, NV, October, 1985.

51. Stone WJ, Kroll WA: Sports Conditioning and Weight Training. Boston, Allyn and Bacon, 1986.

52. Walsh WM, Blackburn TA: Prevention of ankle sprains. Am J Sports Med 5:243, 1977.

53. Walsh WM, Huurman WW, Shelton GL: Overuse injuries of the knee and spine in girls' gymnastics. Clin Sports Med 3:829, 1984.

54. Yamamoto SK, Hartman CW, Feagin JA, Kimball G: Functional rehabilitation of the knee: A preliminary study. J Sports Med 3:288, 1976.

55. Zinovieff AN: Heavy resistance exercise the Oxford technique. Br J Phys Med 14:29, 1951.

15 Injuries to the Shoulder and Elbow: Office Evaluation and Treatment*

BRIAN C. HALPERN, M.D.

Shoulder and elbow injuries are common in athletics today. While such injuries are not as prevalent as knee injuries, the absolute nature and diagnosis of the problem often leave the examiner more perplexed. When examining a patient who complains of "generalized shoulder pain," the first step toward making a diagnosis is to determine, by history, whether the injury was a contact or noncontact type of injury. Following this determination, the key to the diagnosis usually lies in the physical examination.

Most complaints are categorized as bursitis or tendinitis and treated as such; and yet the true anatomy and cause of the problem remain unknown to the examiner. For this reason, cases often become recalcitrant and an early referral to another physician often occurs. Most injuries to the shoulder are of the soft tissue type and, therefore, will be the emphasis of much of this discussion.

Soft tissue injuries occur in the musculotendinous units of the shoulder and elbow. Many times these injuries occur from overuse and poor biomechanics, especially in the case of the throwing athlete. Although professional baseball players, swimmers, and golfers can be afflicted with these syndromes, the recreational athlete is the patient more often encountered. These patients complain of soreness from the inflammatory response to the repeated microtrauma to the musculotendinous units.

Injuries diagnosed early usually respond well to rest, anti-inflammatory medications, stretching and strengthening exercises, and other therapeutic modalities. As the injury becomes chronic, weakness and progressive loss of function may be detected, making an early, accurate diagnosis and treatment on a biomechanical basis imperative.

SHOULDER INJURIES

As always, the examiner must begin with the history. Has the patient had a traumatic injury that precipitated the pain? Pain pattern, character, duration and eliciting factors need to be assessed. A dull aching discomfort, often felt at night, corresponds with rotator cuff tears; whereas a stabbing, burning pain is more typical of bursitis or tendinitis.

Location of the pain can be diagnostic. Pain over the acromioclavicular joint might suggest degenerative disease and, if associated with trauma, the examiner should suspect an acromioclavicular joint sprain. Pain deep in the shoulder may come from rotator cuff involvement, synovitis, or a glenoid labrum tear.

A popping or catching noise inside the joint often indicates a glenoid labrum tear.[1] A history of the shoulder "giving away" or "going out" suggests subluxation or dislocation of the joint. Dislocation is more commonly caused by a contact injury, but subluxation anteriorly or posteriorly can be caused by contact or non-contact injuries. If the stability of the shoulder is affected by either trauma or fatigue, such intra-articular structures as the labrum can be torn by traction of the biceps tendon or impingement between the humeral head and glenoid cavity. These types of injuries often result from a

*This work was supported in part by the Hughston Sports Medicine Foundation, Inc., 6262 Hamilton Road, Columbus, Georgia 31995.

combination of acceleration and deceleration forces and internal and external rotation velocities of the humerus.[10] Therefore, it is essential to question the patient as to the phase of the throwing motion (wind-up, cocking, acceleration, release and deceleration, and follow-through) during which the symptoms occur.

Physical Examination

Although the history is often helpful, the definitive diagnosis usually lies with the physical examination. Begin with an anterior inspection of both clavicles and acromioclavicular joints. The uninjured shoulder must always be examined as a "normal" comparison. Look for asymmetry, ecchymosis, swelling, and atrophy.

Palpate over the acromioclavicular joint for pain, crepitus, and dislocation. Test the stability of the clavicle by pushing down on its distal one-third. Dislocation of this joint can occur in the anterior, posterior, or superior direction. Perform the "cross-over test" by placing the hand of the injured shoulder on the uninjured shoulder (Fig. 1). If the patient can perform this maneuver with minimal or no pain, a Grade I sprain is probably indicated. If this motion is painful, yet the

patient can resist pressure when the examiner pushes the elbow into the torso from this flexed position, a Grade II sprain is probably indicated. If the patient cannot resist at all, a Grade III sprain is indicated.[4]

Next, inspect and palpate the three posterior rotator cuff muscles (supraspinatus, infraspinatus, and teres minor). Also note the trapezius and latissimus dorsi, which accentuate the rotator cuff. By having the patient push against the wall, note any winging of the scapula signifying injury to the long thoracic nerve or serratus anterior muscle.

Assess the patient's range of motion beginning with abduction. This motion occurs with glenohumeral and scapulothoracic movement in a 2 to 1 ratio. For every three degrees of shoulder abduction that occur, two degrees occur at the glenohumeral joint and one degree occurs at the scapulothoracic joint.[7] Check internal and external rotation in the sitting and supine positions with varying degrees of abduction.

To test for anterior stability of the shoulder, hold the patient's arm with the shoulder in 90 degrees of abduction and the elbow in 90 degrees of flexion (Fig. 2). Externally rotate the shoulder with some extension. Any apprehension or pain felt by the patient suggests subluxation or prior dislocation. This

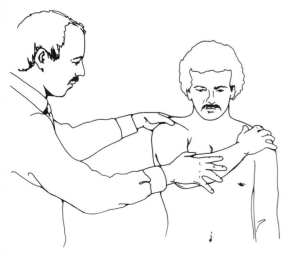

FIGURE 1. Cross-over test. Testing for a sprain of the acromioclavicular joint.

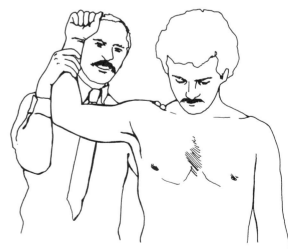

FIGURE 2. Apprehension test. Testing for anterior stability.

"apprehension test" could also indicate a rotator cuff or glenoid labrum tear.[1]

Injuries to the rotator cuff are best assessed by applying downward force to the shoulder at 90 degrees of abduction, 30 degrees of forward flexion, and full internal rotation (Fig. 3). Weakness or pain can indicate injury to the supraspinatus muscle or the suprascapular nerve.[1] Test for strength of the subscapularis muscle by having the patient resist internal rotation with maximum adduction of the arm (Fig. 4). Having the patient resist external rotation with maximum adduction of the arm tests the strength of the infraspinatus and teres minor muscles (Fig. 5).

An impingement test is positive when pain is elicited by internal rotation of the humerus in the forward-flexed position (Fig. 6). This maneuver tends to drive the greater tuberosity under the coracoacromial arch. As this syndrome progresses, refractory tendinitis, wearing of the supraspinatus and biceps tendon, and partial or complete thickness rotator cuff tears can occur.[5]

Additional instability testing is done with the patient supine. With the patient's shoulder abducted to 90 degrees and the elbow flexed to 90 degrees, place your hand on the glenohumeral joint with the fingers palpating the humeral head posteriorly and the thumb, anteriorly. Your other hand supports the patient's arm. With anterior-directed stress to the humeral head, lever it anteriorly (Fig. 7). Repeat this maneuver at varying degrees of abduction, feeling for anterior subluxation.[1]

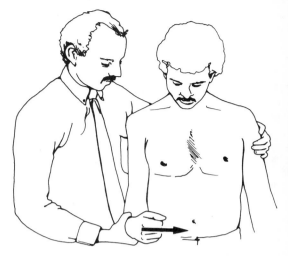

FIGURE 4.   Testing for strength of the subscapularis muscle.

With your thumb on the patient's humeral head, flex the arm forward and direct a posterior stress (Fig. 8). Feel for any posterior subluxation with your posteriorly placed fingers. Posterior laxity is often a normal finding in a throwing athlete's shoulder.[1]

The thrower's shoulder is also prone to glenoid labrum tears, specifically the anterosuperior portion of the labrum. This lesion is diagnosed by the "clunk test" or "labral grind" test.[1] Place your hand posterior to the humeral head while the other hand rotates the humerus. Bring the arm into full overhead abduction while providing an an-

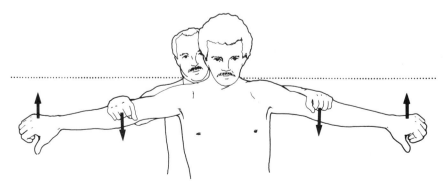

FIGURE 3.   Supraspinatus test. Testing for strength of the supraspinatus and deltoid muscles.

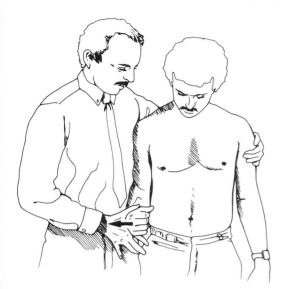

FIGURE 5. Testing for strength of the infraspinatus and teres minor muscles.

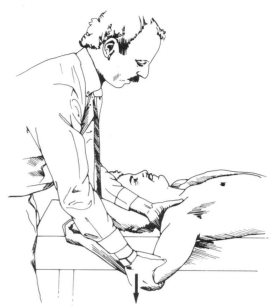

FIGURE 7. Testing for anterior subluxation.

terior force to the humeral head. The "clunk test" is positive when a clunk or grind is felt at the shoulder as the humerus comes into contact with the labral tear (Fig. 9).[1]

The long head of the biceps can be palpated in the bicipital groove while the patient is in the supine position. By externally rotating the humerus, the subscapularis tendon can be palpated and by internally rotating the humerus the supraspinatus tendon can be palpated for tenderness.

An x-ray examination of the shoulder should include an anteroposterior view in internal and external rotation and a transaxillary view.

Injury Patterns

One of the more commonly seen contact injuries is an injury to the acromioclavicular joint. The mechanism usually is direct force onto the point of the shoulder, resulting in a sprain and sometimes a fracture of the distal clavicle. The Grade I sprain involves capsular and ligamentous stretching without frank disruption. Grade II sprains rupture the capsule and acromioclavicular ligament. X-ray films with this grade reveal slight elevation of the clavicle when compared to the uninvolved side. Grade III sprains disrupt both the acromioclavicular and coracoclavicular ligaments causing tenderness and swelling along the ligaments. X-ray films with 10-pound weights in the hands reveal upward drift of the distal clavicle on the involved side.[6] A coracoclavicular distance of greater than 1.3 cm suggests a Grade III

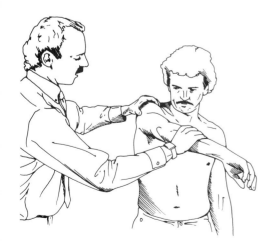

FIGURE 6. Impingement test. Testing for impingement against the coracoacromial arch.

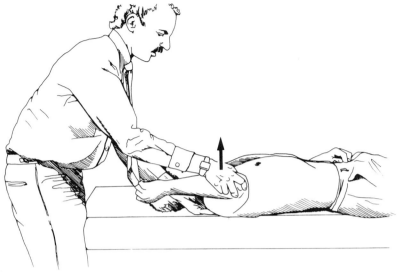

FIGURE 8.   Testing for posterior subluxation.

sprain[2] (Fig. 10). An Alexander view of the joint shows a posterior dislocation that is sometimes missed with a routine AP view.[18]

Treatment of these injuries is controversial. Grade I and II acromioclavicular sprains usually respond well to ice, immobilization in a sling, and early rehabilitation once some of the pain has resolved. For treatment of Grade III sprains, satisfactory results are seen with both closed measures and open surgical reduction.

In their study on shoulder strength following acromioclavicular injury, Walsh, Peterson, and Shelton demonstrated from a standpoint of objective strength that nonsurgical treatment of Grade III AC joint injuries was

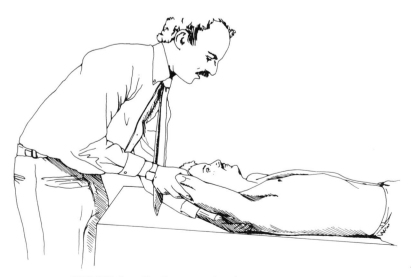

FIGURE 9.   Clunk test. Testing for an anterior labral tear.

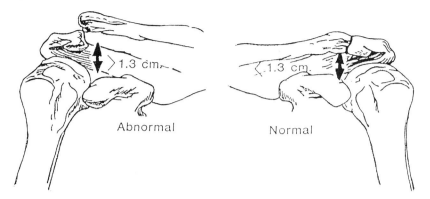

FIGURE 10. Assessing a potential Grade III acromioclavicular joint sprain.

as effective as surgical treatment.[19] The choice remains with the patient and treating physician.

Shoulder subluxation or dislocation is another common contact injury to the shoulder. Subluxation occurs when the humeral head slips over the glenoid rim and then relocates spontaneously; whereas with a dislocation, the humeral head loses contact with the glenoid and lodges along the side of the joint. Subluxation can be so transient that the athlete only feels a sudden pain and the arm "goes dead."[14] Subluxation may occur without contact, particularly in the throwing athlete.

On physical exam, the patient with the more common anterior dislocation is unable to internally rotate the arm and cannot touch the opposite shoulder with the hand of the involved arm. With the less common posterior dislocation, the arm is locked in internal rotation and the patient is unable to externally rotate the arm.[13] An axillary x-ray view is also helpful in diagnosing an anterior or posterior dislocation.

Treatment consists of closed reduction using one of many methods.[11] Following a reduction, three to six weeks of immobilization in a sling, succeeded by an intensive rehabilitation program of muscular strengthening exercises with special emphasis on the internal rotator muscles, is recommended[16] (Fig. 11, except 11H and 11J).

The most common complaint with subluxation of the shoulder is a sudden paralyzing pain as a result of forceful external rotation in the abducted overhead position. The most reliable physical sign is a positive apprehension test. Exercises similar to those used in the rehabilitation of the dislocated shoulder are used for subluxation for at least six weeks with early mobilization of the shoulder.

Most glenoid labrum tears are the result of shoulder instability, the mechanism being forceful subluxation of the humeral head over the fibrocartilaginous labrum.[20] In a throwing athlete, the labrum is more commonly damaged anteriorly and superiorly during the acceleration phase of the throwing act. During this movement, the horizontal adduction and internal rotation places a grinding force on the labrum, and if the posterior stabilizing muscles (posterior rotator cuff) are weak, the anterior force may succeed in damaging the labrum.[10] The most specific test for this lesion is the positive "clunk" or "labral grind" test described previously. Treatment centers around flexibility and muscular strengthening, specifically the posterior rotator cuff muscles, demonstrated in Figure 11 A-L. Often these injuries do not resolve without definitive treatment through arthroscopic surgery.

In contrast to many labral tears, partial tears of the rotator cuff usually respond to physical therapy. These tears are frequently

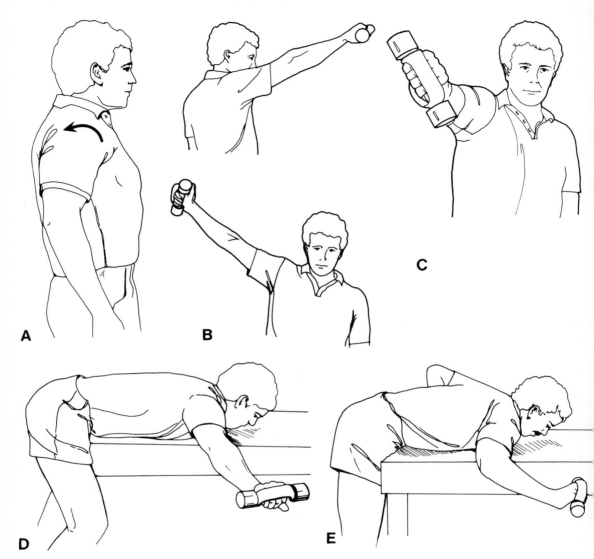

FIGURE 11. *A,* Shoulder shrug with scapular abduction. *B,* The anterior portion of the deltoid muscle is strengthened by forward-flexion exercises. The middle portion of the deltoid muscle is strengthened by abduction exercises. *C,* The supraspinatus muscle is strengthened by internally rotating and abducting the humerus. *D,* Shoulder position for strengthening the external rotators. *E,* Strengthening exercise for the posterior portion of the deltoid muscle and the rotator cuff.

seen in the thrower's shoulder, usually as the result of repeated microtrauma to the supraspinatus tendon. The biomechanical fault is in the deceleration stage, as weak posterior rotator cuff muscles attempt to restrain the forward movement of the humerus. Falling on an outstretched arm is often the cause of a rotator cuff tear in middle-aged males.[3] The partial tear causes pain in the shoulder and is indicated by a positive supraspinatus test. Weakness of the infraspinatus and teres minor may also be demonstrated by physical exam. A complete tear usually results in a loss of active abduction beyond the first 30 degrees, while passive abduction remains full.[3] Although arthrograms are valuable in

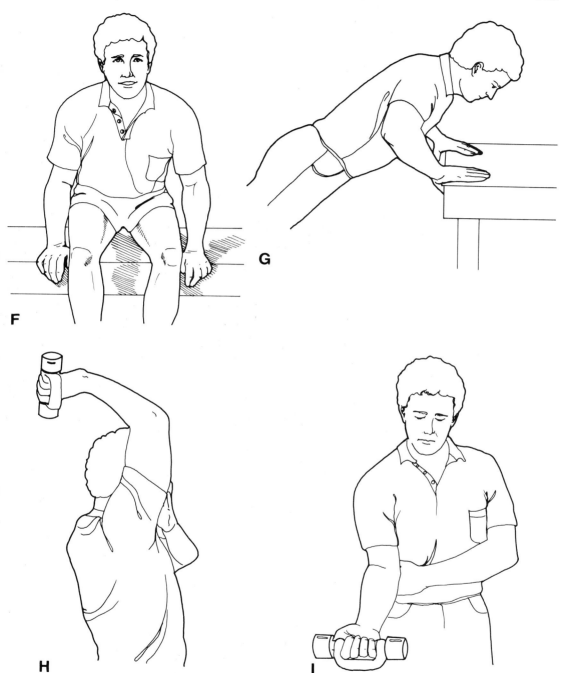

FIGURE 11 (*Continued*).   *F*, Strengthening the shoulder depressor, horizontal adductor and internal rotator muscles. *G*, Modified push-up. *H*, French-curl exercise for strengthening the triceps muscle. *I*, Biceps or elbow curl for strengthening the biceps muscle.

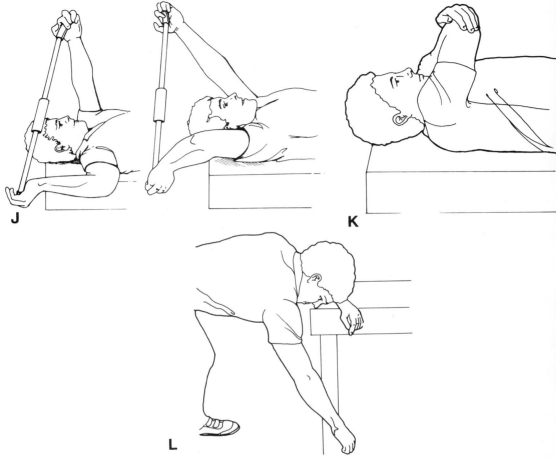

FIGURE 11 (*Continued*).   *J,* External rotation flexibility exercises performed with the shoulder abducted from 90 degrees to full abduction. *K,* Stretching exercise for the posterior shoulder structures. *L,* Pendulum exercises.

the diagnosis of complete tears, partial tears are often missed by an arthrogram.

The rotator cuff muscles are also involved in the impingement syndrome. This chronic inflammatory process of the rotator cuff and, secondarily, the subdeltoid bursa occurs as the muscles impinge against the coracoacromial ligament and the anterior part of the acromion process.[9] This syndrome is more often seen in sports requiring repetitive overhead use of the arm such as tennis, swimming, and baseball. A positive impingement test may be elicited by physical examination accompanied by complaints of pain and, sometimes, weakness.

Treatment for rotator cuff injuries should begin conservatively, except in the instance of a young athlete with an obvious new complete tear. Anti-inflammatory medication, rest, and strengthening and flexibility exercises are the most important elements of conservative treatment (Fig. 11 A-L). Complete rest in a sling will often induce an adhesive capsulitis, adding another complicating factor to the diagnosis and treatment of the shoulder pain. Adhesive capsulitis (frozen shoulder) causes a chronic, persisting pain with decreased range of motion at the shoulder, especially active abduction and external rotation. Shoulder movement and exercises are the key to early recovery for rotator cuff injuries. Strengthening is achieved through a high repetition, low weight program.[1]

Occasionally, steroid injections may be used in rotator cuff injuries but should be reserved for the middle-aged person instead of the young athlete. Arthroscopic surgery of the shoulder is a relatively new treatment option when conservative treatment fails. Many partial rotator cuff tears may be identified and debrided arthroscopically, providing an early return to participation for the athlete. The arthroscopic approach is often utilized after the failure of six weeks of conservative treatment.

Other rotator cuff problems include calcific deposits. When calcification in the tendon becomes painful, it causes a reaction in the overlying bursa, which may itself become inflamed.[15] Common symptoms are severe and incapacitating shoulder pain that presents suddenly and prevents any movement of the shoulder without pain. In these cases steroid and anesthetic injections into the calcium deposit are indicated to decrease the tension in the deposit.[15] Once the acute symptoms are relieved, the patient can progress to range-of-motion exercises, flexibility, and strengthening.

Closely associated with the rotator cuff tendons and the glenoid labrum is the biceps tendon. Anatomically, the tendon has an intimate attachment to the labrum, riding over the top of the humerus close to the capsule and rotator cuff.[15] The long head of the biceps tendon has an important stabilizing function, especially in the throwing shoulder. If other structures like the posterior cuff muscles are weak, then the long head carries more of the load and is susceptible to increasing microtrauma, which results in inflammation.[17] The clinical presentation is chronic pain in the proximal area of the shoulder with palpable tenderness in the bicipital groove. Treatment often revolves around strengthening the posterior cuff muscles and the use of anti-inflammatories. Some authors recommend a steroid injection in the bicipital groove, but, most often, this affords only temporary relief.[15]

ELBOW INJURIES

The biceps tendon is also intricately involved with the elbow joint. A sprain or avulsion of the biceps tendon at the area of insertion can lead to anterior elbow pain. Most other pain at the elbow can be related to the biomechanics of this joint. The common patterns of force overloads to the throwing elbow include tension overload of the medial aspect and compression overload of the lateral aspect of the elbow.[10]

Physical Examination

After taking a careful history regarding the location, nature, duration, and precipitation of the pain, proceed to the physical examination. Inspect for bruising, atrophy, and swelling. Examine for evidence of a possible flexion contracture. Normal flexion should be approximately 135 degrees with extension to 0 degrees. By applying valgus stress to the elbow in full extension and varying degrees of flexion, the integrity of the medial collateral ligament can be checked. This ligament is one of the basic stabilizers for the humeroulnar articulation. Likewise, check for stability of the lateral collateral ligament. Palpate posteriorly for pain and swelling in the area of the triceps insertion and olecranon bursa. Palpate anteriorly along the capsule for tenderness and over the lateral epicondyle for pain as demonstrated in "tennis elbow." Resist extension at the wrist (Fig. 12) to determine discomfort elicited at the lateral epipcondyle, which indicates irritation or weakness of the extensor capri radialis brevis (the major extensor tendon involved in "tennis elbow"). Palpate over the medial epicondyle and have the patient resist flexion at the wrist (Fig. 13). Discomfort indicates inflammation in the flexors of the forearm originating from the medial epicondyle. Finally, perform a neurovascular examination.

Injury Patterns

Several pathologic entities occur about the elbow and many are included in the general diagnosis of Little Leaguer's elbow. These injuries occur to older as well as adolescent athletes. Distraction forces are placed on the medial side of the elbow during the cocking phase of throwing. The result is medial tension, traction on the medial epicondyle, and

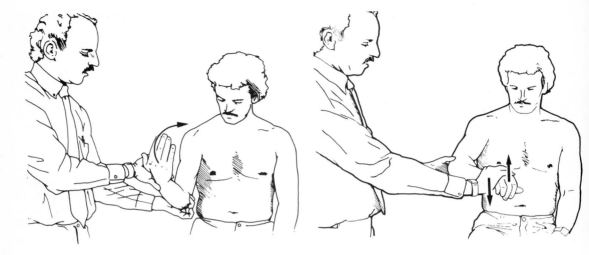

FIGURE 12.   Testing for lateral epicondylitis.   **FIGURE 13.**   Testing for medial epicondylitis.

stress on the flexor musculature with a potential sprain of the medial ligaments.[8]

During the acceleration phase, extreme valgus stress is placed on the elbow. Compression in the lateral compartment, as the radial head abuts the capitellum, may result in fracture of the capitellum or deformation of the radial head, osteochondritis dissecans, or loose bodies in the joint. During the follow-through phase of the pitching act, hyperextension of the elbow can cause injury to the olecranon process causing spurs to form posteriorly.[8]

Little Leaguer's elbow begins with symptoms of pain that can progress to an inability to throw. Palpation can elicit tenderness over the olecranon process, the medial and lateral epicondyles, or the radial head,[8] and x-ray films may show osteophytes or loose bodies. Most cases respond well to rest, anti-inflammatory medications, and flexibility and strength training (Fig. 14). However, in conditions requiring surgical treatment, arthroscopy has become a useful tool.

Olecranon bursitis should first be treated with compression and anti-inflammatories; however, when a pre-existing olecranon bursa problem becomes painful, red, or swollen, aspiration of the bursa contents for Gram stain and culture should be performed.

Treatment for medial or lateral epicondylitis centers around rest from the precipitating activity, anti-inflammatiories, and specific flexibility and strengthening exercises for the flexors and extensors of the wrist.

If this treatment is unsuccessful, a steroid and local anesthetic injection and a tennis elbow splint may be helpful. Resistant cases, however, may indicate a need for surgery.

Elbow and shoulder pain commonly result from combinations of tendinitis, bursitis, muscle strain, and ligament sprain. The key to assessing the injury is a good history but, more importantly, a precise physical examination. Treatment for most of these injuries remains conservative with emphasis on flexibility and strengthening rehabilitation.

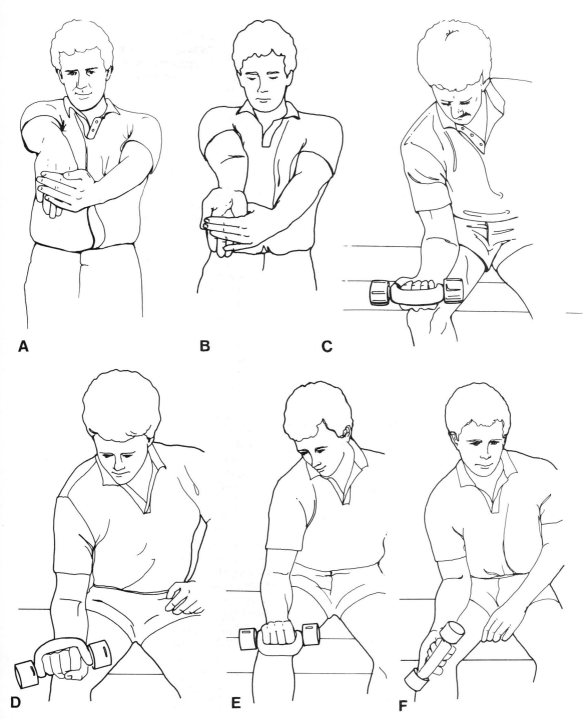

FIGURE 14. *A*, Stretching exercise for wrist extensor muscles. *B*, Stretching exercise for wrist flexor muscles. *C*, Strengthening exercise for wrist flexor muscles. *D*, Strengthening exercises for wrist extensors. *E*, Strengthening exercises for forearm pronator muscles. *F*, Strengthening exercises for forearm supinator muscles.

REFERENCES

1. Andrews JR, Gillogly S: Physical examination of the shoulder in throwing athletes. *In* Zarins B, Andrews JR, Carson WG (eds): Injuries to the Throwing Arm. Philadelphia, W. B. Saunders Co., 1985.
2. Bearden JM, Hughston JC, Whatley GS: Acromioclavicular dislocation: Method of treatment. J Sports Med 1:5, 1973.
3. Booth RE Jr, Marvel JP Jr: Differential diagnosis of shoulder pain. Orthop Clin North Am 6:353, 1975.
4. Halpern C: Diagnosis and treatment of sprains and strains. Ga Acad Fam Phys (GAFP) 7:3, 1985.
5. Hawkins RJ, Kennedy JC: Impingement syndrome in athletes. Am J Sports Med 8:151, 1980.
6. Heppenstall RB: Fractures and dislocations of the distal clavicle. Orthop Clin North Am 6:477, 1975.
7. Hughston JC: Functional anatomy of the shoulder. *In* Zarins B, Andrews JR, Carson WG (eds): Injuries to the Throwing Arm. Philadelphia, W.B. Saunders Co., 1985.
8. Hunter SC: Little Leaguer's elbow. *In* Zarins B, Andrews JR, Carson WG (eds): Injuries to the Throwing Arm. Philadelphia, W.B. Saunders Co., 1985.
9. Leach RE: The impingement syndrome. *In* Zarins B, Andrews JR, Carson WG (eds): Injuries to the Throwing Arm. Philadelphia, W.B. Saunders Co., 1985.
10. McLeod, W.D.: The pitching mechanism. *In* Zarins B, Andrews JR, Carson WG (eds): Injuries to the Throwing Arm. Philadelphia, W.B. Saunders Co., 1985.
11. Rowe CR: Acute and recurrent anterior dislocations of the shoulder. Orthop Clin. North Am 11:253, 1980.
12. Rowe CR: Anterior subluxation of the throwing shoulder. *In* Zarins B, Andrews JR, Carson WG (eds): Injuries to the Throwing Arm. Philadelphia, W.B. Saunders Co., 1985.
13. Rowe CR, Zarins B: Chronic unreduced dislocations of the shoulder. J Bone Joint Surg 64A:494, 1982.
14. Rowe CR, Zarins B: Recurrent transient subluxation of the shoulder. J Bone Joint Surg 63A:863, 1981.
15. Simon WH: Soft tissue disorders of the shoulder. Orthop Clin North Am 6:521, 1975.
16. Simonet WT, Cofield RH: Prognosis in anterior shoulder dislocation. Am J Sports Med 12:19, 1984.
17. Blackburn TA: The off-season program for the throwing arm. *In* Zarins B, Andrews JR, Carson WG (eds): Injuries to the Throwing Arm. Philadelphia, W.B. Saunders Co., 1985.
18. Waldrop JI, Norwood LA, Alvarez RG: Lateral roentgenographic projections of the acromioclavicular injury. Am J Sports Med 9:337, 1981.
19. Walsh WM, Peterson DA, Shelton G, Neumann RD: Shoulder strength following acromioclavicular injury. Am J Sports Med 13:153, 1985.

16 The Spine in Sports

WALTER W. HUURMAN, M.D.

In today's world of increasing physical activity and athletic endeavors on the part of the general population, the spine has joined the knee, ankle, elbow, shoulders and other anatomic areas as a site for athletic related maladies. The athlete who presents with a spine problem needs a physican who understands spinal anatomy and biomechanics as well as a wide variety of pathologic conditions specific to the spine. Owing to the age group of this patient population (young) and general physical profile (more fit), an athlete who develops spinal-related symptoms requires a careful search for specific pathology. Since, in the recreational athlete, response to treatment or eventual recovery is not influenced by compensation considerations, results of appropriate treatment can more frequently be gratifying to both athlete and physician.

As athletic injuries continue to increase in our very active population, those injuries related to the spine increase proportionately in frequency. Many treating physicians feel quite uncomfortable in dealing with problems of the central nervous system and its protective bony enclosures, the cranium and the spine. Dealing with the athlete's physical problems requires a systematic approach. This is particularly true when anatomic relationships are complex and a variety of possible pathologic conditions occur—a situation common to the spine.[10,20] If one approaches the problem with a firm grasp of normal anatomy and biomechanics, the cobwebs regarding specific diagnoses tend to disappear.

For purposes of direct clinical application, the problems of the spine related to athletic activity are best approached in a symptom oriented, differential diagnostic manner. After potential diagnoses are narrowed by an accurate history, the physical examination (Table 1), combined with appropriate labor-atory/x-ray testing (Table 2), further clarifies the problem and allows the primary care physician to make an all important decision: (1) to proceed with treatment or (2) to make a referral to an appropriate specialist.

Neither infallible nor all inclusive, an anatomic approach will simplify the perplexing patient with spinal related complaints.

ANATOMY AND FUNCTION

Composed of 24 articulating segments anchored at one end by the skull and the other by the sacrum, the spinal column functions to provide support for the trunk and extremities and, of equal importance, to provide protection for the delicate and unforgiving components of the axial nervous system. Unique anatomic characteristics within each region (cervical, thoracic and lumbar) provide appropriate amounts of support while providing a varying contribution to the total motion requirements of the body. In its broadest anatomical sense, the spine includes the bony vertebral column, its associated musculoligamentous structures and the neural components—the spinal cord as well as the intra- and extradural nerve roots.

Each vertebral element is composed of a body anteriorly and a complex of lamina/spinous process posteriorly. The two are connected by laterally placed "posts" or pedicles. The space created between the posterior aspect of the body, anterior aspect of the lamina and, laterally, the inner margin of the pedicles constitutes the spinal canal, through which the fragile spinal cord and nerve roots pass (Fig. 1).

Anatomically, the difference among cervical, thoracic and lumbar elements is found primarily in the orientation of the facet joints, which posteriorly provide articulation from one vertebral segment to the next, and

TABLE 1. ELEMENTS OF THE SPINAL PHYSICAL EXAMINATION

Observation:

STANCE
Erect, listing to the side, bent forward

GAIT
Rate (normal, slow, guarded)
Position (normal, flexed, listing)

PALPATION
Tenderness to palpation (generalized, localized)
Muscle spasm (unilateral, bilateral)

RANGE OF MOTION
Active (erect)
 Forward flexion
 Lateral bending
 Trunk rotation
 Extension
 Single stance extension

Passive (performed supine)
 Straight leg raise
 Lasègue's manuever
 Hip flexion, abduction, external rotation
 (Faber)

MUSCLE STRENGTH
Hip flexion (iliopsoas)
Trendelenburg (hip abductors)
Knee extension (quadriceps)
Tip-toe walking (gastrocsoleus)
Heel walking (tibialis anterior)
Toe extension (extensor hallucis)

Elbow flexion (biceps)
Elbow extension (triceps)
Wrist flexion (flexor carpi)
Wrist extension (extensor carpi)
Index finger abduction (first dorsal interosseous)

TENDON REFLEXES
Patellar
Tendoachilles
Biceps

Triceps
Wrist extensors

SENSATION
Dermatomal distribution

---

the size of the anteriorly located vertebral bodies.

Cervical Vertebra. The seven cervical vertebrae provide more motion than found in any other spinal region.[20,26] The facets are located somewhat laterally and are oriented in the frontal plane. With respect to the transverse plane, the cervical facet is tilted in a relatively shallow angle from anterosuperior to posteroinferior. A proportionately large lateral mass is positioned between the lamina and the short, narrow pedicle. On each side the small transverse process contains the foramen, through which the vertebral artery passes in its route from a subcla-

TABLE 2. LABORATORY/X-RAY STUDIES USEFUL IN ASSESSING SPINAL SYMPTOMS

LABORATORY
Urine analysis
Sedimentation rate
HLA B_{27}
Electromyography

X-RAY
Routine plano views:
 Anteroposterior
 Standing lateral
 Oblique

Special Studies:
 Computed axial tomography
 Myelography
 Nuclear imaging
 Magnetic resonance imaging

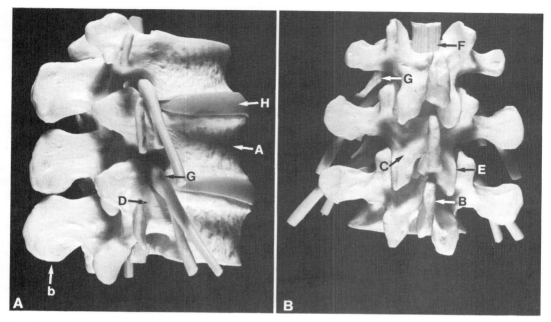

FIGURE 1. *A,* Lateral anatomic view of vertebral elements: **A,** vertebral body; **b,** spinous process; **D,** pedicle; **G,** nerve root exiting from foramen; **H,** intervertebral disc. *B,* Posterior anatomic view of vertebral elements: **B,** spinous process; **C,** lamina; **E,** facet joint, **F,** spinal cord; **G,** nerve root exiting from foramen.

vian origin to the cranial vault via the foramen magnum. The volume of the cervical canal, bounded by the relatively small vertebral body anteriorly, the pedicle and lateral masses laterally, and the lamina posteriorly is sufficient to allow a slight (3 mm) amount of anterior-posterior gliding of one segment upon another without causing damage to the spinal cord.[26]

The volume of the cervical spinal cord does not fill the vertebral canal as much as the thoracic cord does in its location. However, injury to the cervical cord can be more devastating than other neural injuries since sensory and motor innervation to both upper and lower extremity pass through this area.

The anterior intervertebral space at each level in all three regions consists of a semifluid nucleus pulposis and its restraining envelope, the annulus fibrosis. The avascular nucleus acts as an effective shock absorber between bony segments. The enveloping annulus solidly unites the vertebral bodies and consists primarily of fibrous bands arranged in lamellar fashion, much like rings on a tree.

Within the spinal canal, on the dorsal aspect of the vertebral body the continuous posterior longitudinal ligament provides an anterior wall for the canal and blends with the annulus fibrosis at each level. Its ventral companion, the anterior longitudinal ligament, similarly continuously joins the anterior margin of each vertebral body.

Flexion, extension, lateral bending, and rotation greater than found in either of the other two regions predispose the articulations of the cervical spine to degenerative change. The relatively small muscular attachments are less effective in absorbing forces of direct trauma here than in the lumbar spine; the lack of supporting bony attachments make the cervical spine more vulnerable than its ribbed thoracic counterpart.

Thoracic Spine. The thoracic vertebral complex differs from the cervical in that at each level a rib joins the vertebral complex just anterior to its transverse process. The vertebral bodies are somewhat larger than their cervical counterparts. The facet joints are oriented again in the frontal plane but at a more significant angle from the transverse plane. The spinous processes angle inferiorly, actually overlapping to some extent and thus covering the interlaminar space.

The spinal canal through the majority of the thoracic spine is proportionately smaller in relation to the size of the spinal cord than in the cervical spine. There is, consequently, less margin for intervertebral instability. Unlike the cervical and lumbar spine, the bony elements of the thoracic are not left to "fend for themselves" when it comes to providing structural support for the axial skeleton; the rib cage provides needed additional support to protect the thoracic neural elements. The rib pairs provide skeletal protection for the heart, great vessels and lungs, while significantly adding stability to the vertebral column, joining anteriorly via the sternum. Although direct muscular support is again limited, the large posterior thoracic muscle masses (trapezius, rhomboids) significantly absorb forces applied to the thoracic spine.

Lumbar Spine. The lumbar bony elements are relatively massive in comparison to their cervical and thoracic counterparts. The broad, thick vertebral bodies combine with large facet joints, transverse processes, lamina and spinous processes to form a secure base for attachment of larger supportive muscles and ligaments. These soft tissues act as "guy wires" to maintain alignment and affect the strong, coordinated torso movement necessary in most athletic endeavors. The facet joints are aligned in the sagittal plane, most effectively allowing for flexion and extension while resisting rotation. As one approaches the inferior segments of the lumbar spine, anatomic alignment of the facet joints and increasing height of the vertebral bodies anteriorly serves to create a lordotic curve. Although a certain amount of lordosis is necessary for normal, painless function, an increase in this curve will predispose the individual to acute and chronic injuries as described later.[3,11,26]

PATHOLOGY AND TREATMENT

Unlike other areas of the athlete's anatomy, physical complaints related to the spine are not those of instability, giving way, loss of strength, etc., but primarily pain. Among the many characteristics of spinal pain, most important clinically is whether the discomfort is radicular or non-radicular. Continuing in an anatomic fashion, one may look at each segment of the spine in relation to the radicular or non-radicular nature of the pain and begin formulation of an accurate diagnosis.

The Athlete's Cervical Spine

Athletic injuries to the cervical spine are relatively few and, with the exception of thankfully rare but well-publicized trauma resulting in cervical spinal cord compromise,[23,24] are usually transient and treatable. Those injuries that present to the primary care physician, for the most part, include ligamentous sprain/strain or minor bony injury.

Non-Radicular Cervical Pain

Soft Tissue Injuries. Forward or lateral flexion of the neck resulting in the stretch of posterior or contralateral ligamentous/muscular elements may result in fiber disruption. There will be local tenderness to palpation with pain aggravated by motion. Little or no swelling is evident, muscle strength in the upper and lower extremities is normal and neurological testing unremarkable. Routine anteroposterior, lateral and oblique x-rays should be augmented by flexion-extension lateral views to rule out segmental instability. When findings are locally limited and radiographs negative, treatment with analgesics, a soft supportive collar and physical therapy modalities (heat, ice and ultrasound) should suffice to allow complete healing and return to physical activity in two to three weeks.[21,22]

When x-rays reveal sufficient soft tissue damage to allow for abnormal increase in motion between segments, the duration of treatment becomes more prolonged, with 8 to 12 weeks of more rigid immobilization required.[9] Occasionally, if persistent after a course of nonoperative care, surgical stabilization may be required. It is beyond the scope of this discussion to address these problems in detail, and treatment should be rendered by a physician/surgeon well schooled in spinal injury.

Bony Injury. Bony injuries of the cervical

spine are usually caused by violent application of vertical or sheer loading (for example, spearing in football, diving into shallow water, or landing inappropriately in a gymnastic maneuver).[1,23,24,25] If fortunate, the individual may well sustain only minor injury to the osseous structures that does not result in significant neural compromise. Much like minor cervical soft tissue injury, such limited bony injury results in localized tenderness pinpointed by palpation and aggravated by motion; muscular weakness or other neurologic abnormalities are absent. A minor compression fracture of the vertebral body does not compromise stability. It appears as slight wedging on the lateral x-ray and needs be treated much as a soft tissue injury—three weeks of collar immobilization. Similarly, a radiographically visualized nondisplaced fracture of the spinous process with sparing of the ligamentous soft tissues can result from overaggressive neck flexion. In such cases, when an avulsion fracture exists and stability has not been compromised, prognosis for success of nonoperative treatment is greater than when complete ligamentous disruption exists. Three to six weeks of firm collar immobilization will allow for bony union and restoration of stability. When the fracture is accompanied by instability, as documented on the lateral flexion/extension x-rays, treatment is more complex, requiring halo stabilization and/or surgical intervention.[12]

If the patient presents on physical examination with an obvious rotational deformity of the neck accompanied by limited motion, facet subluxation is likely to have occurred. When unilateral, the rotational deformity is more marked than when bilateral. In either case, pain is only moderate and neurologic findings absent; but both rotation and flexion/extension movements are limited. Oblique x-rays are required to make the diagnosis; and occasionally computed or plain tomography will be necessary as well to visualize the pathology.[19,20] Treatment frequently includes surgical intervention and consequently care from an appropriate specialist should be sought.

Radicular Cervical Pain

Indicative of some element of neural compromise, radicular pain most often requires a more aggressive investigational approach and treatment is more involved. One must always assume that the athlete with cervical radiculitis has sustained a potentially devastating injury. Prior to resumption of activity, an accurate diagnosis must be made and pathology sufficiently documented and treated.[10]

Soft Tissue Injury. Recurrent radicular pain aggravated by cervical motion is indicative of neurological compromise due to soft tissue or bony damage. Further athletic participation may result in permanent injury to the spinal cord/nerve roots, therefore, withdrawal from participation is mandatory. In addition to symptoms of extremity pain/paresthesias, the physical examination may show decreased (if the injury is to the nerve root or peripheral nerve) or increased (if the damage is to the spinal cord) deep tendon reflexes. Specific muscle weakness or distribution of sensory disturbance may aid in identifying the vertebral level of injury. Standard anteroposterior, lateral and oblique x-ray views should be augmented by lateral flexion/extension and odontoid images. If these are negative, computed tomography or magnetic resonance imaging may be required to identify fragments of displaced disc material.[13,15,19] Electromyography is additionally helpful in delineating level and degree of injury and may, when repeated, aid in measuring recovery[10] (Table 2).

In the absence of radiographically documented instability, bony injury or soft tissue lesion, e.g., herniated nucleus pulposis, treatment with a soft collar and analgesics should result in resolution of symptoms over a few weeks. The radiculitis in such instances may well be secondary to direct root contusion and with resolution of edema, symptoms will resolve.[22] Failure of this regimen indicates necessity for referral.

Bony Injury. Any fracture that results in mild instability and/or neural compression will usually cause radicular symptoms. Compression fracture of the vertebral body, laminar fracture or lateral mass disruption should be suspected when the force of injury is particularly violent. When not identified on routine x-rays and tomography, technetium bone scanning is helpful in identifying the site of injury.

When an acute fracture is identified and

significant instability (greater than 3 to 4 millimeters of subluxation in lateral flexion/ extension views) is ruled out, treatment in a firm collar for six weeks, if the immobilization promptly relieves radicular symptomatology, may be sufficient.[9] If (1) such a therapeutic approach does not relieve symptoms, (2) symptoms resume after an adequate period of immobilization or (3) the radiculitis is caused by osseous foramenal narrowing, the assistance of a neurosurgeon or orthopaedic surgeon should be sought.

In addition to acute fracture, degenerative disease of the cervical spine caused by repeated trauma may result in osteophyte formation and partial obstruction of the vertebral foramen with resultant nerve root compression (Fig. 2). A frequent problem in athletes who have participated in collision sports, degenerative cervical disease may respond to conservative measures such as immobilization and intermittent cervical traction. However, when motor dysfunction or persistent symptoms exist, surgical treatment is recommended.

Cervical Radiculitis Secondary to Neural Injury. On occasion an athlete will sustain a temporary injury to the neural structures lasting from a few seconds to several minutes or hours. The individual may present on the sideline with complaints of parasthesias, burning or stinging in the upper extremities, or tingling throughout the body. When temporary, such symptoms are usually the result of vertical or sheer stresses, which cause compression of the cord or nerve root by osseous or ligamentous structures not rendered unstable but temporarily distorted sufficient to transmit force to the neural element. Such events, when isolated, are usually inconsequential; but in the presence of continuing symptoms of significant pathology must be ruled out prior to allowing the individual to resume play. Initially, the individual's neck should be placed in a cervical collar until flexion-extension lateral x-rays and oblique views are obtained.

The most recently identified pathology that may cause temporary paresis is congenital narrowing of the spinal canal. Such congenital narrowing has resulted in temporary quadriplegia, an extremely frightening experience. In 34,377 exposed participants, the rate of transient paralysis or paresthesia in one football season was 7.3 per 10,000.[25]

The presence of repeated radicular symptoms ("stingers," "burners") or temporary quadriparesis demands an in-depth evaluation and search for etiology. Tables 3A and 3B outline a recommended approach toward resumption of collision sports in instances of resolved neural compromise. Torg has recently developed guidelines that may be followed should the spinal canal be found to be abnormally narrow.[25] In his review of permanent quadriplegics, of 117 injured between 1971 and 1984, none had experienced prodromal symptoms of temporary paresthesias. Conversely, none of the players who experienced an episode of temporary neurologic symptoms sustained further neurologic injury after returning to play. However, in such instances, this author feels rather strongly that until further evidence is compiled with regard to the natural history of such an anomaly, individuals with documented cervical canal narrowing, should not be allowed to participate in activities in which they are at potential risk.

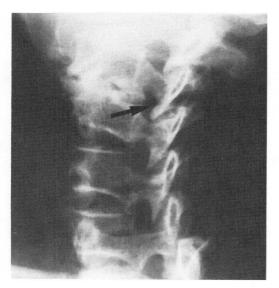

FIGURE 2.   Degenerative changes in C5-C6 with foraminal encroachment are seen best on this oblique x-ray.

TABLE 3A. INVESTIGATION OF RECURRENT CERVICAL RADICULITIS

X-ray studies:
  AP, Lateral, Oblique
  Lateral Flexion/Extension Views
  Pillar Views
Computed tomography
Magnetic resonance imaging

If all studies are negative, treat the symptoms and return to sport activity when asymptomatic.

TABLE 3B. TREATMENT OF PROVEN INSTABILITY

IMMOBILIZE

SOMI Brace × 8 weeks

+

Philadelphia Collar × 4 weeks

↓

Stress lateral flexion/extension x-ray

No instability	<3.5 mm instability	>3.5 mm instability
↓	↓	↓
Return to Activity	Probably OK	Probable fusion candidate

Injuries to the Thoracic Spine

Soft tissue or bony injury of the thoracic spine as a result of athletic trauma is unusual; more often the forces are transmitted along this sturdy mid-line axis to injure the more vulnerable cervical or lumbar elements. Additionally, as a result of significantly less flexibility between its segments, the thoracic spine is protected from degenerative processes to a greater degree. However, inflammatory or neoplastic invasion in this region is not uncommon in the general population. Although we don't often associate such problems with athletes, they (inflammatory and neoplastic problems) must not be forgotten when formulating a differential diagnosis of a spinal complaint.[14,21]

Non-Radicular Thoracic Pain

Soft Tissue Injury. More commonly associated with work stress and tension than athletics, thoracic symptoms of non-radicular pain most frequently represent muscle spasm. Physical findings on examination include point tenderness and soft tissue firmness over the spastic muscle fibers. Motion, particularly truncal rotation, increases the pain; massage temporarily alleviates the symptoms. For those symptoms that are persistent over a number of weeks, anteroposterior and lateral x-rays as well as basic laboratory testing (complete blood count, sedimentation rate or C-reactive protein) (Table 2) should be obtained in search of metastatic disease, occult fracture, infection or noninfectious inflammatory disease processes.

Treatment of non-radicular soft tissue discomfort should be directed toward the symptoms and consists of analgesics, muscle relaxants, and, when persistent, physical therapy. Occasionally an inciting activity can be identified in the history and alterations made in frequency or method of performance.

Bony Injury. On occasion, progressive bony deformity may occur and be the source of non-radicular thoracic discomfort. Most commonly seen in older adolescents, both symptomatic flexible roundback as well as Scheuermann's disease present with localized intrascapular or lower thoracic pain aggravated by prolonged standing, sitting and bending activities.[6,27] Findings on physical examination generally are limited to an increase in roundback deformity, either in the form of a long graceful curve representing flexible adolescent-type postural roundback or a more sharply angulated, rigid kyphosis, as frequently seen in Scheuermann's deformity (Fig. 3). The diagnosis is made on the lateral x-ray, and when the kyphosis as measured between T12 and an upper thoracic vertebra exceeds 40°, the diagnosis of roundback is confirmed (Figure 4). In the case of Scheuermann's disease three successive thoracic vertebral bodies

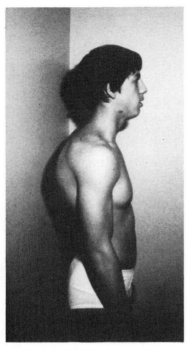

FIGURE 3.   Relatively sharply angled dorsal kyphosis in a 16-year-old male typical of Scheuermann's disease.

must be anteriorly wedged more than 5° each and, on occasion, the vertebral end plate is slightly irregular (Figure 5).

In the case of the former (flexible round back) treatment consists primarily of postural exercise. When severe, treatment similar to that offered for Scheuermann's kyphosis may be carried out.

In the case of Scheuermann's disease, where structural deformity exists, successful, permanently corrective brace treatment is possible (Figure 6).[16]

Radicular Thoracic Pain.   Radicular thoracic pain—that radiating laterally toward the anterior axillary line or distally with gluteal or lower extremity paresthesias—whether due to soft tissue, bone or primary neural causes, should be subjected to in-depth investigation upon first presentation. When physical findings include (1) hypesthesia or hyperesthesia, (2) alterations in deep tendon reflexes, (3) pathologic reflexes (Babinski, clonus), (4) muscle atrophy/weakness, or (5) a change in foot posturing (progressive varus,

cavus, or cavovarus deformities), neural function is compromised.

Introduction of magnetic resonance imaging has shortened evaluation nearly to that single test. Although osseous abnormalities are less well identified, spinal cord compromise by tumor, abscess, or a herniated thoracic disc is readily identifiable on such images; a follow-up CT scan will confirm bony pathology.[13,15] The athlete with such a problem should be referred to a spinal surgeon without delay.

The Lumbar Spine

The athlete has not been spared the curse of pain in the lumbar area, certainly the site of most complaints. The usual degenerative disease of middle age is accelerated in sport participants and, in addition, overuse syndromes are common. Physical activities easily and safely performed by the young adult can cause painful, career-shortening or ending injuries in two other groups of individuals, those who have either not reached bony maturity or who are approaching middle age. A true appreciation of such predisposition by the physician will keep the younger and older athlete actively participating.

Non-Radicular Lumbar Pain

Soft Tissue Injury.   A sudden, violent movement may result in tearing of muscle/ligamentous fibers and cause localized pain, spasm and postural deformity. The event is easily recalled by the individual, and physical examination demonstrates limited motion in flexion, lateral bending or rotation and the presence of palpable, localized tenderness. Prompt treatment with analgesics, physical therapy modalities (ice massage, heat or ultrasound) combined with modifications of activities, will shorten disability to a few days. Return to activity must be gradual and preceded by strengthening and stretching exercises to decrease risk of reinjury.[22,21]

Bone Injury.   Acute failure of the lumbar bony elements is rare. Conversely, overuse compromise of the lumbar skeleton is all too common and increasing in frequency. No

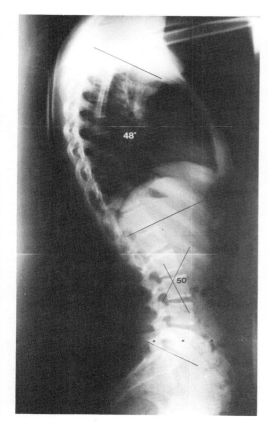

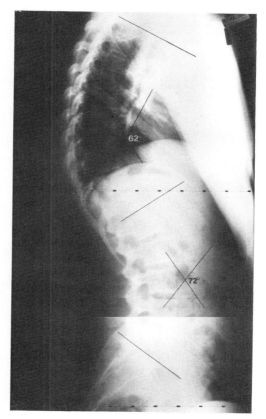

FIGURE 4. Flexible adolescent roundback deformity. Note that there are no structural abnormalities or wedging of the vertebral bodies.

FIGURE 5. Standing lateral x-ray shows slight wedging of the vertebral bodies typical of Scheuermann's disease.

age group is spared, but the adolescent, skeletally immature athlete seems to be particularly prone to these problems. Vulnerability of the young vertebral endplate and pedicle is unfortunately too often ignored by those responsible for junior and senior high school athletes. A training regimen designed for the mature individual will too often result in a functionally impairing injury to the youth's spine (Fig. 7). The physician needs to be aware of these probabilities and to be able to recognize and treat such an injury. Adequate treatment includes communication with coaches, trainers and the athletes themselves regarding appropriate alteration in activity level.

Anatomically, the pedicle (Fig. 1) of the lower lumbar vertebra is prone to overuse failure by virtue of both its size and orientation. Roughly cylindrical, it is best suited to resist stresses directed along its long axis. Unfortunately, the variable degree of lordosis present in the lower lumbar spine orients the pedicle obliquely, placing it in an inopportune position to resist vertical loading.[11,26] Such sheer loading is encountered specifically in gymnasts during dismounts or in any athlete working out with weights during upright lifting activities (military presses, squats, dead lifts). In addition, torsional stress, such as that delivered to the pedicle during other activities (e.g., the tennis serve), also predisposes the area to injury. The result of repeated stress is the development of a "stress fracture" across the delicate, oblique pedicle.[2,3,8]

The symptom of poorly localized pain begins insidiously, gradually increasing in intensity and frequency as long as physical

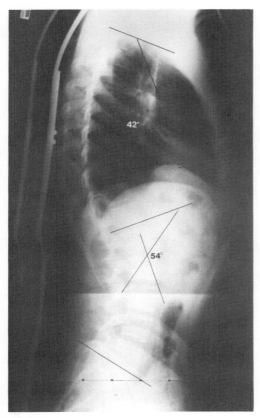

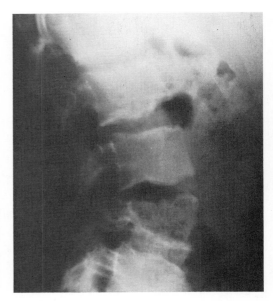

FIGURE 7. Radiographic appearance of lumbar vertebral bodies in a teenage gymnast reveals evidence of repeated end-plate fracture and growth plate irregularities.

FIGURE 6. The same adolescent patient in Figure 5 but with a Milwaukee brace. Note significant passive correction of the deformity.

activity continues. The discomfort is activity related, begins during or shortly after exercise, and lasts for a variable period of time. Physical examination reveals normal neurologic testing (deep tendon reflexes, muscle strength and sensation), a negative straight leg raising test, and only mild limitation of lumbar motion. The athlete has mild restriction of forward flexion; however extension, particularly while standing on one leg (Fig. 8), elicits the discomfort, and the individual is able to localize the pain to the region and side of pathology.

Seen best on oblique x-ray (Fig. 9), the stress fracture or spondylolysis may often also be visualized on the lateral view. Anatomic proximity to the nerve root may occasionally result in radicular symptoms, especially when the deficit is long-standing

and a mass of callus has developed in an attempt at healing. When single leg-stance hyperextension aggravates the symptoms, but plain x-rays are not diagnostic, technetium[99] bone scanning can be extraordinarily helpful in localizing the pathology.[4,18] A three-phase imaging sequence and computerized reproduction of the images further enhances anatomic localization of the problem (Fig. 10A). Computerized and plain tomographic imaging are additional,[7] usually unnecessary, methods of further radiologic evaluation (Fig. 10B). When bilateral spondylolysis is present, there is potential spinal instability, since the anterior structure (vertebral body) is no longer connected to the posterior elements. Under such circumstances, only the anterior and posterior longitudinal ligaments along with the annulus fibrosis serve to secure the vertebral column at the level of pathology. If these soft tissue structures are stretched, the superior vertebral body may displace anteriorly on the one below, creating a spondylolisthesis. In the adult, spondylolisthesis is frequently stable and non-progressive. However, in the

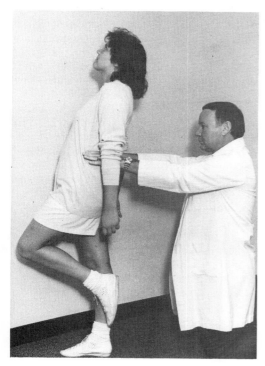

FIGURE 8. Single leg hyperextension test aggravates discomfort in the presence of spondylolysis.

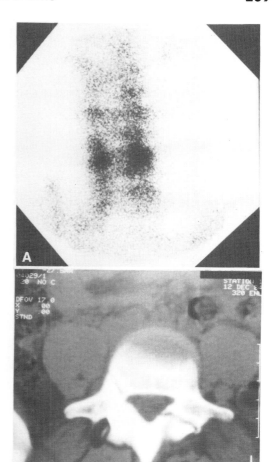

FIGURE 10. *A,* Technetium-99 bone scan demonstrates increased uptake bilaterally in the pars interarticularis region of L4 (same patient as in Figure 9). *B,* CT scan of L4 demonstrates spondylolytic defect on the left and fracture at the base of the pedicle on the right.

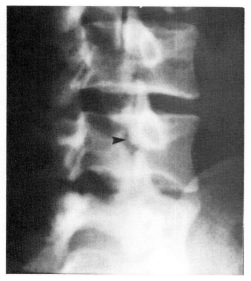

FIGURE 9. Oblique x-ray of the lumbosacral spine demonstrates spondylolytic defect in the L4 pars interarticularis (arrow).

adolescent, not only may the slippage be progressive, but in the supine position it may partially or completely reduce. Therefore, it is imperative that at least one of the lateral x-ray views be taken in the standing position (Fig. 11).

Our approach to treatment of this all-too-frequent problem (spondylolysis) is staged. Like any fracture, the spondylolytic defect will heal if reasonably acute and non-union

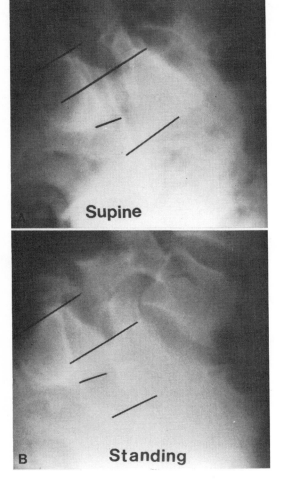

FIGURE 11. L5 on S1 spondylolisthesis increases from Grade II (50%) to Grade III (75%) when the x-ray is taken in the standing position.

back into conditioning, flexibility and finally full activity. If, upon resumption of athletic endeavors, symptoms recur, institution of more complete immobilization, as in any fracture, may allow for healing. Unfortunately, in order to immobilize the lower lumbar spine, the pelvis/sacrum must also be stabilized. This is accomplished with a single leg, pantaloon, body cast (Figure 12). When the lesion is unilateral, the ipsilateral leg is immobilized; if bilateral, either leg may be selected. The athlete is allowed to be ambulatory in the cast, which is worn for 8 to 12 weeks. Upon cast removal, activity is again very slowly resumed. When casting is required, a total of at least six months of rehabilitation is necessary to return the individual to full athletic activities. The bone scan remains positive for up to 18 months, as remodeling continues and the pedicle is increasing in size and strength in order to resist forces to which it is subjected. Consequently,

or pseudarthrosis is not established. The bone scan is helpful in determining the age of the defect—one in which there are active attempts at healing will have increased nucleotide uptake; an established pseudarthrosis in which attempted healing has ceased will be "cold" on the scan.

If the defect is very acute, simple cessation of all aggravating activity for six weeks may result in sufficient bone repair to allow *gradual* return to sport. Over the ensuing six weeks the individual should very slowly work

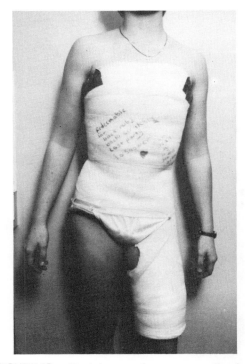

FIGURE 12. Single leg pantaloon cast extending from mid-chest to waist on the right and to the suprapatellar region on the left. Although the patient is ambulatory, the lumbosacral region is immobilized well.

the technetium[99] scan is not a good yardstick by which to measure success of the healing process; non-recurrence of symptoms with resumption of activity is the best indicator.

When nonunion is established or symptoms recur, surgical fusion of the pseudarthrosis is required, and referral to an orthopaedic surgeon experienced in spinal surgery is recommended.

The spondylolisthetic deformity, if stable, does not necessarily require treatment. Certainly if progressive or continually bothersome symptomatology exists, surgical consultation is required. Again, the spinal surgeon familiar with the psychic and physical demands of the athlete's particular interest is the individual best suited to treat such a problem.

The modern day practice of exposing youths to occult spinal injury by subjecting the developing, growing structures to repeated physical impact and stresses may create more long-lasting, less treatable pathology. The vertebral endplate is physiologically constructed much like the physeal plate of the long bones, similarly contributing to growth and development of the part. Microfractures of this "growth plate" may repeatedly occur with on-going trauma of vertical loading, and subsequent growth may be impaired or deformity created. Although symptoms are intermittent and usually last only a few days, subsequent x-rays (Figure 7) reveal the abnormal development and irregular form of the vertebral body portion adjacent to the intervertebral disc. Cessation of inciting activity will prevent formation of new lesions, but residual deformity will persist. The long-term effect of this irregularity in middle or late adulthood is unclear. It would seem most reasonable however, that activity be modified when such a problem is recognized.

Lumbar Radicular Pain

As the athlete increases in age, the usual problems of nerve root compromise seen in the non-athlete similarly become more frequent.[10] Pain radiating into the lower extremity is increased by activity and reduced by rest. Symptoms are similarly aggravated by valsalva maneuvers (coughing, sneezing, and stressing at stool). Physical findings may include protective muscle spasm and limited lumbar spinal motion, but surprisingly often the individual displays a normal degree of flexion, extension and rotation of the trunk. Straight leg raise is positive as is Lasegue's maneuver (passive dorsiflexion of the foot with the extremity just short of the painful position in straight-leg raising). Altered deep tendon reflexes combined with sensory and muscle strength testing will often define the level of nerve root compromise.

Radiographic evaluation, particularly computerized tomography, or magnetic resonance imaging, is particularly helpful in identifying the offended nerve root and source of its compromise (herniated disc, stenotic spinal canal or foraminal narrowing by callus).

Initial treatment should consist of decreased activity. If such an approach, combined with aggressive physical therapy, analgesics and muscle relaxants, fails to relieve the symptomatology, the individual may well require appropriate surgical intervention. Return to athletic activity in the individual whose symptoms resolve may be permissible, but such a decision should be individually made. A wise course would be to modify excessively vigorous endeavors.[22]

Other Sources of Spinal Symptomatology

Infrequently, problems not previously mentioned will be the source of symptoms related to the athlete's spine. Unrelated to athletic activity, the individual's risk of developing a disc space infection, benign tumor such as osteoid osteoma, or non-infectious inflammatory process is no less than in the general population. When the history, physical or radiographic findings, suggest one of the more uncommon sport unrelated diagnoses (e.g., decrease in disc space height, night pain reduced by salicylates, morning stiffness, increased sedimentation rate) treatment is no different than in the nonathlete and other sources listed in the bibliographic references are recommended for specific diagnosis and therapeutic problem approaches to these entities.[22]

Scoliosis. Scoliosis, a condition present to a minor degree in up to 8% of the population and to a more significant degree in 0.3%, has received a great deal of attention over the past two decades due to school screening programs. When it is discovered, questions arise regarding permissable athletic activity. Athletic endeavors have neither a positive or negative proven effect on idiopathic scoliosis of a mild to moderate degree (up to 45°).

When the adolescent's minor curve becomes progressive it is usually necessary to begin non-operative treatment. When such includes some form of bracing, the treating physician must decide the advisability of continued athletic activity. Occasionally the treatment regimen will safely allow enough time out of the brace daily for the individual to participate, but each case must be individualized and decision made by the scoliosis specialist.

REFERENCES

1. Bundens DA, Rechtine GR, Bohlman HH: Upper cervical spine injuries. Orthop Rev 13:556–564, 1984.
2. Ciullo JV, Jackson DW: Pars interarticularis stress reaction, spondylolysis, and spondylolisthesis in gymnasts. Clin Sports Med 4:95–110, 1985.
3. Dietrich M, Kurowski P: The importance of mechanical factors in the etiology of spondylolysis: A model analysis of loads and stresses in human lumbar spine. Spine 10:532–542, 1985.
4. Gelfand MJ, Strife JL, Kereiakes JG: Radionuclide bone imaging in spondylolysis of the lumbar spine in children. Radiology 140:191–195, 1981.
5. Godfrey CM, Morgan PP, Schatzket J: A randomized trial of manipulation for low-back pain in a medical setting. Spine 9:301–304, 1984.
6. Greene TL, Hensinger RN, Hunter LY: Back pain and vertebral changes simulating Scheuermann's disease. J Pediatr Orthop 5:1–7, 1985.
7. Grogan JP, Hemminghytt S, Williams AL, et al: Spondylolysis studied with computed tomography. Radiology 145:737–742, 1982.
8. Jackson DW, Wiltse LL, Dingeman RD, Hayes M: Stress reactions involving the pars interarticularis in young athletes. Am J Sports Med 9:304–312, 1981.
9. Johnson RM, Owen JR, Hart DL, Callahan RA: Cervical orthoses. A guide to their selection and use. Clin Orthop 154:34–44, 1981.
10. Kikuchi S, Hasue M, Nishiyama K, I to T: Anatomic and clinical studies of radicular symptoms. Spine 9:23–30, 1984.
11. Letts M, Smallman T, Afanasiev R, Gouw G: Fracture of the pars interarticularis in adolescent athletes: A clinical-biomechanical analysis. J Pediatr Orthop 5:40–46, 1986.
12. Mazur JM, Stauffer ES: Unrecognized spinal instability associated with seemingly "simple" cervical compression fractures. Spine 8:687–692, 1983.
13. McAfee PC, Bohlman HH, Han JS, Salvagno RT: Comparison of nuclear magnetic resonance imaging and computed tomography in the diagnosis of upper cervical spinal cord compression. Spine 11:295–304, 1986.
14. Micheli, LH: Back injuries in gymnastics. Clin Sports Med 4:85–93, 1985.
15. Modic MT, Weinstein MA, Pavlicek W, et al: Nuclear magnetic resonance imaging of the spine. Radiology 148:757–762, 1983.
16. Montgomery SP, Erwin WE: Scheuermann's kyphosis—long term results of Milwaukee Brace treatment. Spine 6:5–8, 1981.
17. Paris SV: Spinal manipulative therapy. Clin Orthop 179:55–61, 1983.
18. Pennell RG, Maurer AH, Bonakdarpour A: Stress injuries of the pars interarticularis: Radiologic classification and indications for scintigraphy. Am J Radiol 145:763–766, 1985.
19. Post MJD, Green BA, Quencer RM, et al.: The value of computed tomography in spinal trauma. Spine 7:417–431, 1982.
20. Rothman RH, Simone FA: The Spine, Vol. II (2nd ed). Philadelphia, W. B. Saunders Co., 1982.
21. Spencer CW, Jackson D: Back injuries in the athlete. Clin Sports Med 2:191–215, 1983.
22. Teitz CC, Cook DM: Rehabilitation of neck and low back injuries. Clin Sports Med 4:455–476, 1985.
23. Torg JS: Epidemiology, pathomechanics, and prevention of athletic injuries to the cervical spine. Med Sci Sports Exerc 17:295–303, 1985.
24. Torg JS, Das M: Trampoline and minitrampoline injuries to the cervical spine. Clin Sports Med 4:45–59, 1985.
25. Torg JS, Gennario SE, Pavlov H, Torg E: Cervical spinal stenosis with cord neuropraxia and transient quadriplegia. Exhibit, Am Acad Ortho Surg Annual Meeting, Jan. 1987.
26. White AA, Panjabi MM: Clinical Biomechanics of the Spine. Philadelphia, J.B. Lippencott Co., 1978.
27. Wilson FD, Lindseth RE: The adolescent "swimmer's back". Am J Sports Med 10:174–176, 1982.

17 Office Management of Knee Injuries

W. MICHAEL WALSH, M.D.

For most primary care physicians, orthopaedic problems make up a significant percentage of their practices. Many of these orthopaedic disorders may be related to sport, especially if the patient population is young and athletically inclined. The knee continues to present the most nettlesome problems for primary care physicians, and indeed for orthopaedic surgeons as well.

The purpose of this first of two chapters is to present a logical approach to the injured knee that the family physician can undertake in the office. Emphasis is on the evaluation of the acute knee, since this situation usually presents pressing time constraints. Along the way, reference will be made to significant differences in evaluation of the patient with chronic complaints. The second chapter discusses the group of disorders that account for the greatest percentage of overuse injuries of the knee—tracking problems of the patella.

TAKING A HISTORY

Much important information can be gathered before one even begins a physical examination of the knee. The prime question to be answered is, "How did this knee problem begin?" If the patient indicates that the problem started without any single specific trauma to the knee, then we are immediately guided into the realm of overuse injury. Here we will almost invariably be dealing with a certain well-defined group of inflammatory syndromes, most of which involve the extensor mechanism of the knee, that is, the quadriceps, the patella, the patellar tendon, and other related soft tissues such as the synovial plica. More will be said about these entities in the next chapter.

In the youngster with insidious, non-traumatic onset of knee pain, other more unusual explanations must be at least considered, such as osteochondritis dissecans and neoplasm. In older age groups, too, apparent overuse may imply somewhat different pathology. Symptoms of a degenerative meniscus tear, for example, may occur from trauma that is trivial or unremembered. Osteoarthritis or the inflammatory arthritides also may occur without specific trauma. Across all age groups, though, the vast majority of patients who report knee pain, especially bilateral anterior knee pain that is not related to a specific traumatic episode, will be suffering from one of the extensor mechanism syndromes.

If the knee problem is due to a single definite injury, it is important to have the *athlete* specify precisely what occurred. What was he or she doing at the moment the knee was hurt? Was there a direct force applied to the knee by some other object, such as another player's body? If so, where did the force strike the leg and into what position was the knee forced? Was it a noncontact mechanism of injury? What was the athlete doing at that precise moment? Coming down from a rebound or jump shot? Making a turn?

I next press the patient for specific details as to what he or she *felt* when the injury occurred. Did the patient feel or hear a "pop?" Did he or she feel something actually slip out of place? Did the athlete feel immediate pain? If so, where was the pain located?

I next ask the athlete about immediate disability. This is usually the history of falling to the ground and being unable to get up and continue. This situation implies an injury quite different from one in which the athlete is able to continue playing during the game or practice and develops soreness and disability overnight. If the athlete fell to the ground, in what posture was the knee originally held? As the knee was initially flexed, who straightened it out? Was it the coach, the trainer, a teammate, or the athlete himself? If the knee was straightened, was there a sensation of something "going back into place" as this occurred? This history is suggestive of an acute patellar dislocation that was reduced by simple knee extension, whereas a knee that could not be straightened from the moment of injury would lead one to suspect a mechanical blockage to knee extension, such as a displaced bucket-handle tear of a meniscus.

Finally, and very importantly, is the occurrence of swelling. A large swelling that occurs within the first two hours after injury is invariably a hemarthrosis. Few injuries create an immediate hemarthrosis. The most common of these is a tear of the anterior cruciate ligament, which accounts for 80% of the athletic knee injuries that produce the immediate onset of hemarthrosis. The other injury likely to cause hemarthrosis is an osteochondral fracture of one of the joint surfaces. Remember, though, that swelling may not necessarily accumulate within the joint. If one of the capsular ligaments (that is, the actual joint capsule itself) has been torn, any swelling may not be retained within the knee. Therefore, if the rest of the history sounds serious, but the story of swelling is relatively benign, one should not be misled into minimizing this athlete's injury. The same advice goes for the history of pain. Remember that completely torn knee ligaments are generally less painful than partially torn ligaments. Often, the patient with a complete tear will soon be able to walk without significant pain and without instability. However, if the knee ligaments are completely torn, twisting, pivoting, or cutting activity will usually provoke joint instability symptoms.

If the knee injury is chronic, there are some additional symptoms you should ask about. First is the symptom of "giving way." What does "giving way" mean to the patient? Is it a sudden weakness in the leg causing the knee to bend in a direction in which knees normally bend, that is, into flexion or mild hyperextension? If so, this is usually a muscular phenomenon. Any chronically dis-abled lower extremity may eventually experience this reflex muscular type of giving way. On the other hand, is the patient using "giving way" to indicate true joint subluxation symptoms, with "bones going out of place?" This is a far more significant symptom that may indicate laxity of ligaments or patella. Usually joint subluxation does not occur while simply walking straight ahead but rather occurs with twisting, pivoting, or cutting activity.

What about popping? The symptom of popping is so ubiquitous as to be practically useless in terms of specific diagnosis. All sorts of things can create popping in and around knee joints, whether injured or not. However, if either you or the patient can recreate this popping sensation during the physical examination, some usefulness may come from it.

Patients may also complain of locking or catching sensations. What is the difference between these two symptoms? We generally use the term "locking" to mean some mechanical interference with knee motion that is of relatively long duration. Usually this occurs with the knee in flexion, causing inability to fully extend. The patient may eventually learn some maneuver that is performed to "unlock" the knee. A history of true locking is typical of meniscus injury or loose bodies within the joint. If a loose body is the trouble, many times patients will also report feeling a small lump arise in a subcutaneous location that they can manipulate around and eventually see disappear into the confines of the knee joint. Catching, on the other hand, is a much more transient phenomenon. It usually occurs with the knee in extension, causing an inability to flex. It is a sensation for which the patient generally does not perform a specific maneuver to correct. These catching episodes are highly typical of extensor mechanism disorders.

PHYSICAL EXAMINATION

Only after a carefully taken, detailed history should you consider physical examination of the knee. The patient must be adequately exposed. You must be able to see and get to *both* lower extremities, including the feet. Examination gowns are adequate, but gym shorts are ideal. Having a few pair of "loaner" shorts in your office in assorted sizes is extremely helpful. Simply pulling the pants leg up is *not* satisfactory! You must have better access to the entire limb in order to do an adequate examination.

The patient's situation will determine the way in which you proceed. If it's a chronic problem or one of gradual onset, then you should not rush to have the patient assume the supine position on the examination table. Look at the patient in the standing position from both front and side to detect any deformities or asymmetries of the lower extremities. Remember the role that foot deformities can have in creating knee problems. Next, watch the patient walk. Is there a limp? Is there some other evidence of abnormal mechanics of gait? If possible, observing the patient walk or even jog over a longer distance, such as down a hallway, will give you a much better idea of lower extremity mechanics.

Next, in the chronic or overuse problem, have the patient assume a sitting position on the side of the examination table, with both knees flexed to 90°. Here, a number of observations can be made in regard to the extensor mechanism (discussed in the next chapter). Additionally, the earliest and most subtle sign of swelling in the knee joint may be obliteration of the concavity that almost all of us have over the anteromedial part of the knee joints adjacent to the patellar tendon (Fig. 1).

Now and only now, have patients with a chronic knee problem lie flat on their backs. In an acute knee injury, the examination is usually started with the patient lying supine. In either case, one dictate remains firm: start with examination of the uninjured knee first! If both knees are symptomatic, start with the less symptomatic knee first. Try to arrange your office examination table so that both knees can be conveniently examined. If this is impossible, have the patient turn around with his head at the opposite end of the table for each knee. To neglect the normal knee is to miss a vast amount of information! There is a wide range of normal findings in knees. Joints may be more or less lax, depending on our normal make-up and collagen composi-

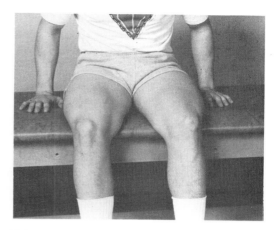

FIGURE 1. Patient sitting with knees flexed 90°. Note normal concavity adjacent to anteromedial joint line, just medial to patellar tendon. Obliteration of this concavity by mild puffiness may be first subtle sign of knee swelling.

tion. One has no idea whether ligament laxity or patellar hypermobility is significant unless one first establishes a frame of reference as far as what is "normal" for *this particular patient*. The other benefit in beginning with the normal knee in the acute setting is that it demonstrates to the patient what to expect when you examine the more painful injured side. By doing a gentle examination with finesse, you set the patient's mind at ease. With a rough examination of the good knee, the response will be, "You're not going to do that to my hurt knee, are you?"

For the sake of brevity, I will not describe the complete examination on the normal side. I believe that will become clear as we discuss the examination of the injured limb.

Observation. Even if you begin the examination with the patient lying supine because it is an acute injury, take a few moments simply to observe the leg. How does the patient hold the extremity? Does the leg lie flat on the table with the knee coming to full extension? Is there some obvious deformity of the leg? Can you visualize swelling that appears to be either inside the joint or in the extra-articular soft tissues? Believe it or not, there are probably some diagnoses that could be made without going any further in the knee examination, just by simple observation. An example would be prepatellar bursitis, in which the prepatellar bursa would be easily visible as a localized "goose egg" sitting superficial to the patella and clearly contained within a bursal structure. The point is to take some time to observe what can be seen.

Initial Palpation. Lay your hands on the patient's knee for a little bit of very gentle palpation. One of the benefits of this approach is to allay fears the patient may have about your manipulation of the knee. Once you make the initial contact in a very gentle fashion, you may often set the patient's mind at ease. About the only thing to really palpate for at this point is effusion within the joint. Use your hand closest to the patient's head to milk any effusion out of the suprapatellar pouch into the subpatellar region where it is most easily felt. So-called ballottement of the patella has always been a mystery to me, but if you believe you can feel the patella float away and then back up against your fingers, ballottement can be done at this time.

Ligament Examination. The most important question you should ask yourself at this stage of examining the acutely injured knee is, "Is this knee stable?" Then, proceed next to the ligament examination. If the injury is extremely painful, and if the patient lacks the ability to fully extend the knee, place a pillow under the knee to hold it in the flexed position while the patient completely relaxes the thigh musculature (Fig. 2). With the patient in this position, perform the Lachman test, which has been proved to be the most reliable indicator of anterior cruciate ligament injury. This test is done by holding the distal

thigh with one hand while applying an anterior drawer type of maneuver to the tibia with the opposite hand (Fig. 3). The test should be done in approximately 15° of flexion, just about the same degree of flexion that is comfortable in most acutely injured knees. Squeezing on sore, injured areas may cause the patient to contract the muscles, invalidating the test. Be careful not to do this. If the test is positive and the subluxation itself is painful, then the patient may allow you only one good chance to perform the Lachman test. One positive response is enough! If the patient is a 280-pound defensive football lineman, and if your hands are relatively small, you may find the Lachman test impossible to perform. In this case, have an assistant stabilize the distal thigh with two hands while you apply the anterior force on the proximal tibia with *both* hands (Fig. 4). John Feagin has described a variation of the Lachman test, done with the patient in the prone position. This is done with the foot and ankle held by your upper arm against your body. It allows both hands to be free and uses the force of gravity to help to create the anterior subluxation of the proximal tibia (Fig. 5). My experience, however, has been that getting into this position with an acutely injured knee is not very comfortable, so this variation has been of greatest help in large patients with a chronic problem.

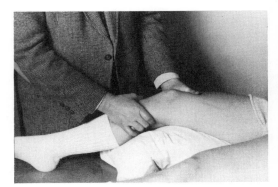

FIGURE 3. A Lachman test in a patient with acute knee injury can be done with the leg on a pillow. An attempt is made to sublux the tibia anteriorly while holding the distal thigh with the opposite hand. This test is done in approximately 15° of flexion. Anterior subluxation of the tibia indicates injury to the anterior cruciate ligament.

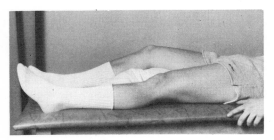

FIGURE 2. A patient with acute knee injury is comfortably positioned on the examination table, with the injured knee in slight flexion on a pillow. The opposite leg and head are flat. All muscles are relaxed.

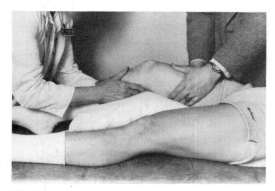

FIGURE 4. Alternative method for performing the Lachman test in a patient with a large thigh. The distal thigh can be stabilized by an assistant while the examiner uses both hands to apply anterior force to the proximal tibia.

Interpretation of the Lachman test, like all ligament stress tests, is based on comparison with the normal knee. The beauty of the Lachman test is that it may help you decide not only whether the anterior cruciate ligament has been hurt but also to what degree. If there is a mild increase in the Lachman test over the normal side, but it still has a good, firm end-point, then there is probably a partial tear of the anterior cruciate ligament. If the Lachman test is markedly positive with a "mushy" feel to the end-point, then most likely the anterior cruciate ligament is completely torn. When the Lachman test is posi-

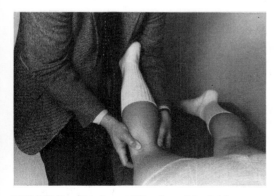

FIGURE 5. Feagin modification of the Lachman test, with the patient in prone position. The examiner holds the foot under his arm. Both thumbs are used to sublux the tibia anteriorly beneath the distal femur. Both index fingers are used to palpate anterior tibial subluxation in relation to femoral condyle.

tive, especially when accompanied by a history that is extremely typical, you may wish to stop the examination here. This is an injury that primary care physicians usually do not want to deal with. The athlete should be sent to an orthopaedic consultant as soon as feasible, probably within 24 hours. On the other hand, if you are seeing the patient soon after injury, you may be able to detect findings that later will not be discernible by a consultant. The patient is also more comfortable than he or she will be later, so you should proceed with whatever further examination is possible.

Next, perform the abduction stress test to check the medial ligaments. This can be done with the knee on a pillow but is probably better done with the thigh lying flat on the examination table and the foot over the side (Fig. 6). One of the examiner's hands grasps the forefoot while the other hand is placed next to the lateral side of the knee. As you get the patient into this position, reassure him or her that you are not going to release the foot suddenly and make the knee bend. The thigh lying flat on the table helps greatly in relaxing the musculature. As with all these ligament stress tests, patients must keep their heads down and be relaxed. If they pick their heads up to see what you are about to do, it is impossible for them to relax their thighs. Now, with the knee at about 30°–45° of flexion, gently stress the knee into a position of valgus, using the hand next to the lateral side of the knee as a fulcrum. What you are feeling and looking for is an opening along the medial joint line, which may actually be visible in a thin, unswollen knee or may be detectable only as a feel. The opening may not be so noticeable as the slight clunk when the medial femur and tibia come back to the neutral position. Done with the knee in 30°–45° of flexion, this is a secure, reliable test for integrity of the medial compartment ligaments. Why do this test with the knee flexed? When the knee is fully extended, it is stabilized by the posterior cruciate ligament. Therefore, one can have a complete rupture of the medial compartment ligaments, and, so long as the posterior cruciate ligament remains intact, the knee will be stable to either abduction or adduction stress with the knee in full extension. This stabilizing effect of the posterior cruciate is relaxed by flexing the knee, thereby allowing the instability created by the medial compartment tear to be felt. If the knee can be straightened comfortably, however, the abduction stress test should be tried in progressively straighter positions until the fullest possible extension is reached. A knee that is unstable in flexion but stable in extension demonstrates that the medial ligaments are ruptured and that the posterior cruciate ligament is probably intact. If significant instability exists both in flexion and in extension, the posterior cruciate ligament as well as the medial ligaments may be ruptured.

Your hands can now be reversed to perform the adduction stress test in both flexion and extension (Fig. 7). If gross instability is present in comparison to the normal knee, this may be a helpful finding. However, realize that the adduction stress test is much less useful overall than the abduction stress test. This is true first of all because most knees will demonstrate a mildly positive adduction stress test in 30° of flexion. Secondly, even

with the knee in flexion, there is a great stabilizing influence of the iliotibial band. Consequently, an adduction stress test that is no different from that on the opposite side should not be viewed with any great amount of comfort. Serious lateral compartment injury may still exist.

Another major point must be raised. The abduction or adduction instability in full extension is a reliable indicator for posterior cruciate injury *only* in the acute setting. It is not reliable in the chronically injured knee, when posterior cruciate injury will be best shown by some of the tests discussed later.

Range of Motion. You have now examined the knee for the two most common ligament ruptures that you will encounter. If these tests are negative, you will wish to carry on with further tests. At this point, determine whether there is enough comfortable range of motion in the knee to allow other manipulations to be done. Gently assist the patient with the acutely injured leg to see how much extension is possible in comparison to the opposite side, followed by the maximum

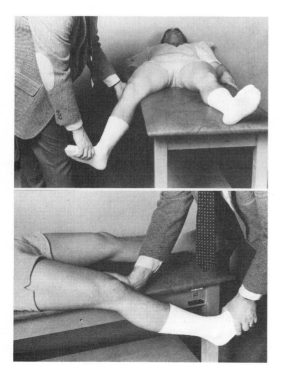

FIGURE 6. Position for performing the abduction stress test in flexion. The thigh rests flat on the examination table, with muscles relaxed. The opposite leg and head must also be flat. A hand placed along the lateral aspect of knee is used as fulcrum, while the opposite hand on the patient's foot applies abduction or valgus. See text for details.

FIGURE 7. Position for performing adduction stress test in flexion. Hand position is opposite that shown in Figure 6. Adduction or varus is applied to the knee. See text for interpretation.

amount of flexion. Lack of range of motion will not provide a specific diagnosis, but if the knee lacks full extension, and has lacked it since the very moment the injury occurred, then you may be dealing with a displaced meniscal tear. It may be of some benefit, especially in the chronically injured knee, to ascertain whether the lack of full extension is accompanied by the "springy" feeling of hamstring muscle spasm causing "pseudolocking" of the knee versus the more solid feel of meniscal or other mechanical blockage to full extension.

Other Ligamentous Tests. If the knee can easily flex to 90°, then you can proceed with the traditional drawer tests. Do these with the patient supine and relaxed, with the head completely flat. The hip is bent to 45° and the knee to 90° (Fig. 8). The foot is then placed flat on the examining table. The most convenient way to stabilize the foot is to sit on the toes gently (watch the Swiss army knife in your pocket!), pinning the foot to the examination table. Both of your hands are then free to grasp the proximal tibia, with thumbs along the anterior aspect of both medial and lateral tibial plateau, flanking the patellar tendon. Your index fingers behind the tibia can easily palpate the hamstring tendons, making sure that they are relaxed. The anterior drawer is then a matter of pulling on the proximal tibia, attempting to sublux it anteriorly beneath the distal femur. The posterior drawer is the simple converse of the anterior drawer. The posterior drawer is performed by pushing the proximal tibia posteriorly rather than pulling it forward.

Several words of caution are in order. These drawer tests can be done with the foot and tibia in various degrees of internal or external rotation. The interpretation is technically somewhat different, depending on the degree of rotation. Simply put, internal rotation of the tibia causes tightening of the cruciate ligaments, whereas external rotation causes relaxation. For your purposes as a primary care physician, do the drawer tests routinely with the foot and tibia in neutral rotation, that is, with the toes pointing straight ahead on the examination table.

Carefully define the starting position for the drawer test, first the posterior drawer test, because if the posterior cruciate ligament has been ruptured, gravity itself may create a posterior sag of the proximal tibia when the knee is first placed in position to perform the drawer test (Fig. 9). Then when you do the anterior drawer maneuver, you will pull the posteriorly subluxed tibia into neutral position and may interpret this maneuver as a positive anterior drawer test, when, in fact, it is the reduction of a spontaneous posterior drawer test. The only way to avoid this pitfall is by careful comparison with the uninjured knee.

Is the anterior drawer test as reliable an indicator for anterior cruciate ligament injury as the Lachman test? Not at all. There are many structures that influence the anterior drawer test other than the anterior cruciate ligament. We commonly see a normal an-

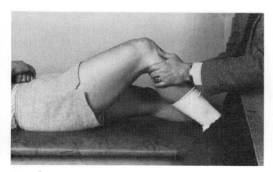

FIGURE 8. Position for anterior and posterior drawer tests. Hip is flexed 45°. Knee is flexed 90°. The tibia is in neutral rotation. Anterior pull or posterior push can be applied to the proximal tibia with both hands. See text for interpretation.

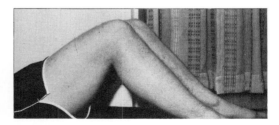

FIGURE 9. Chronic posterior cruciate ligament injury of right knee. Posterior sag in drawer test position is caused by gravity. Attempting the anterior drawer test from this position may give a false impression of positive anterior drawer. The tibia must be reduced first to a neutral starting position in comparison with the other knee before either drawer test is attempted.

terior drawer test when the anterior cruciate ligament has been completely ruptured. Remember, the anterior drawer test alone is *not* a reliable indicator for anterior cruciate injury, even though we continue to do both it and the Lachman test in evaluation of the anterior cruciate.

How do you correlate the posterior drawer test with the instability in full extension discussed earlier? These two tests are both helpful in evaluation of the posterior cruciate ligament, though usually in different settings. Specifically, the positive abduction stress test or adduction stress test in full extension is helpful when the posterior cruciate has been injured along with the medial or lateral compartment ligaments, and the patient is evaluated in the acute period. On the other hand, if the mechanism of injury has been a direct blow to the anterior portion of the flexed knee, as in a dashboard injury, the posterior drawer sign may also be positive immediately following the trauma. The posterior drawer sign, however, is routinely positive in *all* patients with chronic posterior cruciate instability. The best recommendation is to do both the abduction and adduction stress tests as well as the posterior drawer test in all knees you evaluate.

Several other ligament stress tests can be performed on the knee. However, they are rather subtle and more difficult to describe, perform, and interpret. For example, you may be aware that the instability created by an anterior cruciate ligament rupture is really a rotatory type of instability. Usually there is an anterior rotatory subluxation of the lateral tibial condyle in the last 30° or so of extension. This is the phenomenon that produces the symptoms of joint instability that patients report. Tests are available that demonstrate this anterolateral rotatory instability. The two most commonly used are the jerk test and the pivot shift test. These tests are extremely difficult to describe. If you wish to learn the other fine points of knee ligament examination, you should take the opportunity to accompany your orthopaedic consultant to the operating room to examine several knees under anesthesia. It is here that you can easily learn the feel of these more subtle tests. In the meantime, the diagnostic maneuvers described above, if carefully and

repeatedly done, will allow you to identify the vast majority of athletic knee ligament injuries you encounter.

Patellar Stability. By this stage of the examination, you should have already answered the most important question of whether the knee is stable. If the answer is "yes," but the patient has experienced a significant traumatic episode with obvious disability, the extensor mechanism may have been injured. You might reasonably ask yourself next, "Is this patella stable?" That should be fairly easy to determine. First, look for the predisposing physical findings that are discussed in the next chapter by examining the uninjured knee. You can feel confident that, in the absence of predisposing factors, the patient will not have sustained one of the common athletic injuries of the extensor mechanism. On the other hand, the patient certainly could be predisposed and yet the patella may not be the culprit responsible for this acute episode.

After looking for predisposing findings, it is prudent to test for patellar hypermobility. This is best done by positioning yourself sitting on the side of the examination table with the patient's knee flexed across your thigh (Fig. 10). The patient's ankle and foot can then conveniently rest on your other anterior thigh, causing the knee to remain flexed approximately 30–45°. Again, with the patient's head flat and muscles completely relaxed

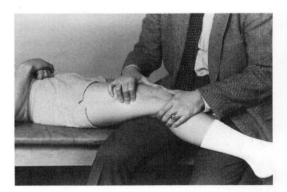

FIGURE 10. Testing for patellar hypermobility. The patient is flat on the table and relaxed. The knee is flexed across examiner's thigh, with the patient's foot and ankle on the examiner's other thigh. Thumbs are placed along medial edge of patella and lateral displacement is applied to the patella.

(especially the quadriceps), position your thumbs along the medial edge of the patella and push firmly, trying to displace the patella over the lateral edge of the femoral condyle. Not only are you looking for hypermobility of the patella in comparison to the opposite side, or in comparison to other knees that you have examined, but you are interested in the feeling of apprehension or discomfort the patient may experience. If a patellar dislocation is the source of the acute knee injury, the patient will usually bolt up off the table, grab you by the wrists, and tell you not to displace the patella again (Fig. 11). Also important is the subjective report by the patients that this is the same sensation they felt when they twisted their knee and something "went out of place."

Meniscal Examination. If you are now confident that this acutely injured knee has neither ruptured ligaments nor acute patellar instability, then you are dealing with a more benign process. Often, this will be an injury to one or both of the menisci. If the knee is not too painful, two tests can be performed that are helpful in the diagnosis of a torn meniscus. The better known of these two tests is the McMurray test (Fig. 12). It is done by acutely flexing the knee as far as possible. The foot and tibia are then either externally rotated to test the medial meniscus, or internally rotated to test the lateral meniscus. While holding the tibia in the appropriate rotation, the knee is brought down from a position of acute flexion into extension. A

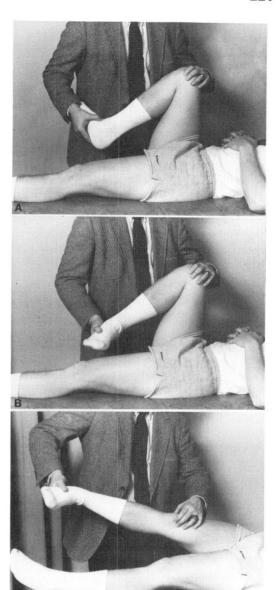

FIGURE 12. McMurray test. *A,* Starting position for testing the medial meniscus. The knee is acutely flexed, with the foot and tibia in external rotation. *B,* Starting position for testing the lateral meniscus. The knee is acutely flexed and the foot and tibia are internally rotated. *C,* Ending position for the lateral meniscus. The knee is brought into extension while rotation is maintained. Ending position for medial meniscus would be same, but with external rotation.

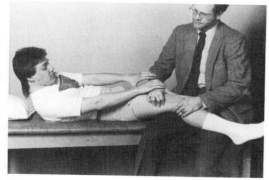

FIGURE 11. Positive apprehension test. Lateral displacement of the patella causes the patient to feel that the patella is about to slip out of place.

classic finding is a painful pop along the appropriate joint line. In other knees, there may be pain over the appropriate joint line without a real pop being felt. There may be a pop that the patient associates with his or her symptoms that is not particularly painful. There may be a painful pop or clicking sensation that comes and goes, or changes with every repetition of the test.

The other test you should be familiar with is the Apley compression test. This is performed with the patient in the prone position and the knee flexed to 90°. The examiner pushes downward on the sole of the patient's foot toward the examination table, compressing the menisci between tibia and femur. Then, with the tibia in either external rotation (for medial meniscus) or internal rotation (for lateral meniscus), the knee is taken through a range of motion while maintaining the compression. The most common Apley test response with a torn meniscus is pain over the joint line on that side of the knee.

Other physical examination is less specific for a torn meniscus. There may be tenderness over the joint line, but this may be present from any condition that causes synovitis in that area. While a torn meniscus may be the cause of an acute episode, it is often seen as the reason for chronic knee disability. In the chronic setting, it is extremely unlikely to find a knee with a significantly torn meniscus that does not have palpable effusion.

Advanced Palpation. Having gone through this entire routine, try to identify other areas of tenderness or localized puffiness that might be present. There are too many potential sore spots to catalogue. Any particular ligament that is torn may be tender or puffy at one of its attachments or along its course. The various bursal structures about the knee may be swollen or tender, including the semimembranosus gastrocnemius bursa, which is best seen when viewing the knee from behind. This is the bursa that, when fluid-filled, is referred to as a "Baker's cyst" or a "popliteal ganglion." In addition to the bursae, any of the tendinous structures about the knee may be tender from an inflammatory process. It is through a thorough knowledge of knee anatomy that these sore or puffy spots become meaningful. Frequent reference to an anatomy textbook, dissection of the knee in a morgue or anatomy laboratory, or watching surgical dissections done by your orthopaedic consultant will facilitate such familiarity.

Other Examinations. Other areas outside the knee joint itself should at least be briefly considered. Muscular findings such as quadriceps atrophy and atonia; weakness of hip flexors and hip abductors; and tightness of hamstrings, heel cords, quadriceps, and iliotibial band are all important. Hip range of motion should be checked, especially in adolescents, where a slipped capital femoral epiphysis may produce referred medial knee pain.

Knee Aspiration. I am often asked about the usefulness of knee aspiration in the evaluation of the acutely injured knee. I aspirate very few knees, believing that through careful history-taking and the thorough but gentle examination described above, I can evaluate most knee injuries. However, many orthopaedic surgeons believe that knee aspiration in the acute setting is a helpful tool. They state rightly that even though there is some risk, it is acceptably small. Consequently, I have no reason to inveigh against knee aspiration, if it helps and if it is done in a precise and careful way. To be completely honest, there are some occasions in dealing with the tense, painful hemarthrosis when I as-

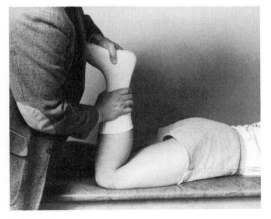

FIGURE 13. Apley compression test. Patient is prone. The examiner applies pressure on the sole of foot toward the examination table. The tibia is rotated externally for the medial meniscus or internally for the lateral meniscus. The knee is then flexed and extended.

pirate the knee for comfort alone. The only error in this line of thinking is that frequently the hemarthrosis reaccumulates, since the cause for the hemarthrosis has not been treated through the aspiration.

If you decide to aspirate a knee joint, it is important to prepare the knee thoroughly with an antibacterial soap, just as one would do in the operating room. Simply swabbing the skin with a little alcohol before performing a knee aspiration would leave you open to liability should complications ensue. The superolateral approach is useful for knee aspiration (Fig. 14*A*). The suprapatellar pouch extends several centimeters above the proximal edge of the patella in most knees. The only pitfall in going too far proximal to enter the suprapatellar pouch is that in some knees the pouch itself is congenitally separated from the knee joint proper, so that you may

not find the fluid you are anticipating. An approach at about the proximal lateral pole of the patella itself is satisfactory. After anesthetizing the skin and deeper soft tissue with local anesthetic, insert a large bore *spinal* needle into the joint, aiming for the interval between the patella and femoral trochlea. It is important to use a spinal needle, since using a needle with an open bore will punch out a plug of skin as the needle passes through, and may deposit that patch of contaminated skin within the knee joint. Using the largest bore possible is important because, in the acute situation, the joint is often filled with early blood clot and it is difficult to aspirate the knee. You may need to flush with sterile saline to aspirate a knee that has already begun to form clots. Using the superolateral approach, the last bit of fluid can be obtained by having the patient carefully flex the knee and externally rotate the hip. The needle and syringe can hang over the edge of the table in a dependent position, encouraging fluid to exit the joint (Fig. 14*B*).

After aspirating the contents with a syringe, squirt any blood into a bowl or basin and look for floating fat droplets on the surface (Fig. 15), which may indicate that there is an obscure bony injury that may not be visible on x-ray. Synovial fluid analysis is beyond the scope of this discussion. It is usually

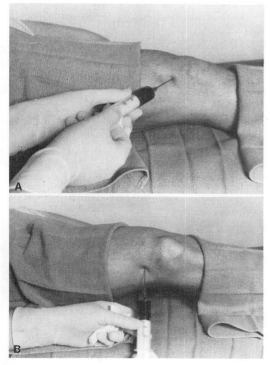

FIGURE 14.   Knee aspiration. *A,* Large-bore spinal needle is used through superolateral approach to aspirate the knee. *B,* Having the patient gently externally rotate the hip and flex the knee over the side of table can help to aspirate the last bit of fluid.

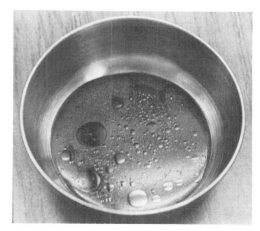

FIGURE 15.   Fat droplets in knee aspirate indicate bony injury and communication of marrow cavity with interior of joint.

helpful only in the chronic knee problems in which there is some question of an inflammatory process. This is usually not the situation in dealing with the injured athlete.

If you go to the trouble of aspirating a knee, you may as well get as much information as possible. Inject 5–10 cc of 1% Lidocaine for some local anesthetic effect. This will not given total anesthesia within the joint but may help facilitate some of the examination discussed previously. Be sure to repeat the Lachman test under the analgesia. Lidocaine and aspiration may allow a better evaluation of this test. Again, remember that the greatest percentage of acute hemarthroses of the knee will be secondary to rupture of the anterior cruciate ligament.

X-ray Evaluation. In all *acutely* injured knees, x-ray examination should be done. Even in chronic knee problems where the diagnosis seems certain through history and physical examination, it is probably advisable to obtain routine x-rays. One would hate to miss osteochondritis dissecans or primary bone tumor in a knee that otherwise seemed to have patellar or meniscal problems. In some patients with typical problems of the extensor mechanism, that is, bilateral knee pain of nontraumatic onset and the presence of predisposing findings, you can treat that athlete for a few weeks to see if the problem can be cured. If unsuccessful, one should certainly go ahead with x-rays if they have not been previously obtained.

A routine anteroposterior and lateral view are used in most acutely injured knees. Oblique views are not obtained unless something suspicious is seen. In chronic problems, other views may be helpful. For example, in a situation suggestive of osteochondritis dissecans, you should be certain to obtain an intercondylar notch view. In the patient with chronic complaints whose knee will flex easily to 90°, I prefer to take the lateral x-ray at that position. This gives the best indication as to the positioning of the patella, as discussed in the next chapter.

In all knees, it is useful to take some type of infrapatellar x-ray. The traditional "skyline" or "sunrise" view is not adequate, though, because these views are made with the knee flexed greater than 90°. Almost all unstable kneecaps will seat in the trochlea when the

knee is flexed this much. Therefore, the infrapatellar view should be made with the patellofemoral joint in more moderate flexion, approximately 30°–45°. It is also convenient and helpful to obtain x-rays of both patellofemoral joints on the same cassette by holding the knees together as the film is exposed. Even if the other knee is not involved, this provides a ready comparison for some of the subtle position changes that one may see on this view.

Stress x-rays are not a routine part of x-ray evaluations of every acutely injured knee. However, in the youngster with open epiphyses, the possibility of epiphyseal fracture exists. It is axiomatic that if you feel apparent knee joint instability in a patient with open growth plates, you should proceed to do a varus and valgus stress x-ray. In many instances, the stress film will show an opening at the level of the growth plate rather than at the joint (Fig. 16). This confirms epiphyseal fracture separation, usually of the Salter I or II type, which should be treated by appropriate immobilization.

The vast majority of times, x-rays of the acutely injured knee will be negative. The most common positive finding in the acute knee is some type of osteochondral fracture. These fractures may occur at any of the joint surfaces but are especially common in patellar dislocation, in which they originate from either the lateral edge of the femoral trochlea or the medial facet of the patella. If a loose osteochondral fracture is seen within the joint, orthopaedic consultation is in-

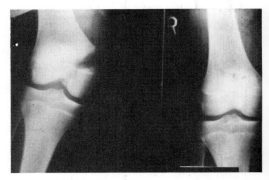

FIGURE 16. Positive stress film in a skeletally immature patient shows opening at growth plate, rather than joint line, when abduction stress is applied.

dicated, even though not all such loose bodies need to be surgically removed. Some small osteochondral fractures may not produce future problems.

Two avulsion fractures that occur around the knee can lead to a specific diagnosis. A small avulsed piece of bone just below the lateral joint margin on the tibia has been called the "lateral capsular sign" (Fig. 17). This bone is pulled off by the lateral capsular ligament, usually along with an anterior cruciate ligament tear. The lateral capsular sign is considered virtually pathognomonic for anterolateral rotatory instability of the knee. A crescent-shaped piece of bone may be avulsed from the most proximal part of the fibular head (Fig. 18). This has been termed the "arcuate sign" and indicates a significant injury to the posterolateral corner of the knee. The musculotendinous, ligamentous, and meniscal complex in the posterolateral knee is referred to collectively as the

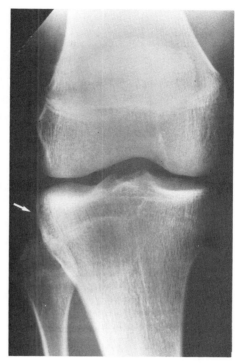

FIGURE 18.   Arcuate sign on knee x-ray. Avulsion fracture from the proximal fibula indicates injury to the arcuate complex and posterolateral rotatory instability.

arcuate complex. Acute injury to this part of the knee causes a posterolateral rotatory instability. Either of these avulsion fractures indicates significant ligamentous disruption and should be referred for orthopaedic consultation.

Currently, we have abandoned the use of arthrography. It was never a very useful part of the evaluation of the acutely injured knee. In the chronic setting, the lack of diagnostic accuracy proved to be more confusing than helpful. As magnetic imaging becomes more refined, it may be supplant arthrography; however, it is only beginning to be used.

INITIAL ASSESSMENT AND TREATMENT

To the non-orthopaedist, this detailed evaluation of one peripheral joint may seem somewhat overwhelming. However, with a little practice, you will spend much less time

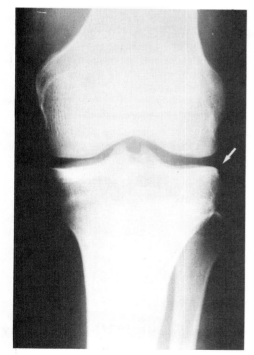

FIGURE 17.   X-ray showing lateral capsular sign. This avulsion is due to bony attachment of the middle portion of the lateral capsular ligament indicative of anterolateral rotatory instability.

evaluating an injured knee than you would in working up a complicated diabetic or heart patient. One item that may help in the initial assessment is the use of a special knee examination sheet or checklist. It not only saves time by allowing you to circle and check items, it also helps you to remember to ask all of the pertinent questions and do all of the pertinent tests, even if it has been some time since your last knee examination or it is late Friday afternoon.

As mentioned earlier, the most significant athletic knee injury that you are likely to en-counter is a grade III sprain of the knee ligaments. A grade III sprain is synonymous with a complete tear of the ligament. By definition, a completely torn ligament causes joint instability. This injury is diagnosed, then, by the presence of instability on one of the tests described earlier. If there is obvious instability in the acutely injured knee, prompt orthopaedic consultation is indi-cated. If you see the patient 24 hours after in-jury and the knee is swollen and painful, you may not be able to decide whether there is joint laxity or not. That's all right. If x-rays are not helpful and orthopaedic consultation is not immediately available, then the right approach is to place the athlete on crutches, with limited weight-bearing on the injured extremity, as well as to recommend elevation of the extremity and application of ice to the knee. The commercially available knee im-mobilizers are not particularly useful except when the patient is extremely uncomfortable getting around on crutches. In most instan-ces, however, the knee immobilizer will not be terribly comfortable, either, because it for-ces the knee into full extension. Some sort of compressive wrap may be beneficial. We use only the white elastic bandages that contain far less elastic than the brown bandages. The white bandages may be wrapped snugly around the knee joint with less risk of con-stricting circulation. A foam rubber or felt pad over the specific area of tissue damage may likewise be helpful. For example, in the common sprain of the medial ligaments from their femoral attachment, there will usually be marked tenderness to palpation over the medial epicondyle of the femur. A foam pad over that area wrapped on with the white elastic bandage may reduce both ede-ma and pain. If you have aspirated the knee, it is important to place the knee in a bulkier compression dressing, including fluffed sponges, combine roll, or perhaps cast pad-ding beneath the white elastic bandage. This is to minimize reaccumulation of fluid.

It is extremely important to start the athlete on some type of early rehabilitative exercises. The simplest of all knee exercises is the quadriceps setting exercise, in which the patient simply tightens the quadriceps and holds it maximally contracted for a count of six seconds, then relaxes it for a count of ap-proximately three seconds. Fifty quadriceps setting exercises should be encouraged each hour the patient is awake. Additionally, while lying with the leg elevated, using ice, the patient should be encouraged to do ankle pumping exercises almost constantly. Simply pulling the foot into maximum dorsiflexion and holding it for a count, followed by push-ing the foot down into maximum plantar flexion and holding it for a count, and doing this repeatedly, is extremely helpful. Both the quadriceps setting exercises and the ankle pumping minimize swelling throughout the limb, which facilitates the repeat examina-tion a day or two later.

The aggressive use of rest, ice, compres-sion, elevation, and simple rehabilitative ex-ercises for a day or two may facilitate your ex-amination. However, if you are still not convinced that the examination is adequate, you can continue the conservative care for another day or two. *Remember,* though, you are dealing with a "golden period" for treat-ing knee ligament tears, which extends for 7–10 days after injury. If ligaments are com-pletely torn and need to be repaired, they should be fixed during this time. If you are running out of time and are still not convin-ced of the adequacy of the examination, the patient must be referred for orthopaedic con-sultation and perhaps examination under anesthesia.

If you are convinced that you have per-formed an excellent examination of the knee, and there is no joint instability, the injury may be only a mild or moderate ligament sprain (Grade I or Grade II injury). These two grades are differentiated only by the rela-tive amount of swelling, pain, and disability that the patient has. In either grade, there should be no joint laxity evident on performing the stress tests described earlier. Do not immobilize mild to moderate knee ligament sprains in the athlete. To do so is to invite increased atrophy and prolonged disability. Instead, manage them with crutches and the simple athletic first aid described above, followed by a rehabilitative exercise program.

If you are convinced that there is no ligament injury, the next most important issue is whether there is acute injury to the extensor mechanism. The management of acute patellar dislocation is described in the next chapter.

If the ligaments and patella have not been injured, a meniscal injury may be present. Suspected meniscal tears are not surgical urgencies and may be managed with limited weight-bearing and rehabilitative exercise.

One thing you must *not* do with the acutely injured knee is to simply hide the leg inside a plaster cast without making a diagnosis. To be certain that there is no ligamentous damage and to decide to manage the patient yourself is quite acceptable, especially if orthopaedic care is not conveniently available. However, to fritter away the "golden period" or to let a patient molder in a cast for six weeks without a diagnosis is not appropriate.

In almost all chronic knee problems, it is reasonable to try conservative care first. Any problem marked by inflammation and swelling can be treated with nonsteroidal anti-inflammatory medication. The most important facet of nonsurgical treatment is an appropriate rehabilitative exercise program. One cannot be "cookbookish" about this advice, because the exercises will be considerably different, depending on the exact diagnosis. For the sake of brevity, the details of individualized rehabilitative exercise routines are not addressed here. Instead, the reader is referred to Chapter 14 for information on general rehabilitation concepts and advice about specific programs.

Certain problems respond better than others to a rehabilitative approach. For example, recurrent locking of the knee caused by a bucket-handle tear of the medial meniscus obviously will not heal through exercise. However, there is really no harm in trying a rehabilitation program. Even if the patient

has to resort to surgical treatment later, this will make it easier to recover from the surgery. If the patient has a degenerative meniscal lesion than is marked more by pain and swelling than by mechanical locking, the entire process may well resolve with anti-inflammatory medication and exercise.

Bracing of the knee is a consideration. The most successful bracing is done for the extensor mechanism. Even a simple neoprene rubber knee sleeve may give enough patellar support to help. This is certainly an inexpensive method to try. Meniscal lesions usually are not affected by bracing techniques. Many expensive custom-made braces are now available for ligamentous instabilities, but it is advisable to send the patient for orthopaedic consultation before incurring the expense (several hundred dollars) of one of these custom-made braces. Generally, bracing by itself is not an acceptable technique, but when combined with rehabilitative exercise it may be of benefit.

SPECIFIC INJURIES

Grade I or II Ligament Sprains. In mild to moderate knee ligament injuries, the athlete should eventually be able to return to sport. These injuries are best managed initially through protection and simple athletic first aid. The rehabilitation program, started early, should progress through more and more complicated exercise techniques and functional activity. Again, the reader is referred to Chapter 14 on rehabilitation.

The only other issue to be addressed is that of confidence. This can probably be determined only by directly questioning the athlete as to whether he or she has total confidence that the knee will hold up to the stress of athletics. The length of recovery time from Grade I or II sprains of the knee ligaments varies so widely as to make it impossible to give the athlete an accurate estimate at the time of the first examination. The physician is well advised to describe briefly the functional goals the patient will have to attain before returning to sport, rather than arbitrarily giving the athlete a specific length of time before he or she may return.

Tears (Grade III Sprains) of the Medial Ligaments. When a complete tear of the medial ligament complex is diagnosed, the athlete should be referred to an orthopaedic surgeon. It is the current thinking that not all medial ligament tears require surgical repair. However, it is necessary to prove that this is an isolated injury of the medial ligaments, with no involvement of the cruciates or meniscal structures. The normal course for these injuries is re-examination under anesthesia followed by arthroscopy of the knee. Any concomitant meniscal injury is treated appropriately. If the injury proves to be an isolated medial ligament tear, many orthopaedic surgeons currently choose treatment with immobilization only. Studies now exist to substantiate the closed treatment approach. Other orthopaedic surgeons, however, believe that direct surgical repair yields the best prognosis. In either case, the knee is generally immobilized for six to eight weeks following a trip to the operating room. Crutches are continued for an additional four to six weeks following removal of the immobilization. This is all combined with an extensive rehabilitative exercise program. Running may be resumed approximately six months following surgery. Because of the need for collagen tissue to mature, return to full sporting activity usually takes place at 9–12 months postoperatively. Regardless of whether surgical or nonsurgical treatment is chosen, the prognosis is quite favorable in tears of the medial ligament complex.

Tears (Grade III Sprains) of the Cruciate Ligaments. Without a doubt, injuries of the anterior cruciate ligament are the most problematic. Factors affecting their prognosis include the amount of ligament tissue torn, location of tear, associated meniscal damage, congenital laxity of the joints, and the athlete's functional goals. All anterior cruciate ligament injuries should be referred to an orthopaedic surgeon. The orthopaedist, along with the patient, should make the final decision about the mode of treatment. Most athletes with an anterior cruciate injury will be treated surgically in some fashion. This usually starts with examination under anesthesia to determine the extent of instability. Most orthopaedic surgeons currently use arthroscopy as the next step in evaluating this injury. After determining the amount of intra-articular damage, a treatment program

can be formulated, and, if surgery is indicated, carried out at the same time. Damaged menisci may require repair or removal. If the injury to the cruciate ligament is only partial, and laxity is mild, the patient may not require surgical repair or reconstruction. If the cruciate has been avulsed directly off of either of its bony attachments, a direct repair may be in order. Usually, though, the tear occurs in the middle third of the ligament, so that the cruciate's tenuous blood supply is disrupted and no direct repair is possible. In this instance, an immediate augmentation or substitution type of procedure may be chosen. Depending on the orthopaedic surgeon, this could mean an intra-articular procedure in which some tissue is placed back through the center of the knee joint to attempt recreation of something resembling a normal anterior cruciate ligament. Other orthopaedists may choose an extra-articular substitution in which lateral joint structures are commonly used to substitute for the anterior cruciate. Any of these surgical repairs or reconstructions is followed by immobilization for some period of time, crutches for an additional length of time, and extensive rehabilitation. One would not expect an athlete with a significant anterior cruciate injury to return to sports sooner than 9–12 months postoperatively. Some residual laxity may persist. Long-term bracing may be necessary as well as modification of life-style. Overall, the prognosis for anterior cruciate injury is not nearly as good as for medial ligament injury.

Acute ruptures of the posterior cruciate ligament are encountered much less frequently. However, their prognosis after direct surgical repair is somewhat better because of a more generous blood supply. Posterior cruciate ligament injuries should certainly be repaired surgically within the first week to 10 days after injury. The length of time to return to sports is about the same as for injury of the anterior cruciate ligament.

Tears (Grade III Sprains) of the Lateral Ligaments. Isolated injuries to the lateral compartment ligaments are not very common in sports. The lateral collateral ligament (or fibular collateral ligament) is in itself not a very important stabilizing structure. Most injuries to this extracapsular ligament alone can be treated nonsurgically. Injuries to the middle portion of the lateral capsular ligament are usually found in combination with tears of the anterior cruciate ligament. When the lateral capsular sign is seen on an x-ray of an acutely injured knee, the problem should be referred to an orthopaedic surgeon as if it were an anterior cruciate rupture. Complete tears of the arcuate complex in the posterolateral corner of the knee, though rare, certainly occur. If an arcuate sign is encountered on x-ray, these injuries too should be referred for orthopaedic evaluation. Direct suture repair may be warranted and carry a good ultimate prognosis. Massive injuries of the lateral ligament complex, though not common in sports, may be associated with damage to the peroneal nerve, which may severely worsen the outcome. The length of time to recover from a repair of the lateral ligaments is about the same as for the medial ligaments.

Acute Patellar Dislocation. The treatment of acute patellar dislocation is described in the next chapter.

Meniscal Injury. Though tears of the menisci are not emergencies, competitive athletes may feel a sense of urgency in having the problem resolved. If so, orthopaedic consultation should be obtained, with the thought in mind of proceeding with arthroscopic evaluation of the knee joint. If an isolated meniscal tear is encountered (that is, one without concomitant ligament damage), a decision must be made as to whether repair or removal is the best treatment. Meniscal repair is a growing trend in orthopaedics. The precise indications and techniques are not completely worked out at the moment. However, most orthopaedic surgeons currently recommend reattachment of a peripheral tear of either meniscus. Though the sutures may be placed arthroscopically, a skin incision is commonly used to retrieve the sutures and to tie them beneath the skin. Immobilization is necessary following meniscal repair. If the procedure proves successful, recovery is expected in about six months. On hearing this time frame, athletes often shy away from meniscal repair, choosing to ignore the potential long-term benefits in favor of a quicker return to sport. Part of the orthopaedic surgeon's job is to counsel the individual athlete regarding the pros and cons of repair versus removal.

The majority of meniscal injuries still require removal of the torn portion of the meniscus. Clearly, arthroscopy has been shown to be the most effective way of doing this. The orthopaedist can actually visualize the joint better with the aid of the arthroscope than with an open surgical procedure—certainly with less trauma to the patient. An arthroscopic procedure can be done as outpatient surgery, with a short period of postoperative disability and often a rapid return to activity.

Osteochondral Fractures. The treatment and prognosis for osteochondral fractures depend on their size and location. Osteochondral fractures detected by the primary care physician should be referred for orthopaedic evaluation. A rehabilitative approach may be undertaken if the fragment is quite small. Some osteochondral fragments never produce symptoms sufficient to warrant even arthroscopic surgical treatment. The majority, however, are treated by some surgical means. Arthroscopic removal is most common. If the fragment is massive, some attempt may be necessary to replace and internally fix it. If the fragment has come from a non-weight-bearing area such as one of the joint margins, no real treatment may be necessary other than removal. However, if it has come from a weight-bearing area, then removal must often be followed by a period of prolonged protection. One never likes to see an osteochondral fracture, especially in a young athlete, because it has been well documented that hyaline articular cartilage does not heal to a normal state. Instead, it is replaced by fibrocartilage, which does not stand up well to the stresses of weight-bearing. In fact, such injury may be a harbinger of degenerative changes to come. Protection on crutches following the osteochondral fracture may need to extend for eight weeks or more. However, immobilization is usually not indicated, since joint motion may actually help to stimulate healing of the defect.

SUMMARY

Office management of athletic knee injuries requires a thorough, thoughtful approach. Although these injuries do not always require surgical treatment, if surgery is indicated, the prognosis is better if it is carried out soon after injury. The role of the primary care physician includes detailed history-taking, thorough examination, institution of a rehabilitation program, and orthopaedic consultation when indicated. Simple athletic first aid and early rehabilitation should always be applied to any knee injury. If orthopaedic evaluation does not become necessary, the athlete's return to sport can be facilitated through a thorough, progressive program of knee rehabilitation and functional retraining.

18 Tracking Problems of the Patella

W. MICHAEL WALSH, M.D.

Of all knee problems presenting to the typical physician's office, the most common are disorders of the extensor mechanism. The term "extensor mechanism" encompasses several anatomic structures: the various parts of the quadriceps musculature; the quadriceps tendon attachment into the patella; the patella and its articular surface as well as the corresponding trochlear surface of the femur; the patellar tendon and its attachments to both patella and tibial tuberosity; and all of the associated supporting soft tissues such as retinaculum, peripatellar synovium, and the structure known as the synovial plica. Any pathologic process involving these structures can ultimately be traced to anatomic predisposition. Without anatomic predispositon, disorders of the extensor mechanism almost never occur, especially in the usual athletic setting. However, predisposition alone is often not enough to create problems unless accompanied by some acute injury process, or, more commonly, repetitive overuse.

Historically speaking, thoughts have changed drastically during the twentieth century about the role of kneecap problems in athletic injuries. Goldthwait,[1] during the first decade of this century, articulated ideas that were to persist as late as the 1960s. Those concepts included the idea that patellar problems afflicted only chubby, knock-kneed, teen-aged females—certainly not the vigorous male athlete. Hughston, in 1968, published a landmark article that helped to change that thinking.[2] He pointed out the prevalence of extensor mechanism disorders in male and female athletes alike. Since that time, much of our thinking in orthopaedics has solidified with regard to extensor mechanism disorders. On the other hand, there are still substantial questions to be answered,

especially with respect to sources of pain and the role of changes in joint pressure in the causation of this pathology.

The purpose of this chapter is to present a logical approach to disorders of the extensor mechanism of the knee, so that the primary care physician can deal with them most effectively in the office. As in the preceding chapter, emphasis is on detailed history-taking, careful physical examination, and nonsurgical treatment.

TAKING A HISTORY

Extensor mechanism disorders may present as a single traumatic occurrence or as a chronic overuse problem. In traumatic injuries, some patients will admit on careful questioning to having had previous mild symptoms. Others report no previous difficulties at all. The most likely acute injuries to the patella are instability episodes and osteochondral fractures. Instability may be in the form of an acute subluxation or an acute dislocation. Obviously these differ only as to the degree of instability. Sometimes it is impossible to tell whether the patella completely left its normal relationship to the femur and spontaneously reduced, or continued to maintain partial contact with the articular surface of the trochlea.

The typical mechanism of injury for any patellar instability is twisting. There may be a force delivered to the knee, usually along the lateral aspect, tending to force the knee into valgus. However, a patella may subluxate or dislocate as a result of non-contact mechanisms as well. In either case, the athlete usually contracts the quadriceps violently. Like any musculotendinous unit, when the quadriceps is contracted it tries to make a straight line from the point of origin on the femur to the point of insertion into the tibial tuberosity. With the knee in valgus and the tibia in external rotation, the quadriceps tends to "bowstring," drawing the patella over the lateral side of the femoral condyle.

As discussed in the preceding chapter, the physician should press the patient for as many details as possible about the sensation experienced at the moment of injury. Most patients report immediate pain along the medial aspect of the knee. Many are able to state clearly that the patella "slipped." The instability usually causes such giving way as to force the athlete to fall to the ground. A knee held in flexion greater than 90° which is accompanied by pain that is relieved when the knee is finally straightened out suggests patellar dislocation. The athlete who happens to lie on the ground in such a way as to see the knee may report that the patella was over the lateral side of the joint. Others do not notice the patella displaced laterally but rather see the uncovered medial femoral condyle and swear that something popped out on the medial side of the knee. When someone finally extends the knee, whether the patient or somone else, there is usually a "clunk" and a sensation of something going back into place as well as relief of the painful symptoms. Of course, in subluxation, reduction on knee extension should be absent.

The history of swelling may vary tremendously, depending to a great extent on the degree of congenital laxity of the patella. A patella may dislocate completely with surprisingly little damage to the supporting structures. In such cases, swelling may not be marked. Large swelling within the joint that occurs within two hours indicates a hemarthrosis and should alert one to the possibility of the presence of one of the common osteochondral fractures occurring with patellar instability episodes.

Acute patellar subluxation or dislocation may present a dramatic appearance and be easier to describe. However, the patient with a chronic or overuse problem of the extensor mechanism is the one most often seen by the primary care physician. These difficulties can be equally disabling and equally challenging to the physician—sometimes more so.

Many of the guidelines provided in the preceding chapter are relevant to taking a history in a patient with a chronic extensor mechanism disorder. The most common complaint will be pain, usually located around the anterior aspect of one or both knees. Swelling may also be noted but usually is relatively mild in comparison to that of acute episodes. Many patients notice cracking, popping, or other noises coming from the region of the kneecap. Transient catching episodes with the knee in full extension are typical of extensor mechanism problems. Instability or giving way of the knee when the athlete twists, pivots, or cuts is likewise common but often difficult to separate from ligamentous instability. Most symptoms reported by patients with tracking problems of the patella are nonspecific. Aside from the occasional patient who clearly states, "My kneecap slips out of place," most patients' complaints could be consistent with a half-dozen different knee disorders.

Two symptoms deserve special mention in dealing with problems of the kneecap: The pain that occurs after sitting for a long period of time with the knee flexed, and pain that is increased by descending stairs or slopes. The greater the degree of knee flexion, the more force is generated within the patellofemoral joint, even when sitting in a non-weight-bearing position. Though the exact mechanism of pain production is unclear, patients with any disorder of the extensor mechanism seem to experience more painful symptoms when forced to sit in a cramped position for any length of time. Back seats of small cars, theatre seats, or airliner seats all wreak havoc with symptomatic patellae, forcing the patient to stand and walk around or seek the aisle seat, where the knee can be extended for comfort. Biomechanically, descending stairs or slopes produces some of the highest forces within the extensor mechanism. The joint experiences force that is not simply equal to body weight but is actually several times body weight, as the extensor mechanism works in an eccentric fashion to decelerate the body's momentum and keep its descent under control. This problem with stairs can become so marked as to force the patient with chronic extensor mechanism problems to choose to live in a ranch-style house rather than a multi-level house.

Most symptoms related to the extensor mechanism of the knee are nonspecific. The spontaneous onset of bilateral anterior knee pain, perhaps accompanied by mild swelling, is highly suggestive of patellar problems, especially if the pain is accentuated by sitting with the knee flexed or by descending stairs. However, the key to diagnosing extensor mechanism problems is artful physical examination.

PHYSICAL FINDINGS

All of the general comments in the preceding chapter about physical examination of the knee apply here as well: the importance of examining the patient in positions other than lying flat on a table; watching the patient walk or run; comparing findings with those of the normal (or more normal) knee; and the gentleness with which the examination is done. Naturally, you will not examine a knee for *either* extensor mechanism problems *or* ligament and meniscal problems. Therefore, the examination process outlined in this chapter and that outlined in the preceding chapter must be integrated in your mind.

Observation on Standing. When examining the patient with a suspected tracking problem of the patella, observe him or her carefully in the standing posture. Look for exaggerated angular deformities from the front and the side view. Extreme valgus of the lower extremities has always been associated with extensor mechanism problems. However, marked varus deformities, especially those in which the varus is sharply localized to the proximal tibia, can also be associated with kneecap problems. When looking at the knees from the side, you are interested mainly in the presence of congenital recurvatum of the knee. This indication of generalized joint laxity would perhaps make you expect to see some relative patellar hypermobility. Look carefully at the feet. Marked pronation may accentuate extensor mechanism difficulties, and treatment of hyperpronated feet may be beneficial to the patellar symptoms. Most important of all the observations in

the standing position is detection of what has been called the "miserable malalignment syndrome." Stan James coined this term[5] to describe the patient who has rotational deformities of the legs and feet. Typically, this is a patient (Fig. 1) with marked femoral anteversion, so that, as the lower extremities come down from hip joints to knees, the femoral condyles are rotated internally, making the kneecaps face inward toward one another (so-called "squinting patellae"). This is most noticeable when the patient stands with feet parallel. The overall appearance of the legs will be that of a varus deformity, with most of the varus sharply localized to the proximal one-third of each tibia. There is also concomitant external tibial torsion bilaterally, so that when the patient stands with kneecaps pointed straight ahead, the feet are externally rotated 45° or more. Finally, there is often pronation of both feet of a rather marked degree. This complicated deformity extending from the hip joints to the feet is indeed a malignant situation for the extensor mechanism, and one that is not easily treated by any method, including surgery.

Observation on Walking. While watching

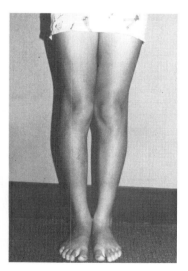

FIGURE 1. "Miserable Malalignment Syndrome." The patient demonstrates femoral anteversion and external tibial torsion. When feet are parallel, kneecaps "squint" toward one another. When patellae point straight ahead, feet are markedly externally rotated.

the patient walk in the hallway, you should pay particular attention to the patella and its movement. Look for any abnormal movements of the patella as it engages or disengages the trochlea. Also observe the position of the lower extremities. Does the patient throw his legs in some abnormal fashion to indicate one of the rotational deformities mentioned above? Also observe the foot mechanics and any part they may play in accentuating the problem.

Examination on Sitting. Next, have the patient sit on the side of the examination table with the knees flexed to 90°. Simply observe the patellae in their positions relative to the distal femora. When viewed from the side, the normal patella should sit very much on the distal end of the femur with the face of the patella pointing toward the wall in front of the patient. A wide range of proximal displacement (patella alta), or, more rarely, distal displacement (patella baja) can be seen in this position (Fig. 2). In patients with extreme patella alta, the face of the patella points almost straight up toward the ceiling. Any degree of patella alta is one of the congenital predispositions to extensor mechanism problems. As the patella is positioned more

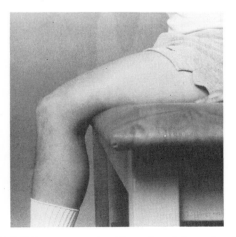

FIGURE 2.   Patella alta. Knee viewed from the side demonstrates more proximal positioning of patella in relation to femur. The top of the patella interrupts the downslope of the thigh to give an appearance much like the lip of a ski jump.

and more proximally, it loses much of the bony support of the femoral trochlea.

Looking at the knees from the front, the normal patella should be very much in the center of the knee as the patient sits with the two knees touching. Again, a spectrum of abnormal lateral postures of the patellae can be seen (Fig. 3). Lateral displacement is also considered to be one of the congenital predisposing findings. Most frequently, one will find a combination of both high and lateral posture of the patellae, the so-called "grasshopper eyes" appearance.

Tibial torsion may also be assessed in the sitting position. By standing above the patient's knees and sighting along the tibial tuberosity and anterior tibial crest, one can assess the relative position of an imaginary line connecting the medial and lateral malleoli of the ankle. Normal external tibial torsion has been reported to range between zero and 40°.

The other observation that is easily made at this time is for Osgood-Schlatter's changes of the tibial tuberosity. Enlargement of the tibial tuberosity is easily seen. Palpate the enlarged tibial tuberosity to ascertain whether it is also tender.

Now have the patient actively extend the knee from a position of 90° flexion to full extension. Carefully watch the tracking of the patella as the knee comes into full extension. Usually, the patella shows a slight lateral deviation in the last few degrees of full knee extension. However, abnormal patellae may show a marked lateral slide on terminal extension. Then palpate the patellofemoral joint as the patient goes through the same range of motion, feeling for crepitation that may be present. Finally, apply resistance to the knee extension with your opposite hand on the ankle while palpating the patellofemoral joint. Often in a patient with a diseased patella, forced knee extension against resistance creates pain.

Next have the patient hold both knees actively in a position of 45° of flexion. This is the best method in which to examine for presence of dysplasia of the vastus medialis obliquus muscle, or VMO (Fig. 4). Dysplasia of the VMO is probably the prime causative finding in all extensor mechanism disorders.

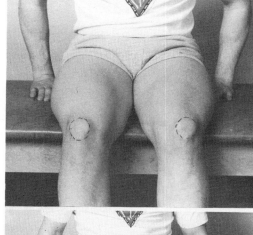

FIGURE 3. Lateral positioning of patellae. Knees viewed from front show lateral displacement of patellae. Kneecaps are tilted away from each other.

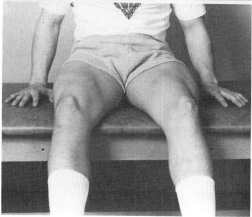

FIGURE 4. Vastus medialis obliquus (VMO) dysplasia. Patient sitting with knees held at 45° of flexion demonstrates lack of normal bulk of VMO along the proximal medial patella.

We certainly consider it to be a major predisposition. If a patient shows a bulky, well-developed VMO in this position, your thinking may rightly be directed away from the extensor mechanism. Again, the presence of VMO dysplasia does not make a specific diagnosis but merely shows a congenital predisposition to the various syndromes affecting the extensor mechanism.

Examination in Supine Position. Many of the findings noted in the previous chapter are also important in the patient with an extensor mechanism problem. For example, you should certainly palpate for effusion and check the range of motion of the knee. However, some findings specifically relate to the extensor mechanism.

Next, compress the patella against the an-

terior aspect of the femur, causing it to glide both medially and laterally as well as proximally and distally. Not only will this give you some indication of the overall mobility of the patellofemoral joint, but it may also create a sensation of crepitation. This crepitation may likewise be painful. Traditionally, it has been taught that painful crepitation from these maneuvers indicates chondromalacia of the patella. This may or may not be true. Flex the knee to 30° over a pillow or bolster, and then repeat this compression test. Often, both crepitation and pain will disappear in this position. If they were caused by true chondromalacia of the patella, they would not disappear. Many times crepitation and pain in the fully extended position come from compressing the patella against the supratrochlear soft tissues, since many patellae lie above the trochlea when the knee is fully extended.

You can next palpate around the entire extensor mechanism. Frequently, symptomatic patellae will be tender along their medial edges. Once again, this has been thought to be due to degenerative changes of the patellar articular surface. However, it is most logical that such tenderness results from the soft tissues being trapped between the examining finger and the patellar surface. By pressing down on the proximal pole of the patella, one can cause the patella to tilt its distal pole upward. Palpate specifically along the entire inferior pole at the attachment of the patellar tendon. Patellar tendonitis is shown specifically by tenderness to palpation in this area (Fig. 5). Less commonly, tenderness occurs along the proximal edge of the patella at the attachment of the quadriceps tendon, indicating a quadriceps tendonitis. In the patient with an acute patellar dislocation, palpation should also be done along the entire course of the vastus medialis obliquus to ascertain the point of injury. If the VMO has been ruptured from its insertion into the proximal medial portion of the patella, you may very easily find a defect in that area that allows invagination of the skin and soft tissues almost into the interior of the joint.

Determine the alignment of the extensor mechanism by measuring the quadriceps angle, known as the "Q angle." The patient's knee must be fully extended with the quad-

riceps *contracted.* Center the pivot point of the goniometer over the patella. The proximal arm of the goniometer points to the anterior superior iliac spine and the distal arm lies along the patellar tendon (Fig. 6). If the results of this measurement are greater than 10° in males, this is considered an abnormal Q angle. Since females normally have more valgus of the knees, up to 15° is considered normal in women.[3]

One should next check for the presence of a pathologic synovial plica by passively flexing and extending the knee from about 30°–90° of flexion (Fig. 7). At the same time, the patella should be displaced slightly medially and the fingers of the examining hand placed in the medial paratellar region. With the quadriceps relaxed, a tender fold may often be palpated that recreates the familiar painful popping sensation that the patient feels.

The remaining part of the examination of the patella itself is the lateral hypermobility test (discussed in the preceding chapter; see Fig. 10). Remember that you are looking not only for hypermobility but also for apprehension, pain, and the subjective report by the patient that this is a familiar feeling that he associates with his knee disability.

Other Examination. Quadriceps muscle tone and bulk may be checked. Circumference measurements of the thigh are not really worth the effort. The muscle status can probably be evaluated best by simply observing the relative bulk of the musculature and palpating for the relative loss of tone.

Inflexibility in certain muscle groups is critically important in dealing with the extensor mechanism. Most common is tight-

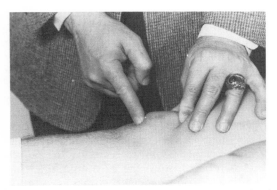

FIGURE 5. Patellar tendonitis. Pressure on proximal patellar pole will tilt distal pole upward. Patellar tendonitis is shown by tenderness along inferior edge at attachment of patellar tendon.

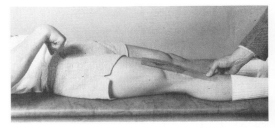

FIGURE 6. Measuring for the quadriceps angle ("Q angle"). Angle is measured with knee extended and quadriceps contracted. See text for details.

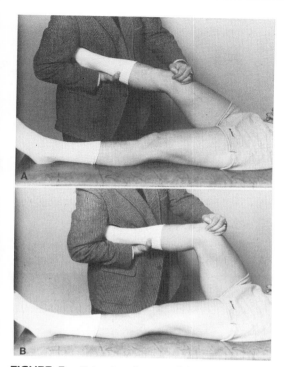

FIGURE 7. Palpation for synovial plica. Foot and tibia are internally rotated. Examiner's hand lies along lateral edge of patella, displacing patella medially. Fingers palpate medial patellofemoral joint while knee is passively moved from approximately 30° (A) to 90° (B) of flexion.

ness of the hamstrings. With the opposite leg fully extended, have the patient flex the hip to 90°. While maintaining the hip at 90°, see if he or she can fully extend the knee so that the entire leg is pointed straight up at the ceiling (Fig. 8). This indicates normal hamstring flexibility, at least in the general population. In certain athletes whose sport places a high premium on flexibility, such as dancers and gymnasts, this is a minimal amount of hamstring flexibility. These athletes should be able to bring the entire leg into more flexion at the hip, with the leg coming toward the head. Lack of normal hamstring flexibility is shown in inability to extend the knee fully with the hip flexed to 90°.

The next most important muscle flexibility measurement to ascertain is flexibility of the gastroc-soleus group along the posterior calf. With the knee fully extended and the foot in a slightly inverted position, passively dor-

siflex the ankle as far as possible (Fig. 9). In normally flexible calves, the foot should come to approximately 15° of dorsiflexion beyond the neutral position.

The third and often neglected flexibility to assess is that of the quadriceps muscle group itself. Turn the patient to a prone position and acutely flex the knee, bringing the heel toward the buttock (Fig. 10). Lack of knee flexion in comparison to the uninjured side, obligatory flexion of the hip joint such that the anterior pelvis rises off the examination table, or simply the patient's report of increased "tightness" along the anterior thigh during this maneuver are all indications of quadriceps muscle tightness that should be stretched out.

With the patient supine, hip range of motion should be evaluated. With the hip flexed to 90°, internal rotation that exceeds external rotation is an indication of some degree of femoral anteversion.

X-Ray Evaluation. Most of the x-ray evaluation is the same as discussed in the preceding chapter. Most recently, however, we have started taking our lateral x-ray views of the knee in 90° of flexion (Fig. 11), which is the same position in which we assess patellar position clinically. A normally placed patella, that is, one with no patella alta, should be placed very nearly on the distal end of the femur, with its proximal pole about in line with the anterior femoral cortex. Deviations from this are most easily seen in this 90° flexed lateral view. Various techniques have been described for measuring an x-ray to determine patella alta and patella baja. The most commonly used is the method of Insall and Salvati, which expresses the greatest diagonal length of the patella as a ratio to the length of the patellar tendon (Fig. 12).[4] This ratio should be very nearly 1.0. Deviations greater than 20% in either direction (less than 0.8 or greater than 1.2) indicate significant patella alta or patella baja. This ratio may be a little difficult to determine because of uncertainties in measuring the length of the patellar tendon on x-ray, especially in determining the point of its attachment into the tibial tuberosity.

The most significant view in dealing with the patellofemoral joint is the infrapatellar view. Many different techniques exist. The

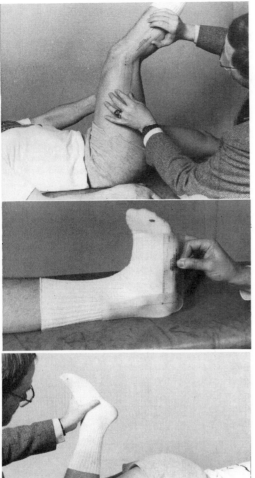

FIGURE 8. Measuring hamstring tightness. With patient supine and hip flexed 90°, knee should extend fully if hamstrings are flexible. If knee will not extend completely, residual knee flexion angle is measured and recorded as hamstring tightness.

FIGURE 9. Heel cord tightness measurement with knee fully extended and foot slightly inverted. Ankle is dorsiflexed as far as possible. Normally flexible gastrocsoleus muscles should allow 15° of dorsiflexion past the neutral position.

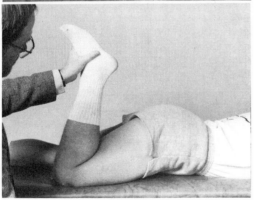

FIGURE 10. Quadriceps flexibility measurement. Patient is turned prone. Knee is flexed to bring heel as close to buttock as possible. Anterior pelvis rising off examination table, sensation of tightness along anterior thigh, or lack of knee flexion compared to opposite side may all indicate quadriceps tightness.

most important point is that this view is taken in approximately 30°–45° of knee flexion. Any of the techniques utilizing knee flexion greater than 90° are not helpful.

Various abnormalities may be seen in the infrapatellar view. These are most easily seen when both knees have been x-rayed together on the same cassette, allowing direct comparison of one knee to the other. Relative deficiency of the lateral femoral condyle, allowing either lateral tilting or lateral subluxation of the patella, may be seen (Fig. 13). Like the clinical findings noted earlier, these

x-ray findings may span a wide range, from mild to severe. Avulsion fractures along the medial edge of the patella are virtually pathognomonic for recurrent patellar dislocation (Fig. 14). Osteochondral fractures may likewise be seen.

Many different techniques for measurement of lateral tilting, lateral displacement, and lack of patellofemoral congruity have been described. These are really not helpful in office practice. Use the infrapatellar x-ray for the information it readily provides. It may alert you to problems within the extensor

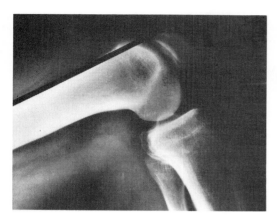

FIGURE 11.   Lateral knee x-ray at 90°. Allows assessment of patella alta or patella baja. Proximal pole of patella should be in line with anterior femoral cortex.

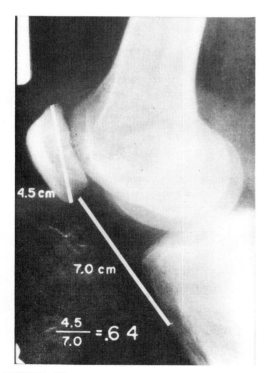

4.5 cm

7.0 cm

$$\frac{4.5}{7.0} = .64$$

FIGURE 12.   Insall-Salvati method for measuring patella alta or patella baja. Greatest diagonal length of patella as a ratio to length of patellar tendon should be 1.0 ± 0.2.[4]

mechanism that you had not suspected. You may be prompted to go back and examine the patellofemoral joint more carefully. It may show congenital predisposition that is present even on the asymptomatic side. However, to spend time drawing lines and measuring angles is generally not worth much. The final diagnosis lies in careful history-taking and physical examination.

SPECIFIC PROBLEMS AND THEIR TREATMENT

Acute Patellar Instability. The athlete with an acute injury may have experienced an acute dislocation that persisted until reduced, an acute dislocation with spontaneous reduction, or an acute subluxation. Diagnosis of this situation is by a typical history (as noted above) and a confirmatory physical examination. Physical examination should show the usual predisposing physical findings (VMO dysplasia, high and lateral patella, increased Q-angle, etc.) on the opposite uninjured knee, as well as swelling, tenderness over the medial supporting structures, and patellar hypermobility with associated apprehension and pain on the injured knee.

Treatment for the first-time patellar dislocation is somewhat controversial. Some authors point out that the injury to the medial supporting structure is like any other acute ligamentous knee injury and recommend immediate surgical repair. I believe that surgery is necessary in only one setting. If the VMO has been ruptured at its insertion, and a defect is palpable along the superomedial edge of the patella, then it is best handled by early surgical repair. This portion of the VMO does not heal well with simple closed treatment. However, in most patellar dislocations, the VMO has been injured either in its mid-substance or at its origin from the femur and medial intermuscular septum. Some patellae can dislocate with surprisingly little acute change in the tissues. Consequently, the majority of first dislocations of the patella can be handled with closed treatment. If a large, tense hemarthrosis develops, the knee can be aspirated for comfort, as described in the preceding chapter. A thick foam rubber or felt pad

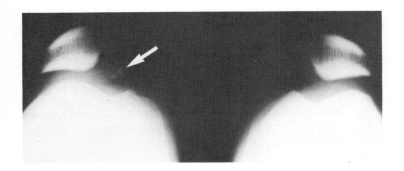

FIGURE 13. Infrapatellar x-ray shows lateral tilting and lateral subluxation of both patellae. Also seen is osteochondral fracture from acute injury (arrow).

should be placed over the area of tenderness in the medial supporting structures to compress them snugly against their femoral attachment. A crescent-shaped foam rubber or felt pad can also be placed along the lateral edge of the patella to displace it more medially. The patient should then be placed in a cylinder cast extending from groin to malleoli with the knee in full extension. Immobilization is continued for six weeks. The patient uses crutches and performs rehabilitative exercises even while in the cast. After the cast has been removed, the athlete should be started on a progressive, detailed rehabilitation program, emphasizing active muscular stabilization of the patella through VMO strengthening, stretching of tight thigh and calf muscles, and functional retraining of the limb. Immobilization treatment for six weeks gives the best chance for the patient to heal without recurrent instability episodes of the patella.

If this is not the first dislocation of the patella, or if we are convinced that this was an acute subluxation rather than a dislocation, we usually do not treat the athlete so aggressively. A cylinder cast is not indicated in these circumstances. Rather, we use a compressive dressing, with perhaps more temporary immobilization in one of the commercially available knee immobilizers. This is continued only for a few days until the acute symptoms begin to subside. Immobilization is followed by all of the detailed rehabilitative techniques for the extensor mechanism.

Osteochondral Fractures. With any acute instability episode of the patella, an osteochondral fracture may occur. Milgram originally described the mechanism by which this occurs.[6] As the patella either leaves or re-enters the femoral trochlea, a segment of bone and overlying articular cartilage may be sheared off, usually from either the lateral lip of the trochlea or the medial facet of the patella. Some of these fragments, if they contain sufficient bone, may be visible on the initial x-ray. In other cases, evidence of such a fracture may only come through finding fat droplets in the bloody aspirate from the knee. Fractures that are purely chondral in nature may not be apparent at all.

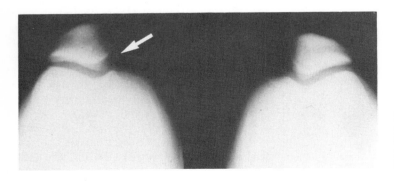

FIGURE 14. Infrapatellar x-ray. Avulsion fracture from medial edge of patella (arrow) is pathognomonic for recurrent patellar dislocation.

If there is a sizable osteochondral fracture visible on x-ray or suspected because of blood in the aspirate, then orthopaedic consultation is indicated. Arthroscopy of the knee may be necessary for large fractures. Occasionally a fragment must be re-attached with internal fixation. Some smaller osteochondral fractures simply can be observed and treated later if necessary. However, this is a decision that is probably best made by your orthopaedic consultant.

Recurrent Patellar Subluxation. Many patients will present to your office with recurrent slipping of the kneecap and giving away of the knee, but they have never experienced an acute episode of major proportions, certainly not a complete patellar dislocation. Examination will show the typical predisposing physical findings as well as hypermobility and apprehension. The patient should be able to associate the feeling of apprehension with the feeling he or she gets when trying to pivot, twist, or cut during sports. The primary care physician may successfully help these patients by prescribing a detailed rehabilitative exercise program as well as the use of a patellar brace. If this problem occurs in a relatively young individual, generalized growth and development with increased muscle bulk may also be a helpful factor. Certainly far greater than 50% of patients with this problem should respond to nonsurgical treatment. If the patient still has significant functional disability after attempting rehabilitation and patellar bracing, then orthopaedic referral is indicated. Various surgical approaches to this problem are available. Arthroscopic lateral release has gained a reputation for providing somewhat inconsistent results. Open methods of extensor mechanism reconstruction have existed for many decades and still tend to be quite helpful in the patient who has not been controlled through nonsurgical means.

Chondromalacia Patella. Even though it has precise pathologic meaning, the term "chondromalacia patella" has come to be applied to any condition that creates painful symptoms around the kneecap, especially crepitation and tenderness. In truth, this is an extremely difficult diagnosis to make with certainty through purely clinical or radiographic means. The term "chondromalacia of the patella" should be reserved for those cases in which objective articular cartilage changes are seen by the orthopaedic consultant, either at arthroscopy or arthrotomy.

The important point, though, is that chondromalacia of the patella does not occur spontaneously. It is a response of the patella to some abnormal mechanical situation, usually one of the syndromes of abnormal patellar tracking. If you believe strongly that your patient has chondromalacia, the appropriate treatment is, once again, a thorough rehabilitation exercise program, the use of a patellar brace, and administration of nonsteroidal anti-inflammatory drugs. Rather than using the term "chondromalacia patella" willy-nilly, it is probably better to use the term "patellofemoral pain syndrome."

Patellofemoral Pain Syndromes. On the opposite end of the spectrum from patients with patellar instability problems are patients with pain but with no symptoms of instability whatsoever. Indeed, even though examination of these patients shows the typical predisposing physical findings, one may not find any true hypermobility or apprehension on testing the patellae. The actual mechanisms of pain production in these syndromes has not been completely elucidated. Logically, however, pain is caused by inflammation of the peripatellar soft tissues such as the synovium. Undoubtedly, these patients are best treated with the three-part approach of rehabilitative exercises, patellar bracing, and nonsteroidal anti-inflammatory medication. Patients who do not respond to this protocol may be candidates for surgery and should be referred. Arthroscopy may be helpful in determining the source of the symptoms and perhaps in treating these problems through such procedures as patellar chondroplasty or debridement of peripatellar synovium.

Synovial Plica. Somewhere in the spectrum of patellofemoral pain syndrome is the entity that has been variously known as the synovial plica, the suprapatellar plica, the medial shelf, and the plica synovialis mediopatellaris. The actual structure is a shelf of synovium extending into the joint and then doubled back upon itself, which is believed to be remnant of the embryological division of the knee joint into three separate cavities: the medial pouch, the lateral pouch, and the suprapatellar pouch. As the embryo develops, these three pouches fuse together, with resorption of the old walls separating them. This resorption process may go on more or less completely. It is believed that the incompletely resorbed wall is what is found grossly as the synovial plica.

There may be a suprapatellar part to this structure. In fact, the suprapatellar pouch may still exist as a totally separate cavity. Usually, however, the more symptomatic part of the plica is the medial portion, which extends along the medial side of the patellofemoral joint. It is not fully known what percentage of the population has such a medial shelf. Arthroscopy has demonstrated that a large percentage of patients have it to a greater or lesser degree. The question remains as to how large a shelf is significant. Some are seen to extend a centimeter or more beneath the medial facet of the patella and are undoubtedly symptomatic. Others are quite narrow and soft and probably cause no trouble.

Diagnosing a synovial plica is as much a clinical challenge as it is merely finding the structure at arthroscopy or arthrotomy. Typically, the patient with a pathologic plica has pain that is greatly increased by sitting with the knee flexed for any period of time. The patient usually learns to extend the knee to relieve the pain. Often, when the knee is extended after sitting, there is a definite "pop" that occurs over the medial aspect of the patellofemoral joint and is associated with relief of the painful symptom. The patient soon learns to extend the knee and pop it to gain relief. There may be a report of mild recurrent knee swelling. Typically, there are also intermittent catching episodes. Occasionally, the patient will find that placing the knee in a slight amount of flexion provides the most comfortable resting position. Because of the nondescript and somewhat bizarre nature of these symptoms, many patients are labelled neurotic before the true diagnosis is finally made.

Physical examination for the plica is as described above. Even though this synovial abnormality could be expected to occur in patients without the other typical predispositions to extensor mechanism problems, it seems that most symptomatic plicae occur in patients with some element of extensor mechanism malalignment. Often the plica is only part of the overall picture in any given patient.

Successful conservative treatment depends on how far the inflammatory process has progressed in the synovial structure itself. Early, mild inflammatory changes may be reversed by anti-inflammatory medication and use of extensor mechanism rehabilitative techniques. Ice massage and hydrocortisone phonophoresis may also be tried. Corticosteroid injection of the plica has also been described, but it is difficult to imagine how one could really be certain of injecting only this synovial fold.

If conservative treatment fails, surgical treatment may be undertaken with good prospect for success. In fact, a plica may be one of the few knee problems for which surgical treatment results in essentially a normal knee. This view is predicated on the thought that this entity is a functionless embyrological remnant. On the other hand, if the plica is present with other extensor mechanism problems, arthroscopic excision may give only partial relief. Most often, even after plica excision, the patient finds it necessary to continue working on the extensor mechanism through rehabilitative exercise and perhaps external support.

Patellar Tendonitis ("Jumper's Knee"). Repetitive jumping in such sports as basketball and volleyball can create chronic inflammatory changes in the patellar tendon. Usually, the symptoms occur at the inferior pole of the patella, where the patellar tendon attaches. Even though the entire patellar tendon may be ultimately involved by some degenerative process, only rarely are the symptoms or findings referred to the body of the tendon itself. Observation would indicate that this patellar tendonitis rarely, if ever, occurs in a knee without the congenital predisposing physical findings we have discussed. Usually, patella alta and VMO dysplasia are prominent findings in the patient with jumper's knee. In addition, many of the factors known to aggravate other extensor mechanism disorders, such as inflexibility of the hamstrings, can greatly accentuate the symptoms of patellar tendonitis. Other than through a history of jumping sports, complaints of infrapatellar pain, and the presence of physical predisposition, the diagnosis of patellar tendonitis is made simply through palpation of the inferior pole of the patella (Fig. 5). Point tenderness in this area confirms the suspected diagnosis.

Chronic patellar tendonitis can be a terribly difficult problem to treat. Traditionally, VMO strengthening and stretching of the hamstrings, heel cords, and quadriceps have been used as rehabilitative techniques to deal with patellar tendonitis. Certainly they are important. More recently, work on the eccentric function of the quadriceps through a bounding program has been emphasized in dealing with this disorder. It has also been pointed out that, through a biomechanical linkage with ankle mechanics, most patients with chronic patellar tendonitis also have demonstrable weakness of the ankle dorsiflexor muscles. Good success in treating patellar tendonitis has been reported with a program of eccentric strengthening of ankle dorsiflexors. So far this appears to be our experience as well.

Beyond rehabilitative exercises, nonsteroidal anti-inflammatories are certainly worth a try. External support for the extensor mechanism using patellar bracing may be beneficial, though we have not found the straps manufactured specifically for patellar tendonitis to be of any help. Ice massage and deep-friction massage to the inflamed area also seem to be helpful. Hydrocortisone phonophoresis or iontophoresis may likewise be tried. However, one should *never* be tempted to use corticosteroid injection into the patellar tendon until all other techniques have been exhausted. To inject a major load-bearing tendon such as the patellar tendon is to weaken the tendon and invite further rupture. We inject a patellar tendon only as a desperate last measure, and only then with the patient's understanding that he or she must refrain from activity for a protracted period of time.

Is there any surgical treatment to offer the patient with intractable patellar tendonitis? None of the reported techniques seems to be very successful. Having been unsuccessful in all attempts to treat patellar tendonitis, you may wish to refer the patient for orthopaedic consultation, realizing that debridement of chronic inflammatory tissue, excision of the inferior pole of the patella, releasing the peritendinous sheath, or some other surgical approach may be the only avenue remaining.

Osgood-Schlatter's Disease. For many years, so-called Osgood-Schlatter's disease was considered to be one of the group of osteochondroses, that is, an avascular necrosis of one of the various growth centers in the immature skeleton. More recent thinking views the Osgood-Schlatter process as one part of the spectrum of mechanical problems related to the extensor mechanism. Almost all young patients with the disease have evidence of some mechanical inefficiency of the extensor mechanism. Most often, this is a significant patella alta. Dysplasia of the vastus medialis obliquus is difficult to judge in the typical age group with the disease because of general lack of musculoskeletal development at that age.

Making the diagnosis is not complicated. Usually there is a history of insidious onset of pain in the region of one or both tibial tuberosities. Occasionally there may be an acute episode superimposed on chronic symptoms, or, uncommonly, acute onset only. Acute onset may represent some additional avulsion of the cartilage along the anterior aspect of the tibial tuberosity apophysis. In the chronic setting, this process occurs more gradually. X-rays may vary from normal, in the early stage, to showing separate bony ossicles loose within the patellar tendon substance later in life. Almost all patients have marked inflexibility in hamstrings, heel cords, and quadriceps muscles.

The danger in treating Osgood-Schlatter's "disease" lies in overtreatment. In the past, casts, cortisone injections, and complete cessation of normal childhood activities have been recommended. In general, none of this is necessary. The mechanical inefficiencies of the extensor mechanism should be treated by appropriate rehabilitative exercises. All inflexibility should be addressed through stretching. As with patellar tendonitis, ankle dorsiflexion exercises are indicated if weakness can be demonstrated. Some sort of simple patellar support such as a neoprene rubber knee sleeve may be helpful. Any local padding over the tender tuberosity can be used to prevent a flare-up of symptoms when the knee is struck against another object. Nonsteroidal anti-inflammatories may help relieve the symptoms. Likewise, liberal use of icing techniques may help. However, throughout all of this treatment, the patient may carry on with whatever physical activity is comfortable. In other words, inactivity should not be enforced but rather should be advised based on any symptoms that might be present. Return to full and normal activity may take place as the symptoms recede. In the worst case, the patient will have persistent enlargement of the tibial tuberosity. This may intermittently become painful in later life. If the patient does develop a painful loose ossicle within the substance of the patellar tendon, excision may be indicated. In the most severe case, simple excision of the ossicle without extensor mechanism reconstruction and correction of the patella alta may not suffice. More extensive reconstruction may be necessary, with a thorough postoperative rehabilitation program. None of these possibilities, however, is affected by letting the early adolescent go ahead with a normal life-style. There is no convincing evidence that the Osgood-Schlatter's lesion leads to a disastrous consequence such as avulsion fracture of the tibial tuberosity.

SUMMARY

Disorders of the knee's extensor mechanism span a broad range, from syndromes characterized primarily by instability to those characterized solely by pain. All of these syndromes are related in origin by congenital predisposition. Some of these syndromes are simple and easy to manage. Most, however, are chronic or recurrent. Primary care physicians should become confident in their ability to assess such problems and have at their disposal a treatment plan that emphasizes rehabilitative exercise, simple physical modalities, anti-inflammatory medication, and bracing of the patella. When such a treatment program is made available to the patient, well over 50% of cases, and perhaps as many as 80–90% of cases, should be correctable.

REFERENCES

1. Goldthwait JE: Slipping or recurrent dislocation of the patella: with the report of eleven cases. Boston Med Surg J 150–169, 1904.
2. Hughston JC: Subluxation of the patella. J Bone Joint Surg 50A:1003, 1968.
3. Hughston JC, Walsh WM, Puddu G: Patellar Subluxation and Dislocation. Philadelphia, W. B. Saunders Co., 1984.
4. Insall J, Salvati E: Patella position in the normal knee joint. Radiology 101:101, 1971.
5. James SL: Chondromalacia of the patella in the adolescent. *In* Kennedy, JC, (ed): The Injured Adolescent Knee. Baltimore, Williams and Wilkins, 1979.
6. Milgram JE: Tangential osteochondral fracture of the patella. J Bone Joint Surg 25:271, 1943.

19 Evaluation and Treatment of the Injured Ankle

RICHARD B. BIRRER, M.D.

The ankle is a key focal point in the transmission of body weight during ambulation. It is capable of the adjustments necessary for fine balance on a wide variety of terrain. Because the joint is subject to the concentrated stress associated with standing as well as movement, the ankle is often involved in static and dynamic deformities that ordinarily do not affect other parts of the body. In fact, injuries to the ankle joint, the majority of which are seen by primary care physicians, are the most common conditions encountered in the treatment of athletic injuries. The prevalence of such injuries has been variously estimated to be between 10–90%, with the highest rate occurring in basketball players.[24,34] At least one study has estimated the incidence to be one significant ankle sprain per day per 10,000 population.[6] Furthermore, ankle injuries are not always minor and are associated with prolonged disability and recurrent instability in 25–40% of patients for several months to several years.[19] Therefore a casual approach (e.g., "it is only a sprain") to the diagnosis and management of these injuries is not tenable. The ubiquitous and unpredictable nature of ankle injuries mandates a precise understanding of the mechanism of injury, a thorough knowledge of the anatomy of the ankle joint, a clear ability to assess the degree of damage, and a solid understanding of appropriate treatment modalities in the acute and rehabilitative phases.

ANATOMY

The mortise (Fig. 1) formed by the distal articulation of the tibia, the fibula, and the dome of the talus constitutes the hinge joint of the ankle. Range of motion is only in one plane, plantar flexion and dorsiflexion. Plantar flexion is somewhat restricted due to the anterior widening of the talar dome. The subtalar joint of the foot allows for the full range of inversion, eversion, supination, and pronation. The two joints often work together as a universal-type joint with modification in one affecting the biomechanics and normal activity of the other. The medial malleolus, formed by the distal tibia, and the longer lateral malleolus, derived from the distal fibula, provide a significant amount of bony stability to the ankle joint through their downward extension along the talar dome. Functional integrity of the hinge joint is therefore sacrificed to structural stability.

Ligaments are the second important element in ankle stability. The larger and stronger deltoid ligament is fan shaped, arises from the medial malleolus, and inserts on the navicular, calcaneal, and talar bones. The medial ligament has both superficial (tibiotalar, tibiocalcaneal, and tibionavicular) and deep (posterior talotibial) components (Figs. 2,3). The ligament, particularly the latter component, stabilizes the joint during eversion and prevents subluxation. There are three distinct lateral collateral ligaments (Fig. 4). The anterior talofibular ligament arises from the anterior tip of the fibula and attaches to the lateral neck of the talus. Its function is to prevent anterior and lateral subluxation of the talus during plantar flexion. Running from the fibula tip to the lateral aspect of the calcaneus in a posteroinferior direction is the calcaneal fibular ligament. This ligament functions to prevent lateral subluxation of the talus during strong adduction of the calcaneus. The posterior talofibular ligament arises from the posterior aspect of the lateral malleolus and inserts on the posterolateral margin of the talus as the

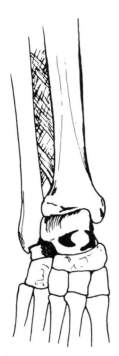

FIGURE 1. The ankle mortise is formed by the distal articulation of the tibia, the fibula, and the dome of the talus.

strongest of the three lateral collateral ligaments. It is responsible for preventing posterior subluxation of the talus during forced dorsiflexion.

The tibia and fibula are joined proximally by the interosseus membrane, whereas distally the two bones are held together by a strong syndesmosis consisting of the anterior and posterior inferior tibiofibular ligaments, the inferior transverse ligament, and the interosseus ligaments. The syndesmosis functions to maintain mortise stability, especially during dorsiflexion associated with weight bearing or the exertion of upward or outward pressure.

The synovial joint capsule also provides additional support, since it encapsulates the entire joint. It is recessed and lax in its anterior and posterior aspects to permit joint motion, although in some individuals it may be thickened anteriorly. The capsule is taut in the medial and lateral aspects, thus contributing to associated ligamentous support.

Lastly, a variety of tendons enhance the stability of the ankle. These are secondary stabilizers, because they transit the joint and have no firm attachments. Their superficial nature, however, makes them vulnerable to injury. The tendons have various locations and are responsible for foot and ankle range

Medial View

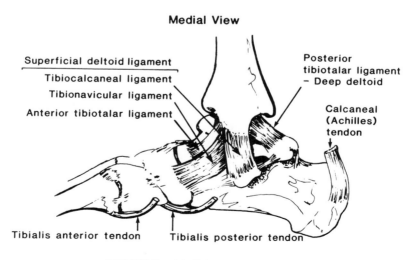

Superficial deltoid ligament
Tibiocalcaneal ligament
Tibionavicular ligament
Anterior tibiotalar ligament

Posterior tibiotalar ligament – Deep deltoid

Calcaneal (Achilles) tendon

Tibialis anterior tendon   Tibialis posterior tendon

FIGURE 2. Medial ankle ligaments.

REAR VIEW

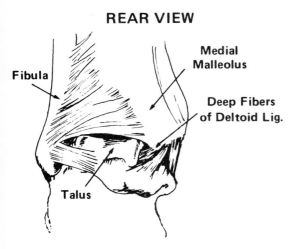

FIGURE 3. Posterior view of ankle demonstrates deep fibers of the deltoid ligament.

of motion. The extensors are located anteriorly whereas the flexors are situated posteriorly. The inverters are located medially and the everters laterally (Figs. 2 and 4).

Additionally there are a number of important soft tissue structures that, although they transit the ankle and are not essential to its structural stability, are important for the functional integrity of the joint and the foot.

The dorsal pedal artery lies on the anterior portion of the ankle and the foot between the extensor hallucis longus and the extensor digitorum longus tendons. In 10–15% of cases it is congenitally absent. It is a secondary source of blood supply to the foot. The long saphenous vein can be palpated medially and just anteriorly to the medial malleolus. The posterior tibial artery, the main blood supply to the foot, is located between the tendons of the flexor digitorum longus and the flexor hallucis longus muscles. It passes posterior and inferior to the medial malleolus and is not easily palpated unless the foot is non-weight bearing and slightly plantarflexed. Immediately posterior and lateral to the posterior tibial artery lies the tibial nerve. Although difficult to palpate as an isolated structure, the neurovascular bundle is joined to the tibia by a ligament that creates the tarsal tunnel. The tibial nerve is the main nerve to the sole of the foot. Posteriorly, the calcaneal bursa lies between the Achilles tendon and the overlying skin. The retrocalcaneal bursa is located between the posterosuperior angle of the calcaneus and the anterior surface of the tendoachilles. The deep peroneal nerve cannot be palpated. Sensation to the ankle is provided by L4 medially, L5 anteriorly, and the S1 dermatome laterally. The following peripheral nerves cover approximately the same area:

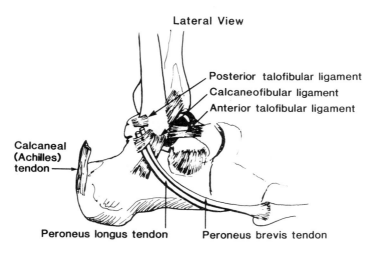

FIGURE 4. Lateral ankle ligaments.

medially, the long saphenous; anteriorly, the superficial peroneal; and laterally, the sural nerve. Finally, lymphatic channels accompany the corresponding vascular bundles. There is a minimum amount of adipose tissue in and about the ankle and a thin amount of elastic skin overlies all of these structures.

GENERAL PATHOGENETIC MECHANISMS OF INJURY

There is 20 to 30 degrees of ankle motion in the sagittal plane during normal ambulation. With further stress, particularly during passive range of motion testing, the hinge joint can achieve 20 degrees of dorsiflexion and up to 50 degrees of plantar flexion; in the coronal plane five degrees of inversion and ten degrees of abduction. Further stress in any of these planes will lead to structural instability.

There are a number of anatomical factors that contribute to ankle injury. Ankle mortise asymmetry creates inherent instability during inversion. The longer lateral malleolus provides a mechanical barrier to eversion ligamentous injury due to its greater surface contact with the talus. In addition, the dome of the talus is appreciably wider anteriorly than posteriorly. During inversion and plantar flexion, the narrow posterior aspect of the talus occupies proportionately less space within the mortise. As a result there is increased ankle joint play, which together with the inherent block to eversion results in predominantly lateral stress forces. Additional complicating factors include tight heel cords and deficient proprioception. Many athletes, particularly females, have tight heel cords that force heel inversion. Regular walking on smooth flat surfaces leads to a proprioceptive deficiency, which is aggravated on irregular rough playing surfaces. Finally, the lateral ligaments of the ankle are smaller and weaker than the medial deltoid ligament. Nonanatomical factors such as surface configuration and footwear are often responsible for injury. Irregular surfaces, particularly those with holes, can produce obvious damage to the ankle. Less obvious circumstances such as banked tracks can lead to repetitive ankle trauma and long-term ankle disability.

Finally, defective, old or inappropriately fitted footwear can result in inversion or eversion stress.

CLINICAL EVALUATION

History. The following items should be carefully investigated in all ankle injuries:

1. What was the position of the foot and direction of stress when the injury occurred (e.g., eversion, inversion, flexion, extension, or a combination)?
2. Was there immediate disability or did symptoms occur at a later time?
3. At the time of injury were there any snaps, pops or crunches noted?
4. When and to what degree were pain, swelling, and discoloration noted?
5. Were there any preexisting problems associated with the joint (i.e., previous injury or systemic disease)?
6. Was medical care sought out? What did the evaluation show? Was treatment initiated, and if so, what were the results?
7. Did the injury ocur acutely or from overuse?
8. What is the functional capacity of the joint at present?
9. What were the surface conditions at the time of injury?

As a final comment it should be understood that a careful history usually will identify the site of pathology and severity of tissue trauma. There are situations, however, where a misdiagnosis can result.

Examination. The clinical examination begins with an inspection of the contour and alignment of the joint, particularly noting any swelling, abrasions, lacerations, or discolorations. The patient should then be asked to demonstrate the overall functional capacity, strength, range of motion, and agility of the joint (i.e., while sitting, standing, walking, running, and at rest). The ankle should be carefully examined for painful trigger points, crepitance, temperature, passive range of motion, and neurovascular status (e.g., sensation, strength, reflexes, and pulses). The abnormal ankle should be compared with the normal ankle throughout the entire examination. A thorough ankle evaluation includes examination of the foot and footwear, leg, knee, hip, and lower back. Occasionally, a local anesthetic injection of 1% lidocaine is useful.

Once the patient's confidence has been gained, the joint should be stressed in a number of maneuvers. The anterior drawer test, which is performed with the patient lying on the examination table with the ankle at 90°, consists of drawing the calcaneus and talus anteriorly while stabilizing the tibia (Fig. 5). Sliding of the talus anteriorly by more than 3–5 mm or a difference of greater than 0.5 mm between ankles is abnormal. A soft endpoint or the perception of a "clunk" may be appreciated and is considered a positive anterior draw sign. The talar tilt test is performed by stressing the ankle laterally (inversion) and medially (eversion) while stabilizing the patient's leg (Fig. 6). A tear of the deep deltoid ligament will produce a palpable gap on the medial aspect of the ankle mortise. Gapping or rocking of the ankle mortise on the lateral side during lateral inversion stress indicates tears of both the anterior talofibular and the calcaneofibular ligaments. The normal angle of inversion talar tilt is up to 15°, although some individuals with ligamentous laxity may tilt up to 20° without a tear. A difference of 5° between ankles is highly suggestive of a tear, and 10° is diagnostic.

Stress films are the best way to confirm equivocal physical findings. Routine xrays include anterior, lateral, and oblique mortise films. Routine films should be supplemented by passive stress test radiographs when the clinical findings are inconclusive. Soft tissue should be examined for swelling and foreign bodies, joint spaces for widening or narrowing, and bones for dislocation or fractures (avulsion or osteochondral).

It is occasionally advisable for the purpose of diagnostic accuracy that radiographs be taken of the normal side for comparison. If the stress films are positive, further evaluation is unnecessary. If stress films are inconclusive and there is a strong clinical suspicion of a complete tear, an arthrogram may be ordered. After a sterile prep and drape, the test is performed on the anterior portion of the joint opposite the area of suspected injury. After initial aspiration, a 10 ml solution consisting of 1 ml of lidocaine and 9 ml of contrast material (e.g., 25% Hypaque solution) is slowly injected and then AP, lateral, and oblique films are obtained. Although the dye may enter tendon sheaths surrounding the ankle and may flow even to the subtalar joint, dye appearing outside the joint capsule or the surrounding tendon sheath is abnormal. The incidence of false negative examinations rises significantly due to healing after the first week following injury. Arthroscopy can also help detect tears and debris.

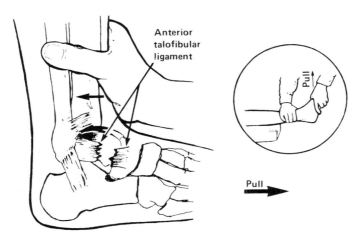

FIGURE 5. Anterior drawer test.

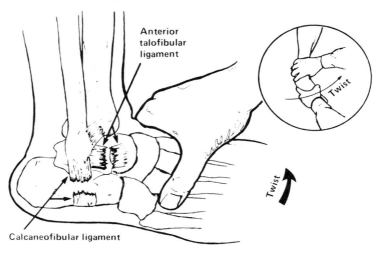

FIGURE 6. Talar tilt test.

ON FIELD MANAGEMENT OF ANKLE INJURIES

Clearly the results of an ankle evaluation will depend on the time of presentation and the time lapse between injury and the subsequent evaluation. Unfortunately, the majority of injuries are perceived as mild, and the athlete does not seek help for several days until the amount of swelling, functional disability, and spasm are maximum. The initial 20–30 minutes following injury have been termed the "golden period." During this period there is usually no discoloration, swelling or disability evident. Pathogenetically, the acute inflammatory process is still in its initial biochemical phase. Therefore, immediate evaluation of an injury through palpation will be extremely valuable in eliciting point tenderness before diffuse swelling, discoloration, and pain prohibit visual identification of the precise location of injury. It is possible to actually palpate the gap in a torn tendon or ligament during the early phase of an injury. Remember to compare and contrast results to the uninjured side in order to estimate deviation from normal ligament tightness. After inspection and palpation, active and passive range of motion should be evaluated and the stress tests (vide supra) performed.

The immediate treatment for all acute ankle injuries consists of the RICE regimen.[10] R stands for rest; I stands for ice and immobilization; C stands for compression; and E stands for elevation. Ice should be applied for 15–20 minutes (i.e., ice cubes in a plastic bag or a crushed ice slurry) every two hours for the first 24 hours. The ice should not be placed in direct contact with the skin. Cryotherapy should be continued for 48–72 hours and can be discontinued once edema and inflammation have subsided.[10] Immobilization is best achieved by taping with adhesive surgical tape or a posterior splint made from fiberglass or plaster of paris. An elastic wrap can be used for compression, but it is an inadequate support device. At least one study suggests that a 24-hour period of immobilization and compression followed by rapid mobilization will achieve full functional mobility in 99% of patients in two weeks with soft tissue injuries.[7]

Return to play is perhaps the most difficult area for a team physician. In the acute situation only those with the mildest ankle injuries (i.e., no edema, no pain, no spasm, and no functional disability) should be allowed to return to competition, with the understanding that the ankle is to be taped and cryotherapy regularly applied during rest periods. For more severe injuries or injuries that have not been completely evaluated, the athlete should be removed from play. In general, an athlete should not be allowed to return to play until the range of motion and strength of the injured ankle is equal to that of the uninjured side.

SPECIFIC INJURIES

Contusions. The most commonly bruised areas of the ankle are the malleoli.[26] The usual mechanism of injury is a direct blow or fall on the exposed surface. The differential diagnosis should consider a sprain or a fracture, especially the former since many sprains will produce maximal tenderness on the malleoli themselves. Radiographs are usually negative, although that does not necessarily mean that the injury is only a contusion. Functional pain or slow healing should make one suspicious of a concommitant incomplete or fissure type fracture. Unless there has been a severe crush injury, ankle function is disturbed very little in an ordinary contusion. Thus it is imperative to carefully inspect and palpate the injured ankle, noting any complications of the blow (i.e., tenosynovitis of the tendoachilles, dislocated peroneal tendons, etc.). The initial treatment is the RICE regimen followed by sterile aspiration of any large hematomas present, and the fitting of a protective appliance such as a sponge, or felt donut. Full recovery should be expected within several days to a week and return to play is therefore rapid.

Peroneal Subluxation/Dislocation. The peroneal retinaculum can be torn with a direct blow to the back of the lateral malleolus while the tendons are taut in eversion and dorsiflexion.[20,29] Powerful contraction of the peroneal muscles, particularly in maximal dorsiflexion, occurs most often in wrestling and down-hill or cross country skiing. Acute subluxation of the peroneal tendon is relatively uncommon and is most often confused with simple lateral ligament sprains. The tenderness and swelling, however, are centered behind the lateral malleolus and extend proximally over the tendons. They are absent over the anterolateral ankle capsule, where they would usually be found in a typical lateral sprain. One or both of the peroneal tendons may pop out of the groove onto the lateral aspect of the malleolus. Reduction is usually spontaneous. Differential diagnosis should include an ankle sprain, contu-

sion, and tenosynovitis. Palpation will reveal direct tenderness over the tendons, which may be confused with tenosynovitis. With acute dislocations it is not possible to displace the tendon during the examination. Treatment consists in relocation, if necessary by directing pressure on the tendon posteriorly and then casting the ankle in slight pronation and flexion. The plaster should be carefully molded to apply firmly to the contour of the lateral malleolus or a J-shaped piece of felt used to compress the tendon in place. Surgery should be considered for failed conservative therapy or for the serious athlete in whom lost time would be critical.

Untreated acute episodes or congenital weakness will result in chronic or recurrent subluxation of the peroneal tendons. There is usually a history of an acute injury, with appreciable soreness for many weeks followed by the recurrent feeling of something slipping out of place at the posterior portion of the ankle during foot eversion. There may be sharp pain and considerable stress noted with the condition. On physical examination, the retinaculum is usually thickened and the groove shallow. It is often possible to manually sublux or dislocate the tendons. Treatment once again is surgical.

Sprains

Mechanism. Sprains of the ankle constitute the most common form of ligamentous injury and are one of the most common injuries that the orthopedist, emergency room physician, or primary care physician manages.[4,9] Sprains can be classified clinically and pathologically. Grade I (mild) is a completely stable ligament with less than 25% of fibers torn. Grade II (moderate) is an unstable ligament with a solid end point and represents tearing of 25–75% of the fibers. Grade III (severe) is synonymous with an unstable ligament having no or an extremely mushy end point (tearing of greater than 75% of the fibers). Although the grades are based on the clinical findings and the result of diagnostic stress tests and radiographs, grading is nonetheless somewhat of a subjective exercise.[11]

INVERSION/INTERNAL ROTATION INJURIES. Eighty-five percent of ankle sprains occur to the lateral collateral ligaments during plantar inversion. The usual scenario is an athlete who has been running (i.e., football, basketball, etc.) or skiing and who changes course in the direction of the ankle in question either losing his balance or being disturbed by an external force, resulting in marked supination.[16] In 85% of situations the anterior talofibular ligament is injured[4,6] This represents 65% of all ankle sprains. With continued force in external leg rotation, supination, and mild dorsiflexion, the calcaneal fibular ligament will also be injured. Twenty percent of all ankle sprains represent combined injury to these ligaments. The posterior talofibular ligament is injured in 1% of cases due to further forced dorsiflexion.

EVERSION/EXTERNAL ROTATION INJURIES. Ten to fifteen percent of ankle sprains involve the medial collateral or tibiofibular ligament complexes. A sharp cut-away from the involved ankle with severe pronation of the foot and internal leg rotation is the usual mechanism of injury. (Fig. 7). Initially the anterior portion of the superficial deltoid ligament (i.e., tibial navicular ligament), the anteromedial capsule, and the anterior smaller portion of the deep deltoid are involved. The mortise remains stable. With progressively more stress, sequential injuries occur to the anterior inferior tibiofibular ligament, the interosseus membrane and ligament, the remaining portions of the superficial deltoid ligament, and the deep deltoid ligament (i.e., the inferior transverse ligament and posterior inferior tibiofibular ligament), resulting in complete diastasis of the tibia and fibula.

Clinical Presentation. A careful history (vide supra) will elicit a history of a twisting motion applied to the weight-bearing joint usually in association with internal rotation, adduction, and the foot flipping under the ankle.[31] Such relatively low force activities are running, walking, or stepping off curbs are typically recalled; the mechanism of injury in high velocity competitive conditions often are unknown. The athlete usually complains of a sudden intense localized transient pain. Three-quarters of patients will be able to bear weight on the injured ankle and one-third will give a history of previous sprains. Unless seen during the "golden period," the degree of edema generally increases with time and may involve the entire ankle. Grade II and III sprains are characterized by hemarthrosis in 60-70% of cases and ecchymosis in 50-60% 24 hours after injury. The edema and distortion tend to be more severe in individuals who continue to be physically active following their injury. Although the area of ligamentous injury is always tender, 30-

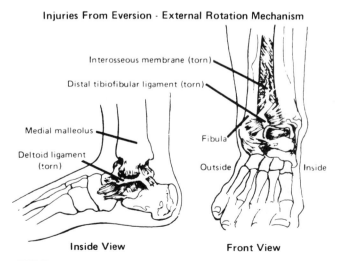

Injuries From Eversion - External Rotation Mechanism

Interosseous membrane (torn)

Distal tibiofibular ligament (torn)

Medial malleolus

Deltoid ligament (torn)

Fibula

Outside   Inside

Inside View   Front View

FIGURE 7. Injuries from eversion external rotation mechanism.

45% of patients will complain of tenderness in uninjured adjoining ligaments. Thus, palpation should always begin in the injured ankle farthest from the suspected site of injury. Remember to always compare the clinical findings to the normal side. In addition to evaluating individual ligaments by palpation, the integrity of the fibula and tibia should be checked. Point tenderness or crepitus should raise the suspicion of an associated fracture. Active range of motion, particularly that reproducing the mechanism of injury, will predictably reproduce pain. This can be confirmed by passive range of motion and stress testing.[31]

INVERSION/INTERNAL ROTATION INJURIES. The anterior drawer test will demonstrate anterior displacement with tears of the anterior talofibular. If there is clinical suspicion of a significant tear of the anterior talofibular ligament in a patient with a negative or equivocal anterior drawer test, anterior drawer stress x-rays should be performed.

The lateral (inversion) talar tilt test will demonstrate tears of the calcaneofibular ligament. Since the calcaneofibular ligament can only be torn when there is a concurrent tear of the anterior talofibular ligament, the anterior drawer test should be positive whenever there is a positive lateral talar tilt test. If there is clinical suspicion of a significant tear of the calcaneofibular ligament in a patient with a negative or equivocal lateral talar tilt test, talar tilt stress xrays should be performed.

EVERSION/EXTERNAL ROTATION INJURIES. Medial stress films will assess the integrity of the deltoid ligament complex. Widening of the space between the talus and medial malleolus of greater than 2 mm indicates an unstable tear of the deep deltoid ligament. If there is separation of the distal tibia and fibula, a tear of the anterior-inferior tibiofibular ligament and interosseus ligament is also present. Similarly an anterior displacement of greater than 3 mm indicates a complete tear of the anterior talofibular ligament during anterior drawer stress radiographs.

Treatment. A Grade I sprain is indicated by the absence of functional or anatomical instability. Treatment is purely supportive and is aimed at the rapid restoration of normal ankle motion and stength.[15,32] The RICE regimen should be utilized for the first 24–48 hours and thereafter as needed during the rehabilitative process.[10,13,28] Crutches or a cane should be utilized if there is any swelling or pain on weight bearing. The cane should be used on the contralateral uninjured side and single crutches are not recommended. Active range of motion exercises within the limits of pain should be encouraged once edema has subsided. This should be supplemented by passive range of motion (ROM) and progressive resistance exercises (PRE).[30] Utilizing an elastic bandage or neoprene inner tube, isometric strengthening exercises can also be used. Although complete anatomical healing will require four to six weeks, strength and range of motion exercises will usually permit return to play in one to two weeks. It is advisable that in the competitive situation adhesive surgical strapping be utilized to strengthen the ankle.[21]

The RICE regimen, which is usually continued for longer periods of time (48–72 hours), is also adequate for Grade II sprains. To assure immobilization, a posterior splint, Unna boot, or adhesive surgical strapping may be applied with the ankle in approximately a 90 degree position until edema and pain has subsided.[18] Thereafter weight bearing, ROM, and PRE exercises, utilizing supplemental adhesive strapping are initiated and supplemented by ice water or contrast soaks in order to promote the rehabilitative process.[3,30] Supplemental adhesive strapping should be utilized during training.[22] Several weeks to months should be allowed for complete healing, and return to play should only be initiated once there is return of full range of motion and strength. It should be noted that some practitioners prefer cast immobilization for short periods of time. Such an approach may be useful in unstable injuries, although its routine use in stable sprains results in considerable amount of athletic deconditioning and disuse atrophy.

Some ideal treatment for third degree sprains (i.e., nonoperative versus operative) is controversial.[1] The Grade II regimen or the application of a cast for six weeks followed by an additional six weeks of ankle protection (e.g., cane, crutches, or adhesive strappings) represents the nonoperative approach.[5,8] The rehabilitative process (e.g., ROM and PRE exercise) begins after cast removal and is continued until full strength and range of motion are achieved, which may require three to six months from the time of injury. Whereas conservative intervention is a reasonable option for Grade III sprains of the lateral ligaments, significant tears of the deep deltoid require surgical intervention.

The operative approach for Grade III ankle sprains consists of accurate anatomical reapposition of the torn ligaments and in the case of the deep deltoid, is considered the best way to maximize joint function and restore ligament strength. Primary surgical intervention should occur within the first seven to ten days postinjury. There is a risk of postoperative complications, and secondary reconstructive repairs are always possible for patients who have significant chronic symptoms. Following surgery, management is similar to that of the nonoperative approach for about three months. Although the incidence of chronic ankle instability in patients treated by surgery is difficult to determine, it appears to be approximately 5%.

Several words of caution are necessary concerning the management of sprains. In general it is best to err on the conservative side when it comes to diagnosis and be liberal when it comes to treatment and rehabilitation. One of the greatest mistakes is to allow an athlete with a Grade II sprain to return too early to competition and suffer reinjury or a Grade III sprain. In addition to misdiagnosis, rehabilitation is most commonly overlooked as a priority area. Specific ankle exercises (eversion, inversion, flexion, and dorsiflexion) should be known and taught by the practitioner. Proper warm-up and the recommendation of using a high-topped shoe or sneaker for routine activity as well as training should be a regular part of the physician's armamentarium. Remember to utilize serial evaluations if the degree of injury is unclear. Finally, it is important to consider the patient's chronological age and functional capacity when deciding the most appropriate therapy. Nonoperative approaches are usually utilized for middle-aged individuals or occasional athletes, whereas surgery is reserved for the young active person or older competitive athlete.

Strains of the Ankle.   Because the ankle is subject to static and dynamic forces, strains of the joint are very common in a wide variety of sports. Strains may be classified in a similar fashion as sprains. The ankle joint per se is not involved in strains. The simple switching from street shoes, which have a firm medial support and heel with a strong contour, to an athletic shoe, which has no heel, minimal support, and weak contour, can cause a static strain of the tibial muscles. Medial strains involve the tibialis anterior, whereas the tibialis posterior is usually vulnerable at its attachment to the tuberosity of the naviculus or vulnerable under its medial side due to its dual roles in effecting inversion and plantar flexion, as well as supporting the foot arch. Tenderness will usually be palpable at the medial border of the arch, with some spread under the arch and the back of the medial malleolus. The tendoachilles can be strained at its site of attachment to the calcaneus, along the tendon's course, or most frequently at the musculotendinous junction. It is usually associated with a tenosynovitis.

Stronger forces in a middle-aged weekend athlete, particularly a forceful drive, push-off, or landing in forceful dorsiflexion, as in basketball, racquet sports, or broad jumping, can result in spontaneous rupture of the tendon.[19] The differential diagnosis should include strain of the calf musculature, contusion, or an ankle sprain. The individual will often complain of a sensation of being accidently kicked or struck by a ball in the back of the calf. A slight limp may be noted on examination, with variable amounts of edema and tenderness on palpation. If seen during the "golden period," a palpable gap will be noted and the Thompson squeeze test will be positive. If the injury is seen several hours after the trauma occurred, swelling may obscure the gap. Active range of motion will still preserve plantar flexion due to intact peroneal, tibial, and toe flexor muscle groups. For younger active individuals surgical repair is indicated. Nonoperative results are usually excellent and are reserved for the older athlete whose primary interests are return to work and everyday routine activities, rather than athletic performance.

Tibio-Talar Impingement Syndrome. Repeated microtrauma to the neck of the talus due to impaction with the anterior edge of the distal tibia when an athlete "drives" off of his planted foot will in time produce a proliferative bony spur and eventual impingement. Such spurs are commonly observed at the neck of the talus and the anterior lip of the tibia, although they have been noted to occur elsewhere about the ankle or with different types of impingement. The complaint of vague ankle pain, particularly during running, cutting, or pushing off at full speed, in association with some point tenderness and swelling over the anterior aspect of the ankle should suggest the diagnosis. Limited or forced dorsiflexion-producing pain is confirmatory. Radiographs will visualize the spur. Initially rest and oral anti-inflammatory agents are recommended, and surgery is reserved for resistant symptomatic cases. The differential diagnosis should include sprains and marginal osteophytes from degenerative joint disease. The latter do not respond well to surgical removal.

Fractures. Significant ligament injuries are often associated with fractures. For instance, a deltoid ligament rupture may avulse the medial malleolus and lead to a spiral fracture of the distal fibula, the most frequent ankle fracture. Similarly, rupture of the lateral collateral ligament can lead to a vertical fracture of the medial malleolus. Such fractures must be accompanied by a lateral fracture or Grade III sprain of the lateral collateral ligament. Tibiofibular ligament damage can be accompanied by a medial malleolus fracture due to eversion. Any distal tibiofibular fracture at the joint line should suggest deltoid ligament injury. Displaced malleolar fractures are often accompanied by ligamentous injury. Avulsion injuries cause transverse malleolar fractures, whereas compression of the talus will result in vertical malleolar fractures. Compression forces that injure the ankle may also damage the spine and calcaneus. Such associated trauma should be suspected and diligently searched for. Results of the clinical evaluation may be very similar to those associated with a sprain of the ankle. AP, lateral, and mortise views are usually adequate to make the diagnosis.

Stable injuries resulting from a single fracture or ligament tear require no reduction and can be treated with a posterior splint and the RICE regimen, followed by a walking cast for four to six weeks. Unstable injuries due to a sprain, a fracture, or various combinations thereof, require reduction.[33] Initially closed manipulation may be successful; however, open reduction is often required. Isometric exercises and plaster cast or early range of motion exercises in a hinge cast will minimize the harmful effects of immobilization (e.g., stiffness and muscle atrophy). Internal fixation devices should generally be removed before the athlete is allowed to return to play in contact sports. Unstable injuries tend to have a very high incidence of complications (e.g., traumatic arthritis, persistent talar instability, Sudeck's atrophy, or ossification of the interosseus membrane).

Small fragments of subchondral bone and overlying articular cartilage can be separated from the talar dome due to compressive or repetitive shearing-type loads, particularly in forced plantar flexion.[12,14,23] The lesion may be located anywhere on the talar dome. There is a gradual onset of pain, which becomes worse over weeks or even months, intensifies with exercise, and usually causes ankle stiffness or locking. Although special radiographic views may visualize the lesion, radiosotope studies or a computerized axial tomogram will produce the best results. Once the diagnosis has been made of a loose fragment in this area, orthopedic consultation should be considered.

Repetitive microtrauma from running can lead to a stress fracture of the distal fibula. Lateral ankle pain may suggest a peroneal tendonitis or a sprain, but the onset of localized firm swelling should suggest the diagnosis. Rest, with a slowly progressive training program within the limits of pain, is the treatment of choice.

Tenderness and soft tissue swelling about the distal fibular epiphysis must be considered a Type I Salter-Harris fracture in a youngster following trauma.[21] Although radiographs may be normal, immobilization in a short leg cast for four to five weeks is appropriate.

CONCLUSION

The majority of ankle injuries will present to the primary care physician. With a solid understanding of anatomy, mechanism of injury, and intervention techniques, most of these injuries will resolve and return to play will be successful. Consultation is advised if the diagnosis is unclear, or symptomatology or clinical findings persist, or the rehabilitative process is nonprogressive. A solid differential diagnosis will avoid misclassifying osteochondral fractures as chronic sprains or mistaking a strain or tendinitis for a fracture. Finally, the continuous care provided by a family physician will identify a problem before an irreversible or poor result is established.

REFERENCES

1. Balduini, FC: Historical perspectives on injuries of the ligaments of the ankle. Clin Sports Med 1:3, 1982.
2. Boccanera, L., Laus, M., Lelli, A.: Chronic lateral instability of the ankle. Ital J Ortho Traumatol 8:315, 1982.
3. Bonci, CM: Adhesive strapping techniques. Clin Sports Med 1:99, 1982.
4. Brostrom, L.: Sprained Ankles, 3: Clinical Observations in Recent Ligament Ruptures. Acta Clin Scand 130:560, 1965.
5. Cetti R.: Conservative treatment of injury to the fibular ligaments of the ankle. Br J Sports Med 16:47, 1982.
6. Connolly, JF: Mechanisms of injuries: The management of fractures and dislocations. Philadelphia, W.B. Saunders, 1981.
7. Crean, D: The management of soft tissue ankle injuries. Br J Sports Med 15:75, 1981.
8. Drez, Jr., D., et al.: Nonoperative treatment of double lateral ligament tears of the ankle. Am J Sports Med 10:197, 1982.
9. Guise, ER: Rotational ligamentous injuries to the ankle in football. Am J Sports Med 4:1, 1976.
10. Hocutt, JE, Jr., et al.: Cryotherapy in ankle injuries. Am J Sports Med 10:316, 1982.
11. Hutson, MA, Jackson JP: Injuries to the lateral liga-

ment of the ankle: Assessment and treatment 16:245, 1982.
12. Israeli, A., et al.: Traumatic osteochondral lesions of the talus. Br J Sports Med 15:159, 1981.
13. Kay, DB: The sprained ankle: Current therapy. Foot ankle 6:22, 1985.
14. Keene, JS, Lange, RH: Diagnosis dilemmas in foot and ankle injuries. JAMA 256:247-251, 1986.
15. Landry, ME: The common inversion sprain and its treatment in the athlete. J Am Podiatry Assoc 66:266, 1976.
16. Leach, RE, Lower, G: Ankle injuries in skiing. Clin Orthop 198:127, 1985.
17. Lindenbaum, BL: Ski boot compression syndrome. Clin Orthop 140:109, 1979.
18. MacCartee, CC, Jr.: Taping treatment of severe inversion sprains of the ankle. Early return to functional activities. Am J Sports Med 5:246, 1977.
19. Mack, RP: Ankle injuries in athletics. Clin Sports Med 1:71, 1982.
20. McLennan, JG. Treatment of acute and chronic subluxations of the peroneal tendons. Am J Sports Med 8:432, 1980.
21. Micheli, LJ, Smith, AD: Sports injuries in children. Curr Probl Pediatr 12:1, 1982.
22. Nemeth, VA, Thrasher, E: Adhesive strapping techniques. Clin Sports Med 2:217, 1983.
23. Paulos, LE, Johnson, CL, Noyes FR: Posterior compartment fractures of the ankle: A commonly missed athletic injury. Am J Sports Med 11:439, 1983.
24. Sando, B: Injuries to the ankle. Aust Fam Phys 13:581, 1984.
25. Scheller, AD, Kasser, JR, Quigley, TB: Tendon injuries about the ankle. Orthop Clin North Am 11:801, 1980.
26. Sinton, WA: The ankle: Soft tissue injuries. J Sports Med 1:47, 1973.
27. Smart, GW, Tautin, JE, Clement, DB: Achilles tendon disorders in runners: A review. Med Sci Sports Exerc 12:231, 1980.
28. Starkey, JA: Treatment of ankle sprains by simultaneous use of intermittent compression and ice packs. Am J Sports Med 4:142, 1976.
29. Stover, CN: Recognition and management of soft tissue injuries of the ankle in the athlete. Primary Care 7:183, 1980.
30. Teow, G: Physiotherapy in the management of sports injuries. Med J Malaysia 33:277, 1979.
31. Turco, VJ: Injuries to the ankle and foot in athletics. Orthop Clin North Am 8:669, 1977.
32. Vegso, JJ, Harmon, LE: Nonoperative management of athletic ankle injuries. Clin Sports Med 1:85, 1982.
33. Walsh, WM, Hughston, JC: Unstable ankle fractures in athletes. AM J Sports Med 4:173, 1976.
34. Weiker, GG: Ankle injuries in the athlete. Primary Care 11:101, 1984.

20 Bicycling Injuries: Prevention, Diagnosis, and Treatment

JEFFREY W. HILL, M.D.
MORRIS B. MELLION, M.D.

The popularity of the bicycle both as a recreational vehicle and mode of transportation is skyrocketing. In 1980, 27% of the adult population rode a bicycle at least once a week.[26] Since Americans won four bicycle gold medals in the 1984 Los Angeles Olympics and American Greg Lemond won the 1986 Tour de France, bicycle fever has risen even more in the United States. Not only are there traditional single, three and ten speed bicycles, but now there has been an explosion of racing bikes; 15, 18, and even 21 speed touring bikes; all terrain bikes; triathlon bikes; and city bikes. Bicycles are traversing all kinds of terrain in all kinds of weather. TV coverage of bicycle events is now commonplace.

With an increase in riding enthusiasm there is also an increase in injuries. In just one year, between 1973 and 1974, there was a 24% increase of bicycle-related injuries. Bicycle deaths increased 24% between 1967 and 1974, 90% of those being involved with a motor vehicle. One study showed 12 to 20% of all bike injuries are associated with a collision with a motor vehicle, with associated death rates of 0 to 14%. Accidents occur most commonly between the ages of six and sixteen, with 77% in one study in this age range. The most common bicycle types associated with injury are the single-speed and ten-speed bicycles, probably because these are the most common types in use. Mechanical failure accounts for 14 to 20% of injury. The most common traumatic injuries are associated with the face and head, wrist, knee, ankle and foot, with the majority of these being soft tissue injury.[6]

The primary care physician will also be faced with the challenge of diagnosing and treating non-traumatic problems arising from this recreational activity. The focus of this chapter will deal with these non-traumatic or overuse syndromes associated with bicycle riding, with limited emphasis on traumatic injury. In order to treat and rehabilitate the injured cyclist, the physician needs a working knowledge of bicycle anatomy, proper technique for fitting the bicycle to the rider, proper riding techniques and bicycle safety equipment. The first section of the chapter focuses on these issues. The second section will be devoted to the common overuse problems encountered, focusing on diagnosis and treatment (mechanical as well as medical).

THE MODERN BICYCLE

Most individuals in today's bicycle buying public are fairly sophisticated and know what they want, what they need, and how much they should spend. This is vastly different from the earlier bicycle boom in the 1970s. Today there are over 400 new models of bicycles introduced every year.[30] The major types of bikes include racing, sport touring, triathlon, city, long distance touring, and all terrain bicycles, each designed for different purposes and terrain. Bicycle selection should be guided by the type and amount of riding a person plans to do. Probably the most important aspect of bicycle buying is the type of frame. Most component parts of the bicycle can be changed, but a good frame is essential. Materials are changing drastically in frame composition. The old steel frame is being replaced by lighter, more resilient and durable chrome-magnesium alloy, aluminum, and even carbon fiber compositions. All of this adds up to a stronger, lighter, better-handling bicycle.

The primary care physician needs to have a working knowledge of the "anatomy and terminology" of the bicycle. (Fig. 1). Treatment of overuse syndromes not only involves medical therapy but most importantly an awareness of the bicycle's fit to the rider. Without knowledge of the relationship of the improperly adjusted bike to overuse syndromes, rehabilitation can be prolonged unnecessarily, causing much frustration and "doctor shopping" from displeased patients.

Fitting the Bicycle. There are five basic adjustments that need to be made in fitting the bicycle to the rider.[7,26] These include the frame size, seat height, seat position, handlebar height and reach. The proper frame size is a critical item, being determined easily be straddling the top tube of the bicycle with both feet flat on the ground (Fig. 2). The correct frame size allows 1 to 2 inches between the crotch and the top tube. If the groin touches the tube the frame is too large, and if there is greater than 3 inch clearance between the groin and top tube the frame is too small.

Seat height is determined by putting the pedals at the six o'clock and twelve o'clock position with the ball of the foot on the pedal; there should be 10 to 15 degrees of flexion of the knee of the extended leg (Fig. 3). Generally speaking, in patients who complain of posterior knee pain, the seat is usually adjusted too high, and if there are complaints of anterior, medial, or lateral knee discomfort, the seat is too low. It is important to note that if seat height is improper, adjustments need to be made in small increments over several weeks allowing the knee to adjust to the new position.

Seat position is determined by putting the pedals at the three o'clock and nine o'clock position, with the ball of the foot firmly in the pedal (Fig. 4). A plumb line is dropped from the forward knee, at the middle of the knee cap. This line should drop straight through the axle of the pedal. The seat should also be parallel to the top tube or very slightly angled upward anteriorly.

Handlebar height should be adjusted, so that the handlebars are equal to or just below the level of the top of the seat (Fig. 5). Reach is defined as a distance from the front of the saddle to the transverse handle bars. This can be determined by placing the elbow at the front of the seat, with the olecranon touching the anterior aspect of the seat. The

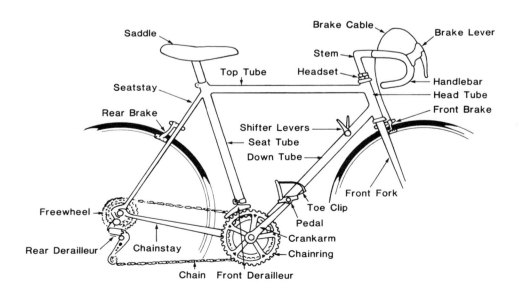

FIGURE 1.   Anatomy and terminology of a modern bicycle.

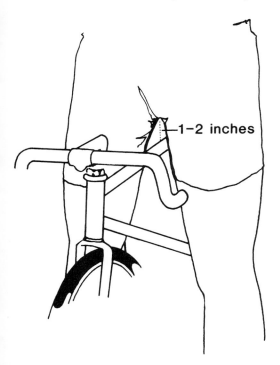

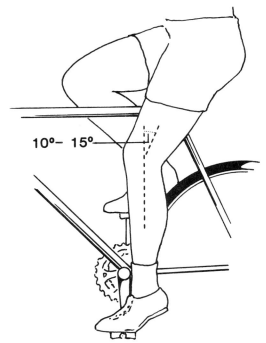

FIGURE 2. Proper frame size. Allow 1–2 inches between crotch and top frame tube.

FIGURE 3. Proper seat height is determined by putting the pedals at the six o'clock and twelve o'clock positions with the ball of the foot on the pedal; there should be 10–15° flexion of the extended leg.

tips of the fingers should just touch the handle bars for proper distance. Reach can be adjusted by exchanging the handlebar stem for one with a longer or shorter extension (Fig. 6). Excessive leaning causes increased neck discomfort from hyperextension, increased back fatigue, and increased hand problems from pressure.

Pedalling and Gearing. Next to improper bicycle fit as the cause of overuse syndrome in cyclists comes riding with inappropriate gear ratios and improper cadence (pedal revolutions per minutes).[1,28] Inexperienced or overzealous riders tend to ride in gears that are too high with a cadence that is too low for the rider's strength and ability. The resulting forces on the legs cause a variety of overuse injuries.

The human body can cope successfully with only a narrow range of resistance to the effort of bicycling. Hills form the most obvious resistance to the cyclist. Wind resistance is more subtle but often just as severe. About 90% of the energy expended

riding at 20 mph on a calm day is used to overcome the "wind resistance" produced by the motion of the bicycle and rider against the still air. This effect is magnified when riding into a head wind. The third factor to consider is the rider's energy level. A tired rider has reduced muscle efficiency and strength and can pedal well only against a lower resistance.

The modern bicycle allows the cyclist to pedal comfortably with a relatively constant pedal resistance at a rather uniform cadence by shifting through a range of 10 to 21 "speeds" or gear ratios. It does so with front gears attached to the "crank," or axle, around which the rider pedals. In racing or "sport" bicycles there are two front gears known as the large chain wheel and the small chainwheel. Touring and all terrain bicycles have a third considerably smaller front chainwheel called a "granny" for use on steep hills, in strong winds, or both. Mounted on the same hub with the rear wheel is a cluster of 5

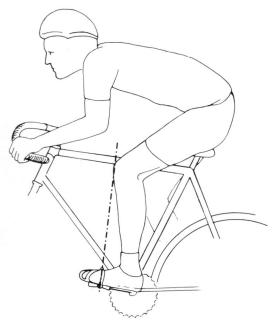

FIGURE 4. Seat position relative to the pedals is determined by putting the pedals at the three o'clock and nine o'clock position with the ball of the foot firmly on the pedal. A plumb line dropped from the middle of the forward patella should fall on the pedal axle.

to 7 toothed cogs (gears) known as the freewheel. The chainwheels are connected to the freewheel by a chain composed of evenly spaced links. Figure 7 illustrates the gearing. To change the gears in use, the rider moves shift levers (Fig. 1). The front shift lever controls the front derailleur, which in turn moves the chain from one chainwheel to another. The rear shift lever controls the rear derailleur, which moves the chain from one cog of the freewheel to another.

Since gear teeth must be uniform in dimension and evenly spaced in order to mesh with the links of the chain, the size of the gears may be expressed by the number of teeth they have. Gear ratio is the ratio of the size of the chainwheel in use to that of the freewheel cog in use. It can be expressed by the formula:

$$\text{Gear Ratio} = \frac{\text{\# of teeth on chainwheel}}{\text{\# of teeth on freewheel cog.}}$$

A higher gear ratio, therefore, results in higher pedal resistance in a given riding condition than a lower gear ratio. Traditionally,

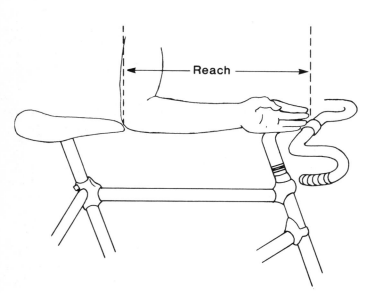

FIGURE 5. Handlebar height should be adjusted so that the handlebars are equal to or just below the level of the top of the seat. Proper reach is determined by placing the elbow at the front of the seat with the fingers extended; the finger tips should just touch the handlebars.

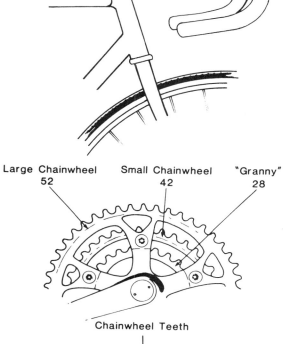

FIGURE 6.   Extension is the horizontal length of the handlebar stem. It can be changed only by replacing the stem.

FIGURE 7.   *A,* Modern bicycle gearing. This example is from a touring bicycle with 3 chainwheels on the crank and 6 cogs on the freewheel. *B,* Calculation of some typical gear ratios using the gearing illustrated in Figure 7 A.

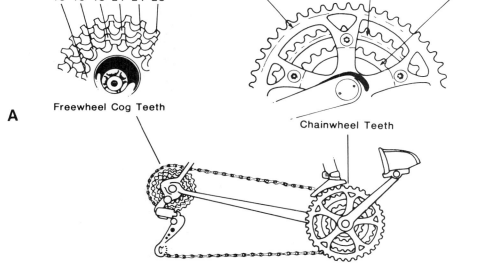

	GEAR RATIO	GEAR INCHES
EXAMPLES	$= \dfrac{\text{\# of teeth on chainwheel}}{\text{\# of teeth on freewheel cog}}$	= gear ratio x wheel dia.
VERY HIGH GEAR	$\dfrac{52}{13} = 4$	4 X 27 = 108
LOWER GEAR	$\dfrac{52}{26} = 2$	2 X 27 = 54
VERY LOW GEAR	$\dfrac{28}{28} = 1$	1 X 27 = 27

racers and other serious bicyclists have multiplied the gear ratio by the diameter of rear wheel to obtain a ratio called gear inches:

Gear Inches = Gear ratio × rear wheel
           diameter

To complete the sequence and obtain the distance travelled per pedal revolution, simply multiple gear inches by π (3.1416):

Distance = Gear inches × π

Table 1 provides general guidelines for selection of proper gears.

High gear ratios require greater muscle strength and conditioning and cause increased stress on the cyclist's hips, knees, and feet. The inexperienced or less-fit cyclist will find it easier and safer to ride at a more moderate gear ratio and, perhaps, slightly higher cadence. Research has shown that the optimal cadence for cyclists in terms of both cycling efficiency and perceived exertion is between 60 and 80 rpm.[5] The individual cyclist should establish over time a comfortable cadence in this range and shift gears to stay at his or her most naturally efficient cadence. Needless to say, for downhill riding or racing there will be times when much higher cadences are employed. Indeed, many experienced cyclist pedal regularly at 80-100

rpm; but maintaining a cadence in this range without injury requires already established fitness and good technique.

The most common advice physicians will need to give bicyclists about pedalling is to ride in a lower gear at a higher cadence. Proper gearing allows for the most efficient pedalling utilizing the least strength necessary.

CLOTHING AND PROTECTIVE EQUIPMENT

The brightly colored clothing and the specialized protective equipment that bicyclists use are much more than a display of fashion. These items are designed to help prevent injury. The uninitiated may think that the rider's garb is merely a form of in-group identification symbol; but, in fact, the helmet, riding pants, and gloves may be just the protection a beginner needs for his or her first long ride. The bright colors are more than fashion. They are designed to "advertise" the rider's presence in traffic or on the highway in order to avoid accidents. Reflective tape may be added to helmets and clothing worn at dawn or dusk and for night riding.

The helmet.   The most important device for a bicyclist to own and wear is a protective helmet. Three-fourths of the bicycle related deaths in the United States are due to head injuries, and in the vast majority of these cases the riders are not wearing hardshell helmets. There are two national safety organizations that test helmets, the American National Standards Institute (ANSI) and the Snell Memorial Foundation. As of January 1, 1986, the United States Cycling Federation instituted a rule that all racers must wear hardshell helmets certified by one of these two organizations.[20]

Modern bicycle helmets consist of a hard plastic shell, which spreads the shock of impact over a wider area, a foam liner which absorbs the shock, and a strapping system, usually with a quick-release chin strap. The key to its function is the liner, which is made from high density expanded polystyrene (EPS) or polyurethane foam, which crushes to absorb the shock of a severe impact. The

TABLE 1.   GENERAL USE OF GEAR RATIOS

GEAR INCHES	USE
27-35 (or lower)	Very low gears. Used for climbing steep hills. Also used for touring hilly terrain with a heavily loaded bicycle.
36-44	Low gears. Used for climbing hills or riding into a severe headwind.
45-60	Slightly low gears. Used for gentle hills or mild headwind.
61-85	Standard gears. Used for riding on level ground. Effort may be maintained for a long time.
86-108	High gears. Used for high speed riding. Used when riding downhill or riding with a strong tailwind.
> 108	Special gearing, not available on most bicycles.

crushable foam appears to be safer than more resilient materials in which recoil may add to the trauma.[4] Needless to say, if a liner has been crushed while protecting a rider, it should be replaced so that the helmet is as good as new.

Bicycle helmets are aerodynamically designed to reduce drag and to entrain air under the front edge and through exterior vent holes for a cooling effect.

Most bicycle accidents produce relatively low velocity impact to the head. If the rider is wearing a helmet, it is highly likely to protect him or her from major trauma.

Mirrors. There is a variety of mirrors from which cyclists may choose in order to see overtaking traffic. Several models mount on the handlebars, attach to the brake lever housing, or plug into the handlebar tip. These generally work well on upright bicycles, but they may not provide good visibility for bicyclers with dropped handlebars. Another option is a small adjustable mirror, similar to a dental mirror, which can be attached to the side of the helmet or clipped on to glasses or protective eyewear. Because it moves with the rider's head, this mirror provides good rear vision with the rider in a variety of positions on the bicycle.

Protective Eyewear. With the broad range of protective eyewear currently available, cyclists can shield themselves from dust, bugs, stones and other flying objects that may jeopardize their eyesight as well as avoid the discomfort caused by sun, rain, cold air, and allergens. There is even some evidence that proper eye protection may benefit performance in competitions.[32] For general sports activities, wraparound or semi-wraparound models are generally recommended, but goggles are better for more extreme conditions. Plastic or polycarbonate lenses and frames avoid potential injury from shatter or sharp edges.

Cycling Clothing. Cycling clothes are designed to attract attention to the rider's presence, maintain appropriate body temperature, and to be relatively streamlined. Bright colors and reflective materials make the rider highly visible. In summer heat singlets, mesh materials, lycra and a variety of new synthetic fabrics allow for cooling. In cooler seasons polypropylene and wool wick perspiration away from the skin while still insulating the body and preventing extreme heat loss. Cycling clothes are form-fitting to prevent flopping or slapping in the breeze.

CYCLING SHORTS. Bicycling racing shorts have now become standard "equipment" for most serious riders. They are tight fitting, knee-length shorts made of lycra, wool, or polypropylene stretch materials with a padded seamless crotch pad made of natural "chamois" or synthetic materials. Their main purpose is to protect the inner thighs, groin, and buttocks from chafing and pressure trauma, and they perform extremely well. Riders who try them once rarely ride again without them. For those who are embarrassed to appear in public in these flimsy elastic shorts, baggier touring shorts are available. Both styles are worn without underpants because the seams of the underwear may chafe and cause blistering and traumatic ulceration. Natural chamois crotch liners should be treated periodically with lanolin to maintain their softness. Synthetic materials work just about as well, wash easier, and dry faster.

SADDLE PADS. Some riders find that, even with a good pair of shorts, they need more seat padding. They may choose from padded seat covers made of an elastopolymer material in a closed-cell neoprene cover or synthetic fleece seat covers. Recently, some manufacturers have begun to market some saddles with extra padding built into the surface.

GLOVES AND HANDLEBAR PADDING. Bicycle gloves are designed to cushion the rider's palm from the pressure and vibration of the handlebar on the long or intense ride. Some of the better gloves contain shock-absorbing elastopolymer or neoprene padding in the palms. Summer gloves are fingerless with a leather palm and net back. Winter gloves incorporate the fingers and contain insulation as well as padding. In addition to padded gloves many riders choose to wrap their handlebars with a wide variety of handlebar padding tapes or to use cushioned slip-on handlebar pads for protection.

SHOES. One of the most underrated pieces of bicycle equipment is the shoe. There are two types, touring shoes and racing shoes. What they have in common is a stiff midsole that distributes the pedalling forces over the entire foot and helps prevent overuse syndromes in the foot and ankle. Touring shoes resemble court shoes and have a similar feel. The toe is roomy on the inside but small enough to fit in the toe clips that are popular on most racing and touring bikes. Some have transverse grooves to grip the pedal in order to generate more power through the entire pedal revolution. Racing shoes carry this principle even further by employing a cleat that fits snugly into a "cage" formed by the racing pedal. The cleated shoe allows the rider to apply force to the pedal throughout the 360° revolution in order to ride faster. Cleats that are not adjusted properly can result in painful knees and ankles.

INJURIES AND OVERUSE

Head Injury

Head trauma carries significant morbidity. In Calgery, Alberta, 67% of all persons hospitalized with a bicycle injury received a head injury.[10] In a study done in a pediatric hospital of 880 consecutive admissions for head injury, the most common mechanism was a fall from a bicycle. In a Florida study of 173 fatally injured bicyclists, the head or neck was the region most seriously injured in 86%.[9] The more serious injuries usually involve a motor vehicle.

Neck and Backache

Symptoms related to the neck and shoulder are quite common, especially in long distance riding. In one study involving long distance touring, 66.4% of all riders reported some discomfort, 20.4% of those reporting significant symptoms.[30] The trapezius muscle was the commonest site of pain, primarily left sided, this being attributed to looking backward to check for traffic. It also occurred in the riders using small rearview mirrors attached to their glasses or helmet. Backache was the third most common complaint in a major bicycle tour.[21]

Neck and back problems are created from the increased load placed on the arms and shoulders to support the rider, especially the weight of the head and upper chest. This is accentuated with the use of drop handlebars. This type of constant load is very fatiguing. Increased "reach" (Fig. 5) is the primary mechanical problem causing these overuse syndromes. This causes hyperextension of the neck to see the road. Changing the cycling position to put more weight at the rear of the rider is the important mechanical change needed. This can be accomplished by moving the seat forward, using randonneur handlebars with less drop, using a stem with a shorter extension (Fig. 6), or raising the height of the stem. Changing hand positions on the bar frequently, wearing padded gloves, using padding on the bar, and riding with the elbows "unlocked" will help absorb road shock. Switching to an upright bicycle may be the only other solution if these mechanical adjustments and riding technique change fail to relieve the problem.

Therapeutic exercise, consisting of a strength and flexibility program for the neck, back and shoulders, is the foundation of medical therapy. Ice massage, occasionally alternated with heat, aspirin and non-steroidal anti-inflammatory drugs, and skeletal muscle relaxants may be useful adjuncts. Pain and spasm which fail to respond to therapy may warrant further evaluation for underlying degenerative disk disease, osteoarthritis, or radiculopathy.

Handlebar Problems

Ulnar Neuropathy. One of the most common overuse problems in bicyclists is ulnar neuropathy, more commonly referred to as "cyclist's palsy" or "handlebar palsy." Almost 10% of the riders in an 8-day, 500-mile tour reported uncomfortable hand problems, and 63% of these experienced paresthesias in the ulnar nerve distribution.[30] It is not a new problem; Destot first described it in 1896 as a problem for some of the competitors in the Paris-Brest-Paris bicycle race.[11,16,24]

Clinically, the bicyclist will experience the insidious onset of numbness and tingling and/or weakness and difficulty with fine motor control after several days of intensive touring or racing. The pattern may be loss of sensory or motor function, or both.[29]

There is some debate about the location and mechanism of ulnar nerve damage in cyclist's palsy. Enough has been published that it is safe to say that the exact location is variable. Several authors have adopted a system of three anatomically determined types of lesions for ulnar compression syndromes. Type I involves the ulnar nerve proximal to or within Guyon's canal and involves both the superficial sensory and deep motor branches. Sensation in the distribution of the dorsal cutaneous branch is spared. Type II lesions involve the deep motor branch after the ulnar nerve bifurcates, and sensation is intact. Type III lesions involve the superficial sensory branch without causing motor deficits.[8,24,29] The mechanism of injury is generally nerve compression, but it is likely that in some patients riding with the wrists hyperextended causes a traction on the nerve, which, in turn, contributes to the injury.

Almost all cyclist's palsy problems resolve with conservative measures. Cutting back on the length and intensity of rides is helpful in the short term, but some other changes are necessary to prevent recurrences. The rider should wear well-padded riding gloves and use handlebar padding as well. Frame size should be checked because too large or too small a frame may prevent proper handlebar positioning. Adjustments of the bicycle saddle and the handlebars should be checked so that a disproportionate amount of the rider's weight does not rest on the hands (see previous section on fitting the bicycle). Lastly, the rider should develop a habit of changing hand positions frequently.[3] Occasionally, the cyclist will need to stop riding to allow healing, but only rarely will surgical decompression be necessary.[3,8,11,16,24]

If problems recur in spite of adhering to all the aforementioned suggestions, the rider might be encouraged to use an upright bicycle.

Carpal Tunnel Syndrome. Although ulnar nerve problems are common in cyclists, carpal tunnel syndrome is rarely the result of handlebar trauma alone. As a practical matter, the suggestions for riders with ulnar neuropathy would be helpful for those with median nerve symptoms as well.[17,22]

Saddle Problems

The most talked about bicycle problems are those which result from the interaction between rider and saddle. Modern dropped handlebar bicycles are designed so that most of the rider's weight is born by the ischial tuberosities. This is true even for racers who tend to use extremely narrow saddles for freedom of leg movement. For recreational riding and touring, slightly wider saddles generally are more comfortable. Women generally prefer even wider saddles because the ischial tuberosities are usually more widely spaced in the gynecoid pelvis. Most saddle manufacturers now produce models designed specifically for women.

Ischial Tuberosity Soreness. Many cyclists who have not ridden for a while will report tenderness around the ischial tuberosities for the first few days of regular riding. This problem is generally self-limited.

Skin Problems. Chafing, heat and perspiration can result in a variety of skin problems in the rider's groin, most of which can be prevented by wearing padded racing pants that are washed and dried after each ride. Simple chafing can often be prevented either by the use of talcum powder for drying or the opposite approach of lubricating agents such as Cramer's Skin Lube or Mueller's Lubricant. Treat established lesions with nonfluorinated corticosteroid cream. In more severe lesions that have gone on to blistering or ulceration, shave the area and apply a DuoDerm Hydrophilic dressing. Cover the lesion and a one-inch border on all sides; the dressing should conform fairly well to the contour of the tissue.

Skin infections of the groin are occasional problems. Warm soaks and incision and drainage are standard therapy. If antibiotics are warranted, bear in mind that folliculitis and furunculoses in this area may involve the coliforms as well as the more typical staphylococci.

Pressure phenomena such as subcutaneous nodules or callus formation may develop over the ischial tuberosities on rare occasions.

Pudendal Neuropathy. Male bicyclists may experience numbness and tingling in the scrotum and the penile shaft.[2,7,14,26] This syndrome has been attributed to compression of the dorsal branches on the pudendal nerve between the bicycle seat and the pubic symphysis.[14] This phenomenon usually results from riding on a saddle that has the front angled up too high or one that is too narrow to support the ischial tuberosities. The saddle top should be horizontal or only minimally angled upward in front. Strategies for prevention include changing the seat angle, wearing padded cycling shorts, using a saddle pad, and changing to a wider saddle.

Traumatic Urethritis. Bicycle saddles can induce a range of urinary tract outflow problems in men and boys. The mildest of these is a silent hematuria reported with both 10-speed and BMX (bicycle motocross) bicycles.[23,27] In its more severe forms the urethral trauma may sensitize the outflow tract to infection[15] or obstruction.[7,15,23,25,27] It is important to distinguish saddle-related obstruction from benign prostratic hypertrophy in order to avoid unnecessary prostate surgery. The preventive strategies suggested above for pudendal neuropathy are also helpful in these conditions.

Vulval Trauma. Women may experience a variety of vulval lesions ranging from superficial abrasions and lacerations to deeper contusions and hematomata due to bicycle trauma. Generally, a slight lowering of the front of the saddle ends the problem, but occasionally it is necessary to change to a broader saddle. Bicycle pants and saddle pads are helpful as well.

Torsion of the Testis. Torsion of the testis has been described in relationship to bicycling, but a distinct cause and effect relationship[18] has not been established.[12,13]

Hip Problems

Greater trochanteric bursitis and iliopsoas tendonitis are the two major problems encountered in the hip of bicyclists.[22] Greater trochanteric bursitis develops from repetitive sliding of the fascia lata over the greater trochanter. This produces pain around the greater trochanter in the abductor muscle groups. Treatment includes intermittent ice applications, anti-inflammatory medications, and occasional injection of corticosteroid into the bursa. Seat height adjustment is important in this condition.

Iliopsoas tendonitis or hip-flexor pain is another problem that presents with pain in the medial and proximal aspect of the thigh.

Management includes rest as necessary and anti-inflammatory medication.

Biker's Knee

"Biker's knee" is a general term for problems related to the way the patella tracks in relationship to the femur. These problems, common to many sports ("runner's knee," "breaststroker's knee"), are the subject of an entire chapter ("Tracking Problems of the Kneecap."). The discussion here will focus solely on the specific relationship of these problems to the bicyclist.

There are two sets of bicycle-related predisposing factors for patello-femoral problems, the set-up of the bicycle and the rider's technique. The most common bicycle problem is that the seat is too low or too far forward in relation to the pedals. Even if the seat is the "proper" height according to standard guidelines, raising it in 1–2 cm increments may relieve kneecap pain without a reduction in pedalling power.

The position of the foot on the pedal is also a determinant of the forces on the knee. The kneecap should be pointed straight forward when riding. If a bicyclist uses cleated racing shoes, the cleats should be positioned to allow the proper kneecap alignment. Severe hyperpronating feet and rearfoot valgus may cause knee pain in cyclists. Standard orthotics are rarely effective on the bicycle; instead, a 1/8–3/16 inch medial wedge cemented onto the bicycle shoe may provide a good solution. The wedge should extend across the front and back plates of the pedal.[7]

Technique often contributes to knee pain. Riding at a low cadence and "muscling" the bike up hills is likely to injure the knees, especially early in the spring after a winter layoff. Patients with biker's knee are encouraged to ride at higher RPM with lower gear resistance. In some extreme cases, it is even necessary for the cyclist to change the bicycle freewheel in order to have some lower gears available for recuperation. Riding flatter terrain will also be less demanding on the knees.

In addition to readjusting the bicycle and modifying technique, the rider will benefit from an aggressive rehabilitation program, focusing on stretching the hamstrings and the heelcords, and strengthening the vastus medialus obliquus. Ice and nonsteroidal anti-inflammatory drugs are extremely useful adjuncts.

Foot and Ankle Problems

Ankle and foot problems occurred in less than 15% of the riders in a long distance tour study.[30] The common problems include paresthesias, metatarsalgia, Achilles tendonitis, plantar fasciitis, and traumatic injuries due to spoke problems.[19]

Paresthesia. Foot paresthesias and numbness are relatively common among bicyclists riding long distances, and they generally resolve spontaneously within a few minutes to an hour off the bike. They are often caused by tight toeclip straps. If loosening the straps fails to alleviate the problem, switching to one of the newer "step in" shoe-pedal combinations may be warranted.

Metatarsalgia. Metatarsalgia is due to poor foot position or improperly placed shoe cleats; poor gearing and cadence may also cause increased pedal pressure. A metatarsal pad, cleat position adjustment, and gearing and cadence changes are usually all that are necessary to correct the problem.

Achilles Tendonitis. Achilles tendonitis may be caused by improper saddle height and pronounced dorsiflexion of the foot during the rotation of the pedal. The symptoms include pain and edema around the musculotendinous junction of the Achilles tendon. Evaluation of pedaling technique and seat height are necessary. The therapy usually includes stretching, nonsteroidal anti-inflammatory medications, and ice. Steroids should never by injected into this site, as they cause tendon weakness and degeneration with possible subsequent rupture.

Plantar Fasciitis. Plantar fasciitis may also occur, and pain in the sole usually at the origin of the plantar fascia on the anterior calcaneus is common. The pain can be produced by dorsiflexing the toes and by pressure applied at the plantar fascia origin. Management includes seat height elevation, heel cord stretching, nonsteroidal anti-inflammatory drugs, ice, and occasionally local corticosteroid injection into the painful area.

Spoke Injuries. Traumatic injuries of the foot and ankle commonly are caused by spoke injury. Laceration of soft tissue from a knife like action of the spoke, crushing injuries from impingement between the wheel and frame, and shearing injuries are the major mechanisms. These injuries most commonly occur when a passenger catches a foot in the wheel of a moving bicycle. Most lacerations occur over the malleoli, Achilles tendon, and dorsum of the foot. Prevention is the main emphasis for spoke injuries. Education about proper riding technique and about not using the bike to carry passengers improperly are the basic preventive measures to be taken. Also, riding a bicycle with loose spokes is dangerous.[19]

DEHYDRATION

Cyclists tend to have greater problems with dehydration because their sweat evaporates rapidly as they ride causing them to underestimate their fluid losses. Thirst becomes noticeable only after a significant fluid loss has taken place. Since a 3% drop in body weight can result in a 20 to 30% drop in performance, waiting for thirst to develop is an inadequate way to meet the body's need for fluid replacement. With long-distance riding and racing, conscious maintenance of good hydration for several days in advance, as well as several hours before the event, is necessary. In hot weather the generally accepted guidelines are for riders to drink two water bottles hourly and to pass clear urine at least every one and one half hours. Failure to urinate or passing yellow urine indicates dehydration.

SUNBURN

Sunburn can be a significant problem, especially in long distance touring, because of the time spent on the bicycle. In one study of a long-distance tour, 40% of the riders reported some sunburn problems, with 5.4% of those riders reporting sunburn to be a significant problem altering the way they rode.[30] Common areas of sunburning are the arms, thighs, and lips in decreasing order of frequency.

Sun screens are effective in blocking the

TABLE 2. SUMMARY OF COMMON OVERUSE BICYCLE PROBLEMS MECHANICAL AND TECHNIQUE ADJUSTMENTS TO CONSIDER IN TREATMENT

	MECHANICAL ADJUSTMENTS	TECHNIQUE ADJUSTMENTS
1. Neck and back pain	A. Adjust seat position (move forward) B. Change mirror placement C. Change to handle bar with less drop (randonneur) D. Shorten stem extension E. Raise stem height F. Switch to upright handle bars	A. Changing hand positions frequently B. Riding with "unlocked" elbows
2. Ulnar neuropathy (handle bar palsy)	A. Wear padded gloves B. Add handle bar padding C. Adjust frame size D. Adjust seat and handle bar (decrease reach)	A. Decreasing length and intensity of rides B. Changing hand position on bar frequently C. Riding with "unlocked" elbows
3. Skin problems	A. Using padded riding shorts B. Appropriate use of sunscreens C. Adjust seat type	
4. Pudendal neuropathy Traumatic urethritis Vulval trauma	A. Adjust saddle angle B. Change saddle width C. Consider padded cycling shorts D. Add saddle padding	
5. Hip problems	A. Adjust seat height B. Change frame size	
6. Bikers knee	A. Change frame size B. Adjust seat height and position C. Adjust foot and pedal position	A. Changing cadence B. Lowering gear ratio C. Riding flatter terrain D. Slowly increasing riding intensity and duration
7. Foot/ankle problems Paresthesia Metatarsalgia Achilles tendonitis	A. Adjust toe clips (decrease tightness) B. Change cleat position C. Adjust saddle height	A. Changing foot position B. Changing gearing and cadence C. Adjusting pedalling technique

short ultraviolet burning rays of the sun. However, in one study testing the effects of sun screen during exercise,[31] it was noted that in high heat/low humidity atmosphere, sun screens tended to block water evaporation, causing increased skin temperature. There was an increase in sweating but evaporation was impaired because of the sun screen. The implications of this study are unknown in bicycle riders. This effect could potentially cause problems for riders because of heat transfer problems caused by cycling clothing and helmet use. It would seem prudent to recommend judicious use of sun screens and to make sure that the rider is drinking enough fluids during an extended ride in hot weather.

SUMMARY

The management of bicycle problems requires treating both the patient and the bicycle. Table 2 summarizes many of the common problems encountered in cyclists and recommended management.

REFERENCES

1. Adams RJ: The proper cadence and introduction to gears in basic riding techniques. Emmaus, PA, Rodale Press, 1979, pp 7-10, 13-20.
2. Bond RE: Distance bicycling may cause ischemic neuropathy of the penis. Phys Sportsmed 3:54-56, 1975.
3. Burke ER: Ulnar neuropathy in bicyclists. Phys Sportsmed 9:53-55,, 1981.

4. Buyer's guide to hardshell cycling helmets. Bicycling 27:28-40, 1986.
5. Coast JR, Cox RH, Welch HG: Optimal pedalling rate in prolonged bouts of cycle egometry. Med Sci Sports Exerc 18:225-230, 1986.
6. Davis MW, Litman T, Crenshaw RW, Mueller JK: Bicycling injuries. Phys Sportsmed 8:88-96, 1980.
7. Dickson TB: Preventing overuse cycling injuries. Phys Sportsmed 13:116-123, 1985.
8. Eckman PB, Perlstein G, Altrocchi PH: Ulnar neuropathy in bicycle riders. Arch Neurol 32:130-131, 1975.
9. Fife D, Davis J, Tate L, et al: Fatal injuries to bicyclists: The experience of Dade County, Florida. J Trauma. 23:745-755, 1983.
10. Friede AM, Azzara CV, Gallagher SS, Guyer B: The epidemiology of injuries to bicycle riders. Pediatr Clin N Am. 32:141-151, 1985.
11. Frontera WR: Cyclist's palsy: Clinical and electrodiagnostic findings. Br J Sports Med 17:91-93, 1983.
12. Gibson OB: Bicycle saddles and torsion of the testis. Lancet 1:1149, 1978.
13. Goodfellow RC: Bicycle saddles and torsion of the testis. Lancet 1:1149, 1978.
14. Goodson JD: Pudendal neuritis from biking. N Engl J Med. 304:365, 1981.
15. Hershfield NB: Pedaller's penis. Can Med Assn J 128:366-7, 1983.
16. Hoyt CS: Ulnar neuropathy in bicycle riders. Arch Neurol 33:372, 1976.
17. Hoyt CS: Averting common biking injuries. Phys Sportsmed 4:40-43, August 1976.
18. Jackson RH, Craft AW: Bicycle saddles and torsion of the testis. Lancet 1:983-4, 1978.
19. Kravitz HL: Preventing injuries from bicycle spokes. Pediat Ann 6:53-59, 1977.
20. Kukula K: Helmet safety standards. Bicycling 27:30, 1986.
21. Kulund DN, Brubaker CE: Injuries in the bikecentennial tour. Phys Sportsmed 6:74-78, 1978.
22. Mayer PJ: Helping your patients avoid bicycling injuries: Part 1: What injuries to anticipate this summer. J Musculoskel Med 2:31-40, 1985.
23. Nichols TW: Bicycle-seat hematuria. N Engl J Med. 311:1128, 1984.
24. Noth J, Dietz V, Mauritz K-H: Cyclist's palsy: Neurological and EMG study in 4 cases with distal ulnar lesions. J Neurolog Sci 47:111-116, 1980.
25. O'Brien KP: Sports urology: The vicious cycle. N Engl J Med 304:1367-1368, 1981.
26. Powell B: Correction and prevention of bicycle saddle problems. Phys Sportsmed 10:60-67, 1982.
27. Salcedo JR: Huffy bike hematuria. N Engl J Med 315:768, 1986.
28. Sanders W: Backcountry bikepacking. Harrisburg, PA, 1982, 26-38.
29. Shea JD, McClain EJ: Ulnar-nerve compression syndromes at or below the wrist. J Bone Joint Surg 51A:1095-1103, 1969.
30. Weiss BD: Nontraumatic injuries in amateur long distance bicyclists. Am J Sports Med. 13:187-192, 1985.
31. Wells T: Affects of sunscreen use during exercise in the heat. Phys Sportsmed 12:132-144, 1984.
32. Zahradnik F: Eyewear. Bicycling 27:116-119, 1986.

21 Taping and Bracing

RONNIE D. HALD, P.T., A.T.C.
DENISE FANDEL, M.S., A.T.C.

A frequent question asked by the injured athlete to the sportsmedicine practitioner is "How should I protect this injury once I return to play?" The answer should result from a decision-making process, dependent on several factors. One of these factors is the knowledge and awareness of what is available. In this chapter, the sportsmedicine practitioner is exposed to numerous taping techniques and braces that may be beneficial in meeting the needs of athletic patients. It is not the authors' intent to teach competence in the techniques of taping or the designing of a brace, however, some detailed examples are presented to aid the discussion. The ability of the physician to identify and evaluate the options will facilitate prescription of the optimal method of support and protection. This understanding will also assist in communication to coaches, trainers, and therapists working with the athlete, thus encouraging the team approach, a necessary component of optimal patient care.

SELECTION CONSIDERATIONS

Before considering common methods of athletic injury support, it is helpful to discuss factors to consider in making an appropriate selection, including: (1) diagnosis of injury, (2) goals to be accomplished by taping or bracing, (3) resources available, (4) sport and position of the athlete, (5) the athlete's acceptance, (6) research findings, and (7) personal preferences. The investigation of these factors and how they interact will assist in the process of determining the best solution.

Diagnosis of Injury. The location, nature, and severity of injury often dictate the suitability of providing external support. For instance, most shoulder problems are not helped by taping or bracing since restriction of range of motion leads to decreased function and possibly secondary problems. However, the ankle, with its inherent skeletal stability, may be more readily supported by external support. The acuteness and severity of injury may dictate more aggressive treatment than taping or bracing can achieve. Some chronic injuries may be helped by decreasing the effect of biomechanical forces on repetitive activities (e.g., long distance running, racquet sports). A referral to and input from an orthopedist may be beneficial.

Goals of Taping and Bracing. Taping and bracing can be divided into three main categories: (1) prophylactic, (2) rehabilitative, and (3) functional. Prophylactic supports are used to reduce the incidence or severity of injury to uninjured normal anatomy or fully rehabilitated injuries. Rehabilitative taping or bracing is used to provide protection of healing injuries during their rehabilitation. Functional braces and taping are used to protect against reinjury following rehabilitation and/or surgical reconstruction. A taping procedure or brace effective for prevention may not be suitable as an adjunct to rehabilitation. Taping or bracing does not substitute for the need for complete rehabilitation. A helpful concept is that of "earning the brace" by completing the rehabilitation. Taping may act as an adjunct to help support injured tissues during rehabilitation; it is a means to an end, not the end itself. If taping or bracing cannot provide any additional benefit, it is probably best to do without it.

Resources Available. Even though a certain taping technique may be ideal for a particular problem, it will not help if there is no trainer or other individual skilled in its application available to the athlete. This is a key advantage to many braces. Once the athlete is properly instructed in their application, no additional expertise is needed. Also, there are financial considerations such as the cost of taping (labor and supplies), and the oftentimes considerable investment required to purchase a brace. With custom-made braces, there may be a period of time before the brace is available for the athlete's use. Coaches and trainers should be approached to determine which options are feasible. In the case of younger athletes, parents should be involved when financial or insurance issues need clarification.

Sport and Position. A taping or bracing that is effective for an athlete in one sport may not be suitable for another athlete, or even the same athlete in another sport. Each sport has its own physical requirements, equipment, environment, and rules that will affect, and many times govern, the selection of protective support for injuries. In some sports, an athlete's particular position or event may need to be considered. Taping may have to be tailored to allow the athlete to perform his or her skills, yet provide adequate protection. Braces must be made of materials that do not endanger the other participants.

Athlete's Acceptance. If the athlete feels that taping or a brace is uncomfortable or decreases performance, the attempt to support an injury will fail. Involving the athlete in the decision-making process and providing choices, where possible, reduce the risk of nonacceptance. If an appropriate choice is made, a very real effect of taping or bracing following injury is the psychological assistance to the athlete's confidence upon returning to competition.

Research Findings. Research about what does and does not work is still in the infancy stage. Many methods and devices that have been used for years have never been tested rigorously. With respect to new techniques or products, it is probably best to keep an open mind but to be critical. Until more work is done, clinical experience will have to suffice.

Personal Preference. After gaining clinical experience with various taping techniques and braces, one usually begins to have certain favorites. There is nothing wrong with relying on experience when the athlete is looking for expert answers, as long as each case is viewed individually.

IMPLEMENTATION

Once a method of support is selected, the choice needs to be made known to all parties involved. Information must also be shared. In order to evaluate the effectiveness of the support as part of the treatment plan, a follow-up visit should be scheduled.

Communication. During the selection process, lines of communication have been formed among the physician, the athlete, and the athlete's coach, trainer, and parents. Once a decision is made, the plan should be made known to all involved. This encourages compliance, promotes safe return of the athlete to sport, and encourages good working relationships among the professionals involved. This sort of communication is very helpful to the team physician.

Education. It should be made clear that the taping or bracing is only a part of the total care plan as well as what is to be accomplished by taping or bracing. In some cases the taping procedure will need to be taught to a coach or trainer by an individual familiar with the method. Preventive measures to protect skin from being injured by frequent taping should be encouraged. With bracing, the athlete will need to be shown how to put on the brace properly. This may include an anatomy lesson in locating the joint lines and how straps must be placed in a certain way to make the brace most effective. The athlete must be able to put on and take off the brace independently before leaving the clinic. Instructions about care and preventive maintenance should also be reviewed to maximize the life of the brace. Written instructions on application and care, if not available, should be developed.

Follow-up. An appropriate time to schedule a follow-up visit when an athlete has been cleared to resume the sport is at the conclusion of the season. This allows the physician and rehabilitation team to reassess the effectiveness of the support, determine its continued need, and encourage "prehabilitation" of deficits before the next season. In multi-sport athletes, change in the type of taping or bracing may be necessary. For those involved in research, this also provides an opportunity to acquire data.

TAPING

To be proficient in taping, one must practice, practice, practice. Anyone who has attempted to learn to tape knows how true this statement is. However, exposure to some common techniques can assist the primary care practitioner in providing a complete treatment plan and in being able to communicate with professionals skilled in these methods. After discussing basic principles, a sampling of common taping methods is presented.

Principles of Taping

Application. One of the most common mistakes made by the novice is applying too much tape. Every piece of tape should have a distinct purpose—more is not better. Other common problems are continuous application of tape and forcing the tape to go in a desired direction; these errors may restrict circulation. A better approach consists of tearing strips often and considering the contours of body parts. Learning how to tear tape and adapting two-dimensional tape to a three-dimensional body part are basic skills. A good taper keeps in mind the need to restrict undesired motion yet allow wanted motion. A tape support is made effective by bridging across the injury and duplicating the anatomy needing support; strength is developed by weaving the strips, overlapping by at least one-half the width of the tape.

Tape Selection. Another important principle is the correct selection of the best tape for the job. The size of the body part determines the appropriate width. The tape must have good adherence to the athlete's skin and have adequate tensile strength to provide the necessary support. Some tapes have elasticity to allow increased ease of application or desired movement, yet provide adequate injury protection; of course this increases its cost. Of importance to the taper is how the tape unwinds from the roll and how easily it tears. Learning how to tear tape is the most basic skill learned by the novice taper. Some tapes do not tear and require cutting between application of strips.

Skin Care. Frequent taping of skin can lead to problems that are preventable. Shaving hair not only increases the effectiveness of taping but also reduces the irritation and buildup of residue that can lead to infection. Skin to be taped should be protected by application of a taping base (usually some formula incorporating tincture of benzoin) that also increases the adherent qualities of the tape. A tape underwrap of thin polyester urethane foam decreases skin problems while it increases the athlete's comfort;[5] however, this adds another interface between the tape and the structure needing support. A lubricant placed in areas that may be pinched with movement within the taping, such as the lace and heel areas of the ankle, can prevent or at least decrease irritation. Correct removal of the tape, using appropriate scissors or cutters, should be taught to the athlete. Scissors with pointed tips should be avoided. Following practice, the skin must be thoroughly cleansed and treated if necessary. Failure to do so can lead to skin breakdown and wounds that may prevent further taping. Some individuals may develop allergic reactions to certain products or materials used in taping, and solutions to this problem must be found. If not, taping may need to be abandoned in favor of some other form of support and protection.

Procedures

This section describes and presents some common uses of tape to support athletic injuries. It is not intended to be complete or exhaustive but rather to reflect current practice.

Buddy Taping. This method splints an injured finger to an adjacent finger to restrict varus/valgus forces (Fig. 1*A*). For additional support, felt or foam may be placed between the fingers being taped (Fig. 1*B*). It is important to allow interphalangeal motion and to avoid using the index and little fingers as a splint, unless, of course, either is the finger involved.

Thumb Figure-of-Eight. Hyperflexion injuries are supported by circling around the wrist and the thumb in a figure-of-eight pattern (Fig. 1*C*).

Thumb Checkrein. Hyperextension injuries to the thumb may be aided by the use of a checkrein between the thumb and index

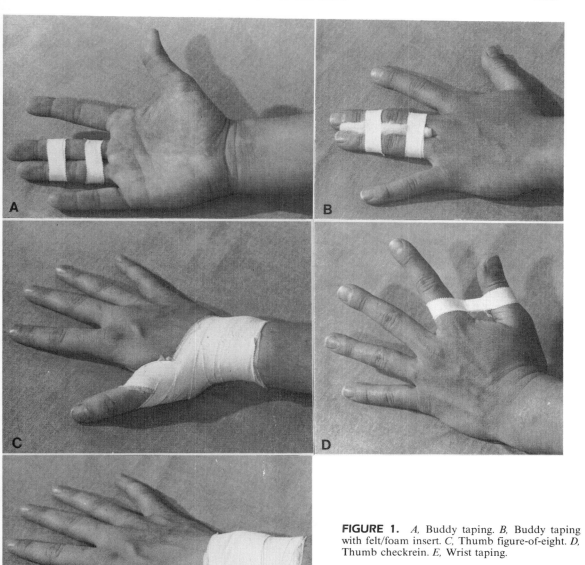

FIGURE 1. *A*, Buddy taping. *B*, Buddy taping with felt/foam insert. *C*, Thumb figure-of-eight. *D*, Thumb checkrein. *E*, Wrist taping.

finger (Fig. 1*D*). Please note that use of this taping can result in injuries to the metacarpophalangeal joint of the index finger.[17]

Wrist Taping. Circumferential strips about the wrist may limit excusion of the carpals (Fig. 1*E*). In cases of dorsal impingement such as in the gymnast or tennis player, the incorporation of a foam "block" into this taping is often helpful.

Elbow Hyperextension Taping. With the athlete's elbow placed in slight flexion, fanning strips are placed anterior to the elbow joint between anchors about the upper arm and forearm (Fig. 2*A*). This taping can be modified to also provide medial (Fig. 2*B*) or lateral support.

Shoulder Taping. Although taping has been and can be used for some shoulder injuries, we feel that the restriction of motion required to provide adequate support decreases function to a point where time and effort are probably spent on rehabilitation.

Hip and Groin Taping. These areas are better supported by the use of elastic wraps using a figure-of-eight pattern about the waist and upper thigh. Since these areas are rarely taped, no further discussion is presented. Again, the question of decreased function to achieve the desired support is important.

Medial (or Lateral) Knee Taping. Fanning strips across the medial (or lateral) aspect of the knee joint across anchors about the thigh and calf may reduce the effect of valgus (or varus) stress. Figure 3 demonstrates a taping to support the medial ligaments of the knee.

The next three taping procedures are presented in a step by step manner. They are not easily demonstrated by a single photograph. They address areas where external support is most often considered.

Knee Anterior Cruciate Ligament (ACL) Taping. The Duke Simpson knee strapping

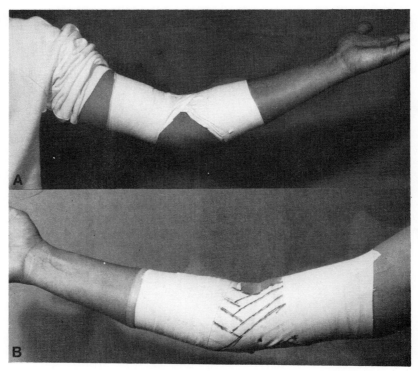

FIGURE 2. *A,* Elbow hyperextension taping. *B,* Medial elbow taping.

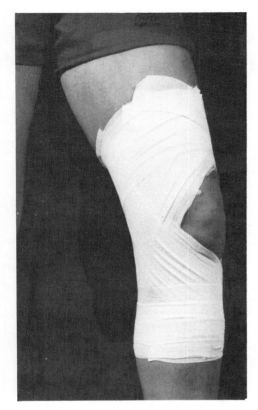

FIGURE 3. Medial knee taping.

has often been touted: "If this strapping fails to hold a knee from further sprain, no brace or other contrivance will."[22] Using a modification of this strapping, Ross[19] developed an effective method to limit hyperextension of the knee, a major factor in anterior cruciate ligament injury. The modification shown here[23] uses a four-tailed piece of neoprene rubber, 15" × 6" with 5" × 3" triangular cutouts (Fig. 4). Tape adherent and underwrap are applied (Fig. 5A), the neoprene sup-

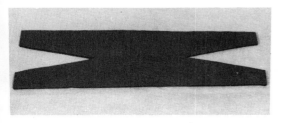

FIGURE 4. Neoprene support for the ACL taping.

port placed in the popliteal space (Fig. 5B), and then covered by underwrap (Fig. 5C). This is done to enable the athlete to reuse the neoprene. Using 3" elastic tape, a circumferential anchor is placed about the calf, revolving laterally. The tape is drawn laterally and upward across the lateral joint line (Fig. 5D). A circumferential anchor about the thigh is then placed. Continuing on the medial side, the tape is drawn downward across the medial joint line (Fig. 5E), around the calf, then upward across the medial joint line again. This creates a medial "X" and covers the neoprene support (Fig. 5F). After passing the tape around the thigh, then down across the lateral joint line, the lateral "X" is completed (Fig. 5G). After passing behind the calf again, the tape is pulled laterally, then upward and posteriorly (Fig. 5H). This should enclose the popliteal space, a practice not usually done due to circulatory problems encountered. The use of the neoprene support seems to counter this problem. After completing a finishing anchor about the thigh, the tape is cut (Fig. 5I), and cloth adhesive tape placed about the thigh and calf to anchor the elastic tape (Fig. 5J). These anchors and the edges of the elastic tape should be applied directly to the skin. Cutting the calf portion of the taping posteriorly allows for expansion of the gastrocnemius musculature (Fig. 5K). This gap is closed with cloth adhesive tape to finish the taping. In order to recover the neoprene support for reuse, this taping is removed strip by strip upon conclusion of activity.

Ankle Taping. Although there are probably about as many taping techniques for the ankle as there are trainers, a basic method that incorporates some of the most common methods will be described. To meet goal of the taping—preventive, rehabilitative, or supportive for a functional return of a rehabilitated ankle injury—the basic steps are adapted by the experienced taper. The athlete's ankles should be positioned at a right angle of plantar/dorsiflexion with neutral inversion/eversion. Hair should be shaved to provide maximal support. Heel and lace pads made of gauze or similar protective material with lubrication are applied to the heel and lace areas to guard against blisters and tape cuts (Fig. 6A). Tape adherent and

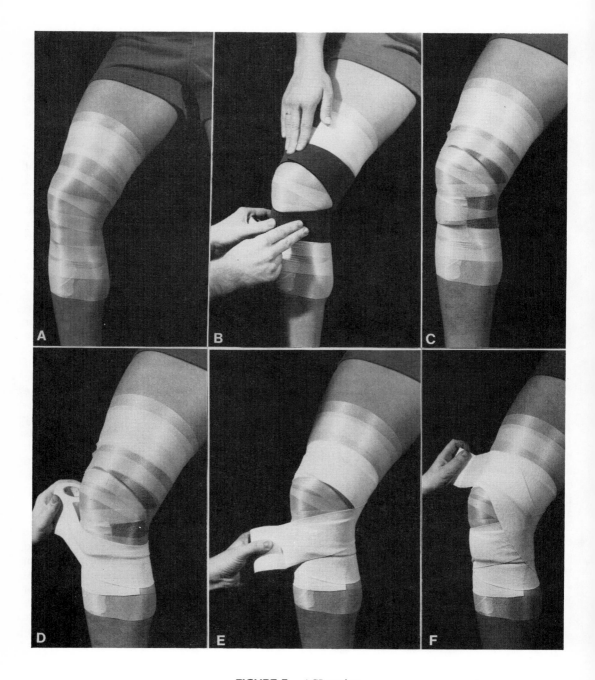

FIGURE 5. ACL taping.

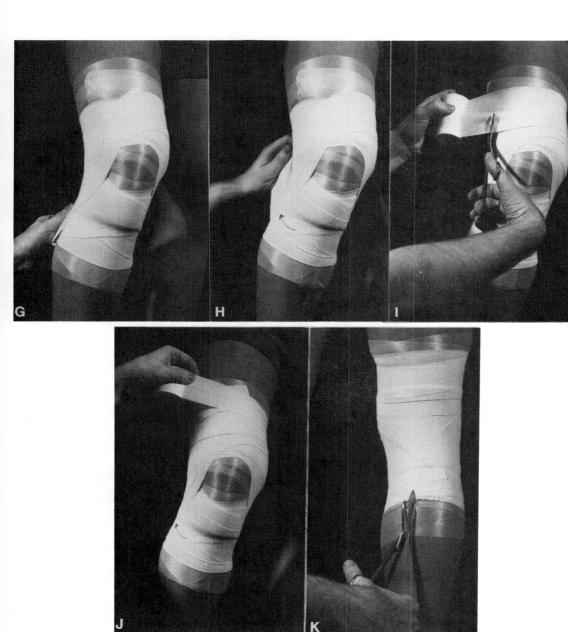

FIGURE 5. (*Continued*). ACL taping.

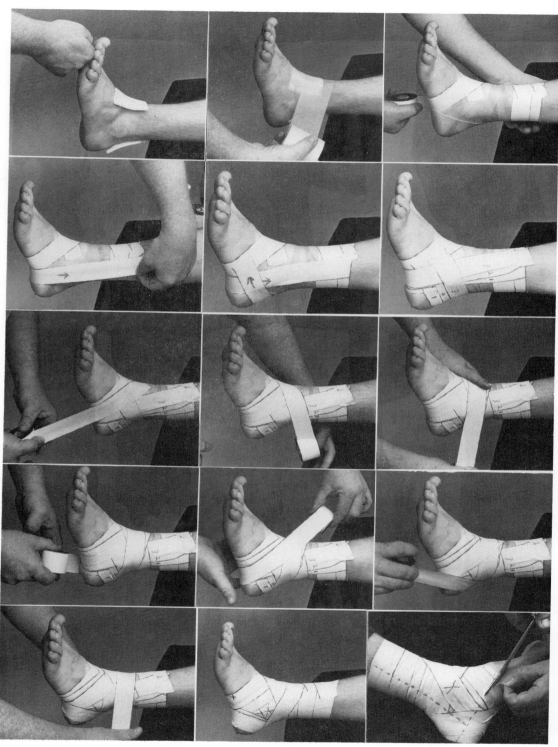

FIGURE 6. Ankle taping.

underwrap are then applied (Fig. 6*B*). Underwrap may be omitted to provide additional support, especially for more acute injuries, but special care of the skin is then required. Anchor strips around the calf at the level of the musculotendinous junction of the gastroc-soleus and around the arch are applied (Fig. 6*C*). The arch anchor must be placed proximal to the base of the fifth metatarsal to avoid discomfort as the foot spreads with weightbearing. A "stirrup" strip is placed on the calf anchor medially, passing beneath the heel posterior to the malleoli, pulling laterally to the other side of the calf anchor (Fig. 6*D*). In an eversion sprain, the stirrup is placed with equal tension medially and laterally. Perpendicular to the stirrup, a "horseshoe" is applied distal to the malleoli, starting and finishing on the arch anchor (Fig. 6*E*). Stirrups and horseshoes are repeated twice more, overlapping the previous strip by one-half. This completes the "basketweave" (Fig. 6*F*). A "figure-of-eight" may be applied to restrict plantar flexion. In the present example, it begins on the outside of the foot, angling under the foot (Fig. 6*H*). "Heel locks" are used to restrict inversion/eversion. A medial heel lock, restricting inversion, begins in the lace area (Fig. 6*I*), angling behind and across the medial aspect of the heel (Fig. 6*J*), then under the heel and returning the lace area (Fig. 6*K*). A lateral heel lock is performed in the opposite direction, angling across the lateral aspect of the heel (Fig. 6*L*). These steps may be repeated as necessary to obtain the desired support. Circular strips are placed about the lower leg, overlapping distal to proximal, to eliminate open spaces that may result in skin irritation or blisters (Fig. 6*M*). Anchors may be repeated to close, thus decreasing the number of free tape ends exposed that may roll up when the athlete puts on socks. The complete job is inspected for wrinkles and gaps, and the athlete questioned as to the adequacy of the support and its comfort (Fig. 6*N*). The ankle strapping is removed by using a blunt-nosed bandage scissors or tape cutter to cut along the medial aspect, posterior to the medial malleolus (Fig. 6*O*). Various padding may be incorporated into the taping, such as a "J" pad along the lateral malleolus for subluxation of the peroneal tendons, or a dorsal "block" in the lace area to restrict dorsiflexion in cases of anterior impingement.

Frequently, questions are asked about the value of preventive ankle taping. A review of the literature by Metcalf and Denegar[14] highlights several points. With exercise, the initial restriction of range of motion is considerably reduced, but does appear to be adequate to restrict the extreme ranges of motion responsible for ankle injury. There are some who feel that the restriction of ankle movement may increase the incidence of knee injuries, but this has been refuted by research. Ankle taping does not affect athletic performance. There is some evidence that the protective effect of taping is due to increased proprioceptive input. It appears that the use of ankle taping to prevent reinjury to ankles previously injured is more easily defended. Also there is some benefit, albeit less, from the use of reusable cloth ankle wrapping[12] or a high-top shoe.[8] The greatest issue is that of cost-benefit. Until it can be conclusively established that the cost of labor and supplies needed to provide protective taping outweighs the cost of preventable injury, the decision of whether or not to tape will rely on professional opinion and budget considerations.

Arch Figure-of-Eight. This taping method may be effective to control excessive pronation, to decrease stress on the plantar fascia, and as an adjunctive treatment for shin splint. Due to the increased perspiration of the soles of the feet, it is almost mandatory to apply this taping without the use of underwrap. An anchor strip is placed loosely around the metatarsal heads (Fig. 7*A*). Half of the figure-of-eight is performed by starting at the base of the great toe, angling across the longitudinal arch, around the heel, and returning the base of the great toe (Fig. 7*B*). The other half is similar, using the base of the little toe as the starting and finishing point (Fig. 7*C*). These steps are repeated once or twice (Fig. 7*D*). Next horizontal strips are placed, pulling medially, from the heel to the ball of the foot (Fig. 7*E*). A "low dye" strip[24] is begun at the base of the little toe, passed behind the heel, and then ended at the base of the great toe (Fig. 7*F*). A closing anchor is placed on the dorsum of the foot over the original anchor (Fig. 7*G*). Care must be taken to ac-

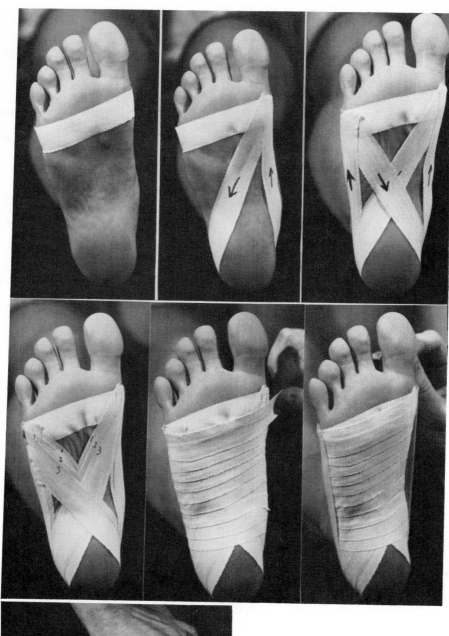

FIGURE 7. Arch figure-of-eight.

count for the expansion of the foot upon weightbearing.

Achilles Tendon Taping. This taping uses anchors around the arch of the foot and the calf with elastic tape to give support to the musculotendinous structure (Fig. 8). The athlete's ankle is taped in a position of slight plantar flexion, thus restricting excessive dorsiflexion.

Turf-Toe Taping. Strips are fanned between anchors around the great toe and the arch to prevent flexion and/or extension of the great toe (Fig. 9).

BRACING

The primary care practitioner can become overwhelmed when attempting to choose a brace. The bracing market is full of claims with no guarantees, just disclaimers of liability. Often the athlete may already have a brace or knows of someone from whom to borrow one. The physician's role is then to evaluate critically the brace's effectiveness. With new products available every day, it is probably more important to recognize certain features of the common braces. After presenting some of the advantages and disadvantages of bracing, a discussion of some presently available functional braces and orthotics follows.

Bracing—Pros and Cons

When compared with taping, there are several advantages to bracing. First and

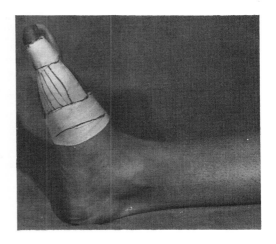

FIGURE 9.   Turf-toe taping.

foremost is ability to provide protection or support to athletes who do not have access to a skilled taper. Also once the initial investment is made, braces may be more cost effective. In certain problems, a brace or orthotic device can provide a means of support not available from taping. Most braces are more convenient, but drawbacks do exist. Because of the additional interface and lack of adhesion to the skin, the problem of migration can occur during vigorous activity. This may lead to failure of the brace to provide support and also cause decreased athletic performance or other problems. The use of tape adherent, anti-migration straps, or specially designed undergarments may help. The most common complaint made by the athlete is the weight some braces require to provide adequate protection. With wear, Velcro fasteners fail to hold fast, straps or buckles break, and elastic stretches out. Waiting for replacement parts does not allow the athlete to participate safely without the brace. Another problem is sizing—what do you do with athletes who are between sizes or have body proportions differing from the brace design? Custom-made braces are available but are generally more expensive. The best advice is to select devices carefully and to be prepared to deal with the problems that may arise from the brace prescribed to protect the patient. This is an area where you may need

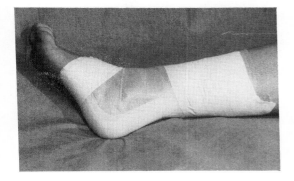

FIGURE 8.   Achilles tendon taping.

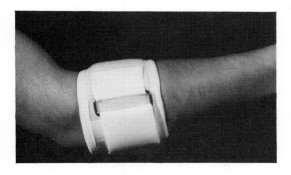

FIGURE 10.　Tennis elbow counter-force brace.

to seek the advice of the trainer, sports therapist, or orthotist.

Suggestions from Our Practice

Tennis Elbow Strap. Epicondylitis is most commonly seen in athletes in racquet sports, baseball, and softball who perform repeated forearm pronation and supination movements. The sportsmedicine practitioner can supplement and augment the rehabilitation program with a Velcro or elastic strap combination brace often called a "tennis elbow strap" or "counter-force brace" (Fig. 10).[15] There are numerous braces of this type on the market designed to reduce the contractile force of the extensor musculature, which causes irritation and inflammation at or near the radiohumeral joint.

Silicone Rubber Wrist/Hand Cast. Some hand and wrist injuries requiring immobilization may be supported so that participation in sports is permitted, even in collision sports such as football. By fabricating a playing cast out of various silicone rubber compounds, the injury can be given adequate protection without subjecting other participants to risk from an unyielding material. Details of their construction are found in the references.[1,3,6]

Lateral Prophylactic Knee Braces. Prophylactic lateral knee braces (Fig. 11), designed to lessen the severity of lateral impact, valgus force injuries, are still in relative infancy both in design and implementation. Recent research has raised questions as to the possibility of "preloading" knee structures and predisposing the wearer to an increased risk of ligament injuries.[10] Brace migration is a major problem as is compliance of the athlete in proper positioning and care of the brace, all essential to the successful success of effectiveness by: (1) shaving the skin as described for taping, (2) using a taping adherent, (3) using audiovisual aids (i.e. videotapes, posters) supplied by the manufacturers in teaching proper application and for daily reminders, (4) daily checking of positioning by coaches and trainers, and (5) weekly checking on upkeep by coaches, parents, equipment managers, trainer, and players.

As with all braces, with lateral prophylactic knee braces there is no guarantee that an injury will not occur, but rather an assump-

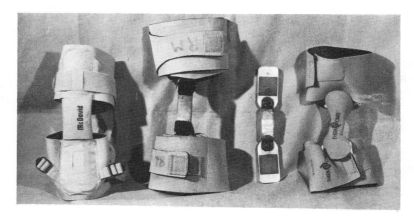

FIGURE 11.　Examples of lateral prophylactic knee braces.

tion that, by design, lateral impact injuries may be lessened in severity. A practical problem faced by the sportsmedicine practitioner is the popularity of the braces based on anecdotal reports of bent braces that "saved" a player from injury, but research has not substantiated this claim. Hewson et al.[9] found that in collegiate football players there appeared to be no reduction in the number of knee injuries since the adoption of lateral prophylactic knee braces and subsequent rule changes. With respect to their effect on performance, Prentice and Toriscelli[18] found that there was a significant decrease in 40-yard-dash times while wearing the braces but no decrease in agility or backward running.

We feel that time and money might be better spent on preventive conditioning than on braces for now, in light of recent research. Lateral knee braces may have a place at the end of a total rehabilitation program, but the popular axiom that the lateral knee braces are "better than nothing," in view of recent research to the contrary for athletes without injury, may require rethinking.

Functional Knee Braces. Another recent surge in brace development is that of functional knee braces. These are designed to provide support knees made unstable by injury or to provide additional protection following surgery to correct these instabilities. Some of these braces are "ready-made," with sizing to provide for immediate fit. Others require custom construction based on some form of cast molding or measurement of the athlete's leg. Considering the conditions being addressed and the cost of these devices, input from the orthopedist is critical. Attempts to support anterior cruciate injuries usually involve some form hyperextension stop through the use of controlled hinges and control of the rotational component through the use of straps or fitted shells (Fig. 12). These braces also provide support to other knee structures. Some studies have investigated the relative effectiveness of these braces,[2,7] but no brace has been found to completely control the knee in all situations.

Knee Braces for Patellofemoral Pain Syndromes. Peripatellar pain and/or dysfunction resulting from anatomical causes, otherwise known as extensor mechanism malalignment (EMM), is being more accurately diagnosed and treated as knowledge of patellofemoral mechanics is increased by research. We have found success with two types of braces in assisting the athlete in return to full function, the Palumbo lateral patella stabilizing brace, and the neoprene rubber sleeve with patellar cutout.

The Palumbo brace (Fig. 13) combines the support of an elastic sleeve with patellar cutout with a lateral buttress strap designed to dynamically decrease excessive lateral

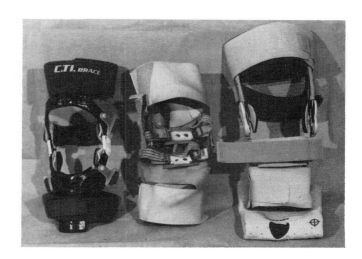

FIGURE 12. Examples of functional knee braces.

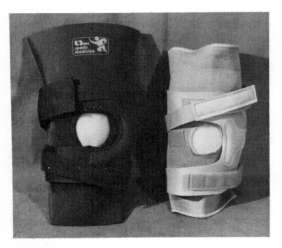

FIGURE 13. Palumbo braces, neoprene (left) and elastic (right).

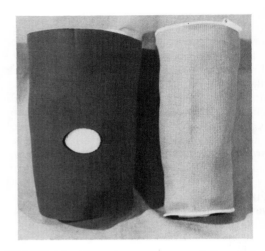

FIGURE 14. Knee sleeves, neoprene (left) and elastic (right).

tracking of the patella, which is commonly responsible for the pain experienced by patients with EMM.[16] Lysholm et al.[13] reported that during isokinetic testing of patients with EMM in braced and unbraced conditions, strength measurements increased while pain decreased during the test with the patellofemoral joint braced.

Neoprene braces provide uniform compression and allow for nearly normal range of motion of the knee (Fig. 13 and 14). It is essential that the athlete with EMM or patellar tendinitis ("jumpers knee") be fitted with a sleeve with a cutout for the patella. This is necessary to allow full range of motion, support, proper tracking, and decrease compression of the patellofemoral joint with activity. There are numerous brands available, some with a lateral buttress, for the physician and athlete to choose from, always keeping in mind the need for a patellar cutout.

Knee Sleeves. Sleeves can be used to provide compression of the knee (Fig. 14) as well as other soft tissue areas, such as the calf musculature and the quadriceps and hamstrings. They are often made of elastic or Spandex and provide even compression and may promote local tissue healing. Neoprene is another material used for these purposes. Its major difference from elastic and Spandex is its ability to retain body heat, thereby increasing the sense of warmth that some-

times makes the athlete who suffers from tendinitis more comfortable. They also provide some pain relief from sensory stimulation. Patients wearing these devices report a feeling of security, probably due to increased proprioceptive input. As discussed previously, when a sleeve is used at the knee it is important to use a brace that has a patellar cutout to decrease irritation to those prone to EMM.

Ankle Braces. Numerous ankle braces are available commercially which provide the sports medicine practitioner variety and flexibility in fitting the individual athlete and to support the injury. Slip-on elastic braces are best utilized when even compression is desired, such as to decrease edema. They do not restrict inversion or eversion significantly enough to be considered prophylactic support.[11] Certain manufacturers (e.g., Stromgren) combine the comfort of even compression using Spandex, elastic, and Velcro strap combinations to restrict inversion or eversion (Fig. 15). We have found them easier to manage with regard to the break-in period and they are a better alternative than the slip-on ankle brace. A third type of prophylactic support for the ankle is a lace-up style (Fig. 16). These braces often have medial and lateral stays, providing increased restriction of inversion or eversion motions. In considering the use of these

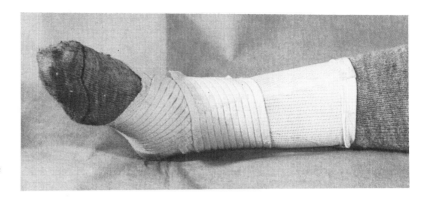

FIGURE 15. Elastic ankle support.

braces, one might also consider them as an alternative or adjunct to ankle taping, especially if a competent, skilled taper is not readily available. Bunch et al.[4] compared the comfort and effectiveness of ankle taping to five different commercial ankle braces. Initial comfort and support were highest in the freshly taped ankle. However, after 20 minutes of inversion exercises, "two of the lace-on braces offered the same level of support as the tape." They concluded that, at the end of their conservative 20-minute test, there was no difference in the level of support for the top two lace-on style braces (Swede-O, Mikros 9-in.) and taping.

Air Cast. The air cast can be of great use to the physician, therapist, and trainer from early in the rehabilitation program to the late stages of return to functional activity for the athlete with a moderate to severe ankle injury. Stover[20] described the use of a semi-

rigid support in case studies of seven athletic patients. The air cast is similar in design and principles for use to the semi-rigid material described (Fig. 17). It provides a milking effect upon weightbearing, which appears to decrease post-trauma edema with the addition of an air bag lining, it allows for an earlier return to functional activities, it decreases unwanted excessive inversion and eversion, and it protects the already injured ligamentous and soft tissues from reinjury or further injury, thereby decreasing rehabilitation time.[21] We have found that air casts are easy to use and fit in most athletic footwear. Their application is easily taught and followed and the athlete's confidence in the brace is increased with use. Even when combined with ankle taping, it does not significantly decrease speed or jumping ability.

SHOE INSERTS

Although not truly braces, orthotics are common devices used to aid in the treatment of athletic injury. Orthotics are defined here as devices placed in the athlete's shoe to balance the foot during activity. External support in the area of orthotics requires careful selection by the practitioner and athlete alike, always being conscious of the demands of the activity, ease of application, and adaptability to the athlete's condition.

Soft Orthotics. Sometimes used until the permanent orthotic returns from the laboratory, some soft orthotics can also be purchased over the counter (Fig. 18). They are

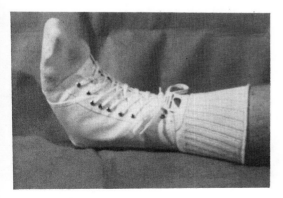

FIGURE 16. Lace-up ankle support.

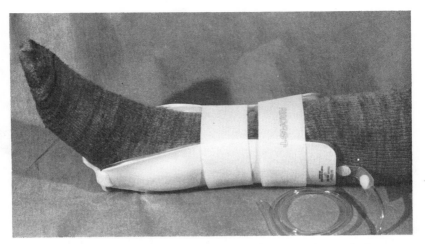

FIGURE 17.   Air cast with pressure adjustment tube attached.

relatively easy to adapt to and have a high compliance among athletes. Care must be taken in not using a "cure for all" orthotic that may treat more than one condition, thus predisposing the normal foot structures.

Hard Orthotics. Sometimes more difficult to get accustomed to initially, these devices are usually custom fit for the individual condition, but some over-the-counter varieties exist (Fig. 18). They hold up well and are often the key to solving the mystery of pain within the kinetic chain of the body. They should be used only in patients involved in straight ahead running.

Semi-rigid Orthotics. These devices attempt to provide the support of hard ortho-

tics but are designed to balance the feet of athletes involved in agility sports (Fig. 18). Since each sport has its own skill requirements, the orthotic selected must reflect these differences.

Sorbothane Insoles. Sorbothane is often used to decrease impact forces (Fig. 19). These insoles are easy to use and do not attempt to correct or alter foot mechanics.

Heel Cups. Soft heel cups (e.g., Tulis) are well recommended for the athlete with a "heel bruise" or "heel pain" when other possibilities have been ruled out. They help to decrease impact and to improve the shock absorption capabilities of the fat pad of the calcaneus.

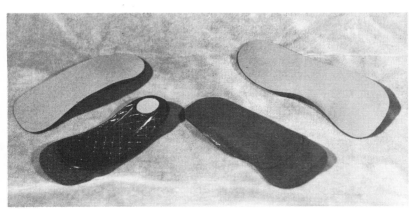

FIGURE 18. Spenco arch supports, rigid (left) and semi-rigid (right).

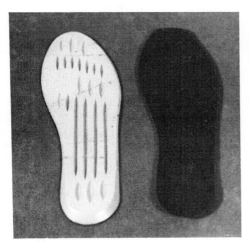

FIGURE 19. Sorbathane insoles.

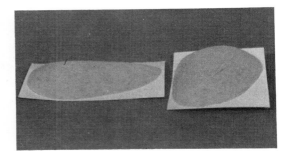

FIGURE 21. Longitudinal arch pads.

Metatarsal and Longitudinal Arch Pads.
Metatarsal (Fig. 20) and longitudinal (Fig. 21) arch pads, when applied to the footwear and not the foot, provide very good support to the ligamentous, bony, and muscular structures that help to form the arches of the feet and also provide some symptomatic relief for painful foot conditions. They can also be applied directly to the skin, following the previously mentioned principles of taping.

Steel Shoe Inserts. These can be used to help manage metatarsal fractures and turf-toe, and in certain brands of football turf shoes are standard equipment as they are incorporated directly into the insole liner (Fig. 22).

CONCLUSION

The need for research and development in the area of external support of athletic injuries is quite evident. Until such rigorous studies are conclusive, selection of taping and bracing will continue to depend on anecdotal information. Being aware of what is available, keeping abreast of new developments and analyzing them carefully, and talking to others who have experience in

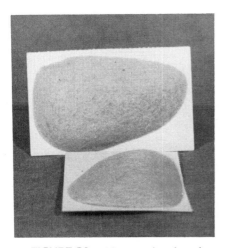

FIGURE 20. Metatarsal arch pads.

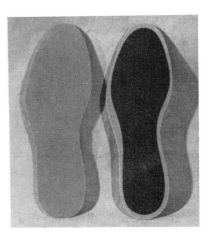

FIGURE 22. Steel shoe inserts.

their use can assist the sportsmedicine practitioner in selecting a method of support. Taping and bracing can decrease the risk of reinjury, especially when performed under the supervision of one skilled and knowledgeable in these methods. Because of the inherent nature of sport, it is paramount that the practitioner imply no guarantees. Placing an emphasis on complete rehabilitation and individualizing the choice of taping or bracing will allow the athletic patient to safely resume activity.

REFERENCES

1. Bassett FH, Malone T, Gilcrist RA: A protective splint of rubber. Am J Sports Med 7:358, 1979.
2. Beck C, Drez D, Young J, et al: Instrumented testing of functional knee braces. Am J Sports Med 14:253, 1986.
3. Bradley JA: The modified rubber playing cast. Physician Sportsmed 10:168, 1982.
4. Bunch RP, Bednarski K, Holland D, Macinanti R: Ankle joint support: A comparison of reuseable lace-on braces with taping and bracing. Physician Sportsmed 13:59, 1985.
5. Distefano V, Nixon JE: An improved method of taping. J Sports Med 2:209, 1974.
6. Doughtie M.: The use of RTV-11 silicone rubber for a carpal navicular fracture. Athletic Training 14:146, 1979.
7. Functional knee braces help stabilize medial collateral ligament. Orthop Today 6:1, 1986.
8. Garrick JG, Requa RK: Role of external support in the prevention of ankle sprains. Med Sci Sports 5:200, 1973.
9. Hewson GF, Mendini RA, Wang JB: Prophylactic knee bracing in college football. Am J Sports Med 14:262, 1986.
10. Knee braces to prevent injuries in football: A round table. Physician Sportsmed 14:108, 1986.
11. Laughman RK, Carr TA, Chao EY, et al: Three dimensional kinematics of the taped ankle before and after exercise. Am J Sports Med 8:425, 1980.
12. Libera D.: Ankle taping, wrapping, and injury prevention. Athletic Training 7:73, 1972.
13. Lysholm J, Nordin M, Ekstrand J, Gilquist J: The effects of a patella brace on performance in knee extension strength test in patients with patellar pain. Am J Sports Med 12:110, 1984.
14. Metcalf GR, Denegar CR: A critical review of ankle taping. Athletic Training 18:121, 1983.
15. Nirschl RP: The etiology and treatment of tennis elbow. J Sports Med 2:308, 1974.
16. Palumbo PM: Dynamic patellar brace: A new orthosis in the management of patello-femoral disorders. A preliminary report. Am J Sports Med 9:45, 1981.
17. Peppard A: Thumb taping. Physician Sportsmed 10:139, 1982.
18. Prentice WE, Toriscelli T: The effects of lateral knee stabilizing braces on running speed and agility. Athletic Training 21:113, 1986.
19. Ross SE: The supportive effect of modified Duke Simpson strapping. Athletic Training 13:206, 1978.
20. Stover C.: A functional semirigid support system for ankle injuries. Physician Sportsmed 7(5):71, 1979.
21. Stover CN: Air stirrup management of ankle injuries in the athlete. Am J Sport Med 8:360, 1980.
22. Thorndike A: Athletic Injuries: Prevention, Diagnosis and Treatment. Philadelphia, Lea and Febiger, 1948.
23. Weber JE: Personal communication. 1987.
24. Whitesel J, Newell SG: Modified low-dye strapping. Physician Sportsmed 8(9):129, 1980.

RECOMMENDED READING

1. Arnheim DD, Klafs CE: Modern Principles of Athletic Training, 5th ed, St. Louis, C. V. Mosby, 1981.
2. Athletic Uses of Adhesive Tape. Johnson & Johnson Products, Inc., 1981.
3. Cerney JV: Complete Book of Athletic Taping Techniques. West Nyack, NY, Parker Publishing Company, 1972.

22 Overuse Syndromes in Runners

WALTER B. FRANZ, III, M.D.

Part I: Approaches to Diagnosis and General Treatment Principles

Physical exertion in America has moved from the workplace to the swimming pools, tennis courts, and tracks of our communities (Fig. 1). During the Industrial Revolution human labor accounted for 30% of the energy used in factories and farms. It now accounts for less than 1%.[59] As work-centered human activity decreased, leisure- and fitness-intensive activity markedly increased. It is estimated that 10 million Americans run recreationally or competitively and approximately 36% of these runners will sustain an injury of some type in their running career.[19] As an entry point into the health care system, the primary care physician is often faced with the diagnosis and treatment of runners' injuries, regardless of his or her specialty or background. In approximately 65% of injuries, if the primary care physician is knowledgeable about this subject, no additional consultation may be needed.[59]

Overuse syndromes are chronic musculoskeletal injuries that occur when an excess of stress over repair exists in exercised tissue. Because tissue repair lags behind tissue inflammation, stresses in tissue can accumulate and an athlete can overload the capacity of tissue to compensate and repair, resulting in injury.[40] Overuse syndromes are not unique to runners. Any sport or occupation involving chronic musculoskeletal activity can result in overuse syndromes, i.e., tennis elbow, ulnar neuropathy in bikers, and shoulder problems in swimmers. All overuse syndromes involve chronic tissue stress which occurs during repetitive activities, and the tissues affected are usually biomechanically critical anatomic structures. The lower extremities in runners are the structures most stressed, since they are responsible for locomotion, shock absorption, and surface adaptation. The capacity of the lower extremities to repair after running-induced stress is limited, however, by daily training routines and by the extensive use of the lower extremities in activities of daily living.

Runners endure injuries and the rigors of training for a variety of reasons, the most notable being to gain physical fitness and decrease cardiovascular risk factors,[33] to reduce stress,[43,46] to attempt to prolong life[49] and to lose weight.[21] In contradistinction, runners stop running more often due to switching to another form of exercise or for personal time reasons rather than injury, since most runners feel that it is better to run while hurting than not to run at all.[32] With the vast popularity of running as well as its strong association with modification and amelioration of cardiovascular risk factors, it is not surprising that runners will avoid any encounter that may decrease their chosen activity. Such encounters may occur in the physician's office as a necessary adjunct to the treatment of overuse syndromes. If the physician is able to diagnose, treat, and return the patient to running as soon as possible, the patient will view the encounter as positive.

GENERAL APPROACH TO OVERUSE INJURIES

The approach to the patient with running-induced overuse syndromes is enhanced by several additions to the customary history and physical examination. To treat these

THE RUNNING DECADE 1972-1982

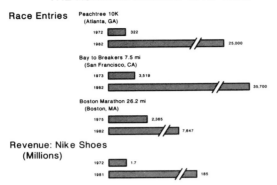

FIGURE 1. Reproduced with permission from Flippin: The Runner 4(11): 20, August, 1982.

TABLE 1   STAGING OF OVERUSE SYNDROMES

Grade I	Post activity soreness Duration of symptoms less than two weeks Generalized tenderness

Grade II	Pain during end of running and
	   immediately after
	Duration of symptoms greater than
	   two weeks
	Localized pain, minimal inflammation

Grade III	Pain during early training
	Duration of symptoms greater than
	   three weeks
	Point tenderness, definite objective tissue
	   inflammatory signs (erythema, edema,
	   crepitus)

Grade IV	Pain with activities other than training,
	   severity of which prohibits training or
	   competition
	Grade III symptoms plus—Disfunction
	   of injured structure, muscle atrophy,
	   tisue breakdown

patients successfully, a physician must know the specific pathophysiology and epidemiology of runners' injuries and the specialized historical factors of training practices as well as possess an appreciation of normal and abnormal biomechanics and an understanding of the functional anatomy of the lower extremity. In addition, the physician must be able to prescribe proper footwear and orthotics when necessary and should know the principles of exercise prescription that allow a patient to reach peak fitness safely as well as how to return a patient to running after a proper course of rest and physiotherapy. Treatment will succeed best if the patient and physician are able to agree on a program to treat the specific injury, maintain fitness, and allow re-evaluation of training goals and formulation of injury prophylaxis for the future.

Pathophysiology of Overuse. Pathologically, overuse syndromes in runners start as microtrauma to localized tissue areas that are under stress. As inflammation develops faster than the tissue's capacity for self-repair, macroscopic irritation and damage culminate in tissue disruption.[26,40] Ideally, at the onset of symptoms in very early overuse (grades I and II), the runner should evaluate his or her training program for possible errors or deficiencies (Table 1). However, the same "drive" that motivates athletes to run likely will encourage an attempt to "run through" the pain. Most patients will not seek medical advice until more advanced degrees of injuries are present, as in grade III or IV

overuse. At this time pain limits competitive effectiveness and some interruption of the patient's training activities is inevitable, in order to allow tissue repair.[40] During this period of enforced rest the patient should be taught the warning symptoms of early overuse and be encouraged not to follow the inappropriate and overused dictum, "no pain, no gain."

Epidemiology of Overuse Syndromes in Runners. Epidemiologically, the most significant factor in overuse syndromes in runners is excessive mileage during training.[6,32,51] There is a linear relationship between injury rate in runners and mileage run.[51] From a practical standpoint, once the 30-mile-per-week training threshold is reached, the yearly injury rate rises to greater than 20% per year for females, 15% for males.[51] Numerous other factors have been epidemiologically examined with respect to runners' injuries, such as age and sex of the runner, the effect of terrain upon running injuries, and the benefit of stretching and warm-up activities upon injury incidence. Although all of these factors may have direct importance in individual cases, the mileage run becomes most important. "Over-mileage," however, may be a relative rather than an absolute concept. For instance, total mileage run per week does not take into account how rapidly this level of mileage was achieved, and although relatively few total miles per week may be run, the pace of advancement may have been excessively ambitious[6]. Specific guidelines on how often and to what degree mileage should be advanced per week may be difficult to find. In general, a greater than 10% increase of mileage per week should be avoided.[1] From a pathophysiologic approach, an increase in training mileage should not be accompanied by more than the lowest grade of overuse symptoms (Fig. 2).

History of Present Injury. The history of a patient with a presumed overuse syndrome should include three basic subunits. The first subunit is concerned with the traditional aspects of any patient encounter, i.e., when the injury occurred, what structure seems to be injured, the characterization of the pain, what treatment has already been provided and the pertinent past medical and orthopedic history. The second subunit of information should include questions about specific training practices and inquiries intended to uncover possible biomechanical abnormalities that may be contributing to the injury. Specific inquiry should be made about the total weekly mileage, as well as recent changes in miles run or intensity of running. Because of differences in shock absorption, the type of surface upon which the runner trained should be known. The surface grade should be noted, because if the patient has recently switched to hill training, ad-

ditional stress may have been placed upon previously unstressed structures. For instance, uphill running may overstress the gastric-Achilles tendon system and downhill running may stress tibial stabilizers such as the plantaris muscle or overstress the anterior tibialis muscle group.

A frequently omitted but important historical item is the side of the roadway on which training occurs. Consistently running on a banked roadway or track will cause excessive pronation of the upper foot and excessive supination of the lower foot (Fig. 3).[61]

Careful scrutiny should be made of "leisure" sports in which the patient participates. Much time can be spent dissecting the training practices of a runner and finding no specific factors that indicate the diagnosis of an overuse syndrome, only to learn that the patient has taken up sports that the patient does not view as competitive or fitness-oriented but that may be contributing to an injury. A typical example is the runner who also participates in racquet sports where excessive strain may be caused by the quick

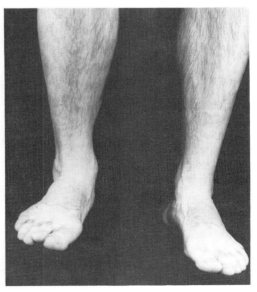

FIGURE 3. Effect of banked surface on biomechanics. Subject is exhibiting internal rotation and pronation of uphill tibia and foot and external rotation and supination of downhill foot.

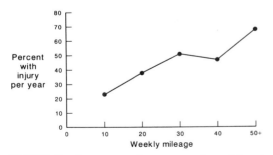

FIGURE 2. Percentage of runners, male and female, injured during one year per weekly mileage run. (Adapted from Koplan J P, et al: JAMA 248:3118, 1982.)

lateral motions necessary. Therefore, a combination of sports may place more strain on a lower extremity structure than any of the individual activities taken alone.

The third subunit of the history involves specific training practices. In the competitive runner, practices such as interval training may be undertaken to build speed and strength, in addition to the long, slow distance training that most joggers prefer. Interval training commonly introduces fast or sprint running at a pace greater than normally utilized in racing. Since the biomechanical strain of sprinting is greater, injury may occur.[5] Many athletes now include resistance training in their personal fitness programs. Such training, especially that involving full quadriceps extensions, squats, or hamstring strengthening exercises, should be noted, since ligamental strain, muscle injury, and tendonitis may result from overzealous resistance work.

The history should also focus on footwear.[15] This includes both the patient's training footwear, specifically how often a patient changes footwear, to what degree wear is apparent before a change, and whether or not the patient trains extensively in repaired rather than replaced shoes. Extensively repaired shoes may lose their shock-absorbing function due to mid-sole fatigue. The use of racing footwear should be noted, because racing flats may have little heel lift or shock-absorbing capacity and should be used primarily for highly competitive situations and not for general training. It is also prudent to question the patient about footwear worn recreationally or during work. Many patients run only a few minutes a day, whereas they may walk, work, climb stairs, dance, and stand for several hours a day in ill-fitting, poor shock-absorbing footwear. The third subunit should also include any systemic effects of overtraining. Systemic signs of overuse syndromes include excessive fatigue after exercise, and especially fatigue and excessive stiffness persisting the day after training. There may be no way to quantitate "staleness" in an athlete; however, when faced with a patient who expresses a history of generalized fatigue and a lack of interest in further training and a wish for additional rest, it is usually safe to assume that these are important signs of generalized overuse.

BASIC BIOMECHANICS OF RUNNING[2,29,30,38]

The forces generated by an average runner during even a leisurely jog are astounding. For each mile run, each foot contacts the running surface approximately 1000 times. At initial foot contact the lower extremity is required to absorb and dissipate forces 2–3 times body weight. Over a one-mile jog several tons of force per foot are accumulated and then multiplied by the several miles per day that many recreational runners train.[16] An exact biomechanical analysis of walking, running, and sprinting is beyond the scope of this chapter, but the basic components of running biomechanics are helpful to the primary care physician in diagnosing and treating overuse syndromes.

There are two basic phases of gait in running, the support phase during which the reference foot contacts the surface, and the recovery phase during which the reference foot is following through in preparation for surface contact. The percentage of the gait cycle delegated to the support phase or the recovery phase varies greatly from walking to running to sprinting. The walking gait generally does not have a prolonged recovery phase because there is no time when a limb is airborne; therefore, the amount of time in the support phase is long and allows for excellent shock absorption and dissipation (Fig. 4). The time available for shock absorption in the runner's support phase is approximately 50% of that of walking, and the recovery phase is lengthened. As speed in-

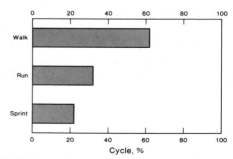

FIGURE 4. Comparison of time available for support phase in walking, running, and sprinting. (Adapted from Mann RA, Hagy J: Am J Sports Med 8:345, 1980.)

creases and a sprinting stance is assumed, the support phase is further shortened to approximately one-third of the time compared to walking.[38] Careful gait analysis of the runner has shown that when speed increases to the point of sprinting, the runner runs continually on his or her toes. Because of the high speed there is insufficient time for the lower extremities to absorb shock other than to absorb some ground contact forces by ankle dorsiflexion. An analogy has been suggested—that the sprinter is using his or her legs as if they were spokes on a wheel rather than a fixed structure.[29]

It is helpful to proceed through a normal running gait cycle, and for reference purposes the right foot will be described (Fig. 5). Starting with the end of the recovery phase, the right foot begins a forward swing that flows into right foot descent. The descent stage is heralded by rearward motion until foot descent terminates with foot strike. At this point, the right foot accelerates to the same velocity as the body. With foot contact the support phase begins. The hip is initially in extension and slight internal rotation. The knee is slightly flexed and in most runners the foot initially makes contact in a supinated position on the outside of the heel. The supinated foot is a relatively firm, rigid base to support further contact and eventual propulsion. The foot then rapidly pronates into an unstable but highly shock-absorbing and flexible structure to allow for surface adaptation. The subtarsal joint needs at least 4 degrees of pronation to be able to adapt adequately for surface contact and shock absorption.[64]

If the foot cannot pronate adequately, an increase in foot strike shock will be transmitted proximally, leading to possible overuse symptoms. On the other hand, if the foot pronates too much, the resulting hypermobility can lead to a variety of overuse problems. Motion is also occurring in the transverse plane during initial surface contact, with internal tibial torsion occurring concomitant with subtalar-joint pronation. The contact stage takes approximately 25% of the time of the total support phase. Midstance phase then begins and encompasses the middle 50% of the support phase. During this time, the center of gravity of the body moves over the foot due to hip extension and forward momentum. The ankle dorsiflexes to shorten the extremity. During the midstance phase the foot should be biomechanically in the ideal neutral position, with the lower tibia in direct line with the calcaneus and perpendicular to the metatarsals. At the end of the midstance phase a 10 degree forward swing occurs on the foot in order to start heel lift for the eventual takeoff stage. During the end of the midstance phase, the tibia externally rotates and the subtalar joint supinates, changing the foot to a rigid structure in preparation for takeoff. During the takeoff phase, the last 25% of contact phase, the heel rises, the knee extends, and plantar flexion occurs at the ankle. The very forceful extension of the knee and plantar flexion of the foot propels the body with the center of gravity moving up and forward. The rigid steady lever generated by supination of the subtalar joint accommodates the intense muscular activity of takeoff. Ideally the pro-

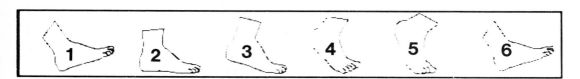

FIGURE 5. *Stylized biomechanics of the running foot.*
1. *Heel strike.* Foot in supinated position, initial surface contact, beginning of support phase.
2. *Midstance.* Foot pronated to adapt to surface and to dissipate shock. Center of gravity over STJ. Tibia internally rotates.
3. *Late midstance.* Center of gravity anterior to STJ. Heel lift with dorsiflexion of foot.
4. *Early toe-off.* Foot re-supinates to allow rigid lever for propulsion. External rotation of tibia.
5. *Toe off.* Propulsion of limb.
6. *Recovery phase.* Foot airborne, begins to swing posteriorly in preparation for new gait cycle.

pulsive forces extend vectorally toward the ball of the foot and first ray.

In this simplistic overview of running biomechanics, it must be appreciated that upper body structures are also playing a role in the running gait cycle. Generally the arms are synchronous with the contralateral limb and the trunk rotates away from the supporting limb. The trunk should be nearly erect, and if not, as occurs with fatigue, there is less time to accelerate the foot backwards during the descent phase and the result is increased forces on foot strike.[38]

PHYSICAL AND BIOMECHANICAL EXAMINATION[2,28,29,50,64]

The physical examination of the runner with an overuse syndrome centers on two major areas: (1) the specific physical examination of the injured structure or anatomic area; and (2) examination of the patient for any biomechanical abnormalities that could have caused the injury or might lead to injuries in the future. The specific findings on physical examination for the most common overuse syndromes will be covered in the second part of this chapter.

A systematic approach is used for the biomechanical examination. With the patient standing, first examine general muscular development, noting the quadriceps, particularly the vastus medialis group. Deficiency in the vastus medialis muscle may lead to abnormal patellar tracking, which is implicated in patellar pain syndrome. Observing the rear of the patient, attention should be paid to any evidence of pelvic tilt, which may suggest a leg-length discrepancy. If there is a question of leg-length discrepancy, the patient may be placed supine and leg length measured from the anterior-superior iliac spine to the medial malleolus. A true anatomically short lower extremity will usually have compensatory supination of the foot on the short extremity and pronation of the foot on the normal or longer extremity. A greater than ¼ inch difference in leg lengths may be sufficient to warrant an appropriate correction.

Again examine the standing patient in the frontal plane to note varum or valgum deformities of the femur and tibia. Generally a valgum deformity of the femur is accompanied by genu varum, and varum deformity of the femur by genu valgum, a contrasting pair of abnormalities. These frontal plane deformities tend to cause considerable alteration of foot planting and side-to-side sway during running. The coxa vara–genu valgum combination is especially problematic with respect to overpronation as well as medial joint strain in the knee. Tibial varum is a relatively common condition found on the biomechanical examination. This will be noted by the patient's knees being far apart when the feet are in juxtaposition. The patient can then be asked to assume his or her most comfortable normal stance. Careful attention should be paid to whether or not the patella are centered toward the examiner, turned in toward each other, or deviated laterally.

Further attention should then be directed to the biomechanics of the subtalar joint (Fig. 6). Ideally the subtalar joint, when in neutral position, should allow the tibia, talus and calcaneus to be in direct alignment, and a line drawn through these structures should be perpendicular to the metatarsals as they contact the supporting surface.[64] To recognize if there is a deviation from the ideal, place the patient prone and palpate medially and laterally over the talus, moving the foot until there is an equal protrusion of the talus on each side. The subtalar joint should be in the neutral or biomechanically ideal position. At this point note the relationship of a line bisecting the calcaneus to the tibia (Fig. 7). In most cases the calcaneus will be in a slight varus position, i.e., no greater than 4 degrees in relationship to the lower leg.[64] The angular positioning of the forefoot from the rearfoot is then determined by providing plantar force to the fourth and fifth metatarsal until resistance is felt (Fig. 8). When resistance occurs, draw an imaginary line from the head of the fifth metatarsal to the head of the first and then determine if this line deviates from a perpendicular relationship with a line bisecting the calcaneus. If the relationship is a perpendicular one, then there is no difference between alignment of forefoot to hindfoot. If there is a forefoot

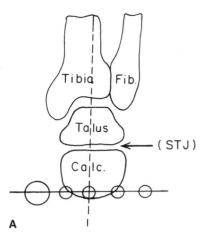

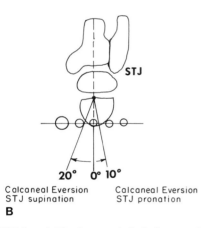

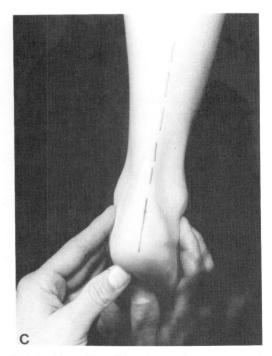

FIGURE 6. *A, The theoretical ideal: the neutral subtalar joint (STJ).* In this position tibia, talus, and calcaneus are in alignment. The metatarsals are perpendicular. *B,* Motions about the subtalar joint (STJ) Total range of motion = 30°. *C,* Determining the "neutral" subtalar joint. The patient is prone and the talar neutral position is being determined.

varus or valgus difference, this should be noted. Forefoot valgus is commonly found in the cavus foot. Forefoot varus may require increased pronation to adequately contact the surface while running.[29,64]

The physical examination of any runner presenting with an overuse syndrome is not complete without an examination of the patient's footwear.[9,16] The patient should always be encouraged to bring along running footwear, which may demonstrate the patient's biomechanics by its specific wear pattern. The normal wear pattern for most biomechanically sound runners includes wear

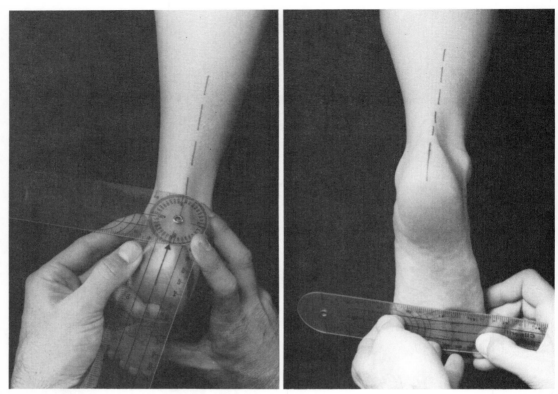

FIGURE 7. The subtalar joint neutral position has been determined and its angular deviation from the perpendicular is measured. This subject shows minimal varus displacement.

FIGURE 8. Determining forefoot angular deviation from the ideal. This subject has a slight varus of the forefoot.

on the outside or lateral aspect of the heel, which represents initial foot strike, and wear over the first metatarsal and ball of the foot, representing normal toeoff.[2] In many runners the wear pattern may be normal, but it may be obvious that the running shoes are badly overworn. Once the lateral heel sole is thin to the point of showing midsole, the shock-absorbing capacity of many shoes will be exhausted. In addition, the overwear of the lateral aspect of the heel will allow excessive supination of the foot at the time of heel contact. It is also important to examine the everyday footwear of the patient, because in many cases the patient will have appropriate athletic footwear but will have overworn everyday shoes, which may lead to exacerbation of previous problems.

GENERAL TREATMENT APPROACHES

The initial step in the general treatment approach to any overuse syndrome in runners is classification of the degree of overuse. Classification of the extent of overuse will help both physician and patient evaluate treatment effectiveness and training modification.[40] The McKeag scale is a useful system.[40] The McKeag scale, which is a classification of overuse in terms of severity and symptoms, goes beyond the simple utility of an accurate record in the patient's history. Involving the patient in noting overuse symptoms, when they occur and to what degree, engages the individual in the diagnosis and treatment of the problem and therefore makes him or her an active participant in therapy and prophylaxis. Such cooperation is essential, since the goal of the treatment of overuse syndromes is to make the patient the prime mover in rehabilitation and modification of training or competitive practices that may have caused the injury.

Rest.[26,30,40,58] Paramount in the treatment of an overuse syndrome is rest, since the basic etiology of overuse injuries is the inability of the normal repair mechanisms to compensate for inflammation generated during activity. Rest, however, is a generic term and must be properly applied and prescribed. The more severe the class of injury, the more likely more stringent rest is needed. Likewise, in the sedentary individual, cessation rather than modification of activity may be necessary, whereas in the elite athlete, "rest" may mean a decrease in training mileage, with modification, not cessation, of running. Both the recreational and competitive runner may benefit from being encouraged to adopt a training activity with less biomechanical strain on a specific body part but one that maintains aerobic fitness and strength. For many runners, this will be a non-weight-bearing activity such as swimming. Bicycling may also be utilized in specific instances if it is pain-free. For athletes who must maintain a high level of competitive performance, training may need to be divided into several smaller training sessions per day, with rest and rehabilitation in between. Whenever rest is prescribed, it must be done with the goals and preferences of the patient in mind. If not, the athlete will view rest as a mandated cessation of a desired activity, perhaps an unwelcome side effect of consulting a physician and therefore a treatment to be avoided. If, however, rest is presented to the patient as a way of decreasing inflammation of an injured structure, and if an ancillary activity is provided that allows the patient to remain active and fit, he or she will likely accept rest as a useful adjunct of therapy.

Cryotherapy.[31,41,58] Application of ice or other forms of cryotherapy to injured structures in overuse syndromes are generally used in any situation involving acute inflammation. Cryotherapy inhibits inflammation directly and increases the tensile strength of injured tissue. The athlete may apply the ice for 20 minutes or to his tolerance for discomfort and then allow tissue rewarming and reapplication. Ice is most useful in the acute and early treatment phase of overuse syndromes to decrease swelling and as an adjunct to decrease pain and inhibit inflammation during rehabilitation. Contraindications to cryotherapy include any medical condition in the patient that inhibits the sensory nerve supply, such as diabetes, vascular disease, during the use of local anesthetic, or with any medical condition that would place the patient at risk of thermal injury. Heat is best used in the rehabilitation stage to increase tissue flexibility and elasticity and to encourage stretching. It should not be applied acutely or in suspected compartment syndromes, since heat may increase compartment volume and further compromise circulation.

Compression and elevation of the injured structure are usually utilized along with cryotherapy. Compression decreases edema and prevents accumulation of inflammatory products in the tissue. Elevation, likewise, will decrease edema, promote venous and lymphatic flow, and localize concentrations of inflammatory debris.

Pharmacologic Treatment. Nonsteroidal anti-inflammatory drugs (NSAIDs) and salicylates are useful both acutely and chronically in overuse syndromes. These drugs basically act by inhibiting prostaglandin synthesis, which interrupts the cascade of inflammatory response in injured tissue. Pain relief during the longer term use of these agents generally signifies decreased inflammation as well as the initial "pain killing" mechanism of action. Use of salicylates or NSAIDs will depend on cost, compliance, and side effects. Agents generally need two weeks for full effect.

Injectable corticosteroids, often mixed with a local anesthetic, are occasionally indicated when more conservative methods of treating some soft tissue injuries have been exhausted. Steroids should not be injected into tendons, since direct injection into these structures may induce structural weakening and ultimately rupture.[52] Since some systemic spillover will occur with injectable corticosteroids, they should be used cautiously. The possibility of introducing infection should always be considered, especially if joint injection is planned, and the risks and benefits of joint injection should be carefully weighed in this situation. The skin should be surgically prepared and scrubbed before injecting corticosteroids into a bursa, a joint, or peritendinous tissue.

Orthotics.[11,16,18,30] Orthotics related to running are inserts of rubber, plastic, or other molded material in the shoe to alter or counteract biomechanical abnormalities thought to be implicated in overuse syndromes.[1] More precisely, orthotics balance the foot and direct its biomechanics toward the ideal neutral position so as to inhibit excessive pronation or supination. The proper fitting and construction of an orthotic are beyond the scope of this chapter. An orthotic will best suit the patient when a definitive biomechanical abnormality is found that is directly implicated in the overuse syndrome being experienced by the patient. Considerable knowledge of orthotics and their biomechanical use is needed in the proper construction and application of devices to limit subtalar joint abnormalities. It is important to realize that many runners will have abnormal biomechanics but will be symptom-free with respect to overuse. In these patients the use of orthotics may cause symptoms in and of themselves, and therefore such treatment of these patients is inappropriate.

Shoes.[2,9,16,20] A component of any treatment program for overuse syndromes in runners is the prescribing of proper footwear. The major footwear problem of most runners derives from overworn shoes, followed by footwear inappropriate for a specific biomechanical abnormality. Runners accumulating more than 25 miles/week should change shoes every three months, less than 25 miles/

week every four to six months.[20] The basic functions of any quality shoe used in running are to enhance shock absorption and foot control, and to provide good traction and protection (Fig. 9). The soles of good running shoes should be carbonated to provide long wear. A waffle style construction of the sole will allow greater shock absorption. A widened heel with a heel lift provides for enhanced shock absorption and less stress upon the Achilles tendon.

The lasting or curve of the sole of the shoe should generally conform to the patient's own foot shape. In general, most patients will do well with a relatively straight last. The runner with a high arch or cavus foot may benefit from a more C-shaped or curved last. The shoes should be comfortably snug, but should allow for a mild increase in volume of the foot as running occurs.

Heel control to limit excessive heel motion can be accomplished by purchasing a shoe with a firm heel counter or cup. A good controlling shoe will not wobble when standing on one foot.[20] Padding around the Achilles tendon in good quality shoes provides less direct trauma to the Achilles tendon. A meshed upper portion decreases heat and moisture buildup in the shoe. Many manufacturers now provide information on shoes that have been selectively designed to limit common foot abnormalities such as overpronation or oversupination at the subtalar joint. If these biomechanical abnormalities are thought to play a role in a particular patient's overuse syndrome, it would be reasonable to prescribe a particular shoe type.

Warm-up and Cool-down Techniques.[34,45,57] It is suggested that, prior to stretching, a warm-up long enough to cause sweating and a mild feeling of exertion take place. During

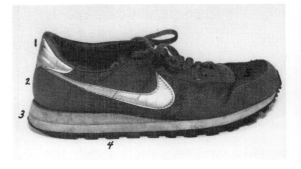

FIGURE 9.   Running shoe anatomy: **1,** Achilles tendon pad; **2,** heel counter for firm heel control; **3,** heel lift to decrease Achilles tendon tension and add shock absorption; **4,** carbonated waffle sole to provide increased shock absorption, traction and excellent wear characteristics; **5,** nylon mesh upper to promote ventilation, decrease shoe weight and provide flexibility.

an appropriate warm-up, increased muscle temperature enhances oxygen release from hemoglobin, increases blood flow by a vasodilatory effect in muscle, and decreases blood viscosity.[34] The proper warm-up also enhances muscular contraction and speed of neuromuscular transmission, which improves the reaction time to stimuli. The final benefit of the warm-up period is that tissue elasticity increases along with decreased viscosity of synovial fluid, thereby allowing greater flexibility and gains to be made from stretching.

Immediately after the warm-up period, gentle nonballistic stretching should be done. Many specific muscle stretching techniques and regimens have been devised, but the best general guideline for any stretching program for runners is to pay careful attention to the hamstring and gastrocnemius muscle group and to the iliotibial band, since excessive tightness in any of these muscles and connective tissues may lead to specific overuse syndromes. Proprioceptive exercises that involve stretching also seem important to facilitate enhanced neuromuscular efficiency.[57] It is important that the stretching be done gently and never past the point of minimal discomfort, since excessive pain may represent tissue injury not enhanced flexibility.[59] Some runners may advocate a gentle warm-up in their training period, followed by stretching at the end of their run. This is permissible as long as the warm-up period is providing appreciable flexibility at the start of the run. An appropriate warm-up in this instance would be alternating a jog for 220 yards with walking 20 yards, for approximately one half mile.[34] Following the training period, an active rather than passive cool-down period is recommended to facilitate removal of lactate from tissue, to allow heart rate and respiration to decrease to pre-exercise levels, and to allow further stretching of warm flexible muscles.

Flexibility, Strength and Stretching.[59,63] Although not directly implicated in overuse syndromes, lack of muscle group flexibility may potentiate other biomechanical abnormalities, which then lead to an injury. Lack of flexibility can also impede rehabilitation of an injury. It is important for runners to realize that running, like any other musculo-skeletal activity, will selectively strengthen certain muscle groups and leave other muscle groups relatively underdeveloped. For the recreational jogger, this would commonly be hypertrophy of the hamstring gastrocnemius muscle group, with concomitant inflexibility of these muscles unless they are stretched appropriately. For example the relative lack of development of the quadriceps, especially the vastus medialis group in the runner, may have a role in abnormal patellar tracking as seen in chondromalacia.[24] Specific exercise of the quadriceps group and especially the vastus medialis will be accomplished with rehabilitation exercises.[2] It is important to recall that the vastus medialis group, which stabilizes the patella medially, will be selectively exercised if resistance is used in the last 15–20 degrees of extension.

Another commonly overlooked muscle group that is important in preventing back pain in the runner is the rectus abdominis group. The rectus abdominis is not ordinarily exercised in the runner unless specific attention is devoted to its development. If rectus abdominis strength is inadequate, remedial exercises commonly suggested are leg lifts, which strengthen the lower rectus abdominis group, and slow sit-ups, especially "abdominal crunches," which exercise the upper portion of the rectus abdominis.

GOALS AND FITNESS PRESCRIPTION

As mentioned in other connections, the most common etiologic factor in overuse syndrome is overtraining.[32,51] When a patient is seen for an overuse syndrome, one of the most important factors related to treatment and rehabilitation is re-evaluation of training practices and goals, which may change greatly the rate of injury recurrence with little or no change in fitness.

Case Report. A 30-year-old male suffered from chronic bilateral Achilles tendinitis of two years' duration. At the time of presentation to his physician, the patient had been running approximately 20–22 miles per week at a 7½ min/mile pace. To increase fitness, the patient was alternating running with competitive soccer. When ased what the basic goals of his personal fitness program were, he listed them as: (1) to maintain fitness and modify cardiovascular risk; (2) to maintain a high enough fitness level to be competitive in soccer; and (3) to continue a fitness program but decrease the chronicity of the Achilles tendinitis. The history disclosed running on hard unyielding surfaces such as concrete roadway and asphalt. His running shoes were of good quality but badly overworn, and his everyday footwear had a badly worn sole and heel. Physical and biomechanical examination disclosed a relatively high-arched foot with severe tenderness of both Achilles tendons and a tendency for the calcaneus to be in varum with the talus in the neutral position. It was suggested to the patient that he decrease his mileage significantly and purchase new street and running shoes, but the patient was reluctant to decrease his training or limit his competitive soccer. The main reason that the patient refused to decrease his training mileage was that he felt he would suffer in terms of cardiovascular fitness. The patient was then asked to undergo a cardiovascular fitness evaluation, which disclosed a functional aerobic capacity of 140% for his age group. With this information, the patient acknowledged that his current program was producing excellent fitness but overuse. The patient agreed to decrease total mileage run as well as limit his soccer to a minimum. A frequent recheck of the patient's fitness level disclosed that his fitness was maintained but the grade 3 overuse syndrome of Achilles tendinitis decreased to grade 1, a minimal level.

In this case no change in fitness was noted with decreasing mileage run per week, whereas the overuse problems rapidly ameliorated. Alternative goals for a similar patient might be to participate in another sport activity such as swimming or bicycling to maintain fitness yet allow the running-induced injury to heal.[58]

Part II: Specific Overuse Injuries of Runners

For the practicing physician overuse injuries will not present as a training problem or as a biomechanical abnormality, but rather as pain or dysfunction of a specific body part which is interfering with running. Any lower extremity structure can be affected in a runner. Therefore, the list of possible injuries is almost inexhaustible. In this section common major overuse syndromes associated with running are presented.

THE KNEE: PATELLAR PAIN SYNDROME[10,24,35,37,42,47,56]

Pain in and around the knee is the most common overuse complaint and site of injury of runners. [6,29,32,42,47] Patellar pain syndrome or "runner's knee" is the most common specific knee overuse syndrome.[6] Many authorities would term this syndrome chondromalacia patella, but true chondromalacia or frank degeneration of the articular surface of the patella with fibrillation of the surface occurs only in the most severe forms of this syndrome.[10,42] The tracking problem is discussed in depth in Chapter 18.

ILIOTIBIAL BAND SYNDROME[2,26,29,36]

Iliotibial band or friction syndrome is the most common cause of lateral knee pain in runners (Fig. 10). Anatomically, the iliotibial band is a fascial band that extends from the iliac crest and inserts on the lateral tibial tubercle, also known as Gerdy's tubercle. The iliotibial band also receives contributions from the tensor fascia lata and the gluteus maximus muscles. With hip flexion and extension, the band is pulled anteriorly and posteriorly, and with repeated movement the band may impinge and develop friction with the lateral femoral condyle.[36]

Biomechanical abnormalities associated with the iliotibial band syndrome suggest

that any abnormality increasing the varus stress about the knee possibly will cause increased iliotibial band friction. Common etiologies include genu varum, cavus feet, footwear excessively worn on the lateral heel, and runners with overpronation leading to increased internal rotation of the knee and increased knee retinaculum tension laterally.[29,36]

The problem may result from a single severe running session or a sudden increase in running distance. Downhill running is often implicated because of the increased stride length of downhill running, which increases lateral tissue tension about the knee. The patient first notes pain laterally around the knee after exercise. This pain is usually not initially limiting and running may be continued. Pain then develops during running, eventually leading to severe cases in which pain occurs during daily activities, especially going up and down stairs and during other sports. The patient often finds that walking with a stiff knee in full extension enables him to ambulate without pain. Physical examination demonstrates tenderness laterally 2 cm above the joint space over the lateral femoral condyle. Crepitus may be noted over the area of pain. Palpation of the iliotibial band with flexion and extension of the hip will reproduce the pain. Ober's test may also be utilized to detect increased iliotibial band tension, which may be causing excessive pressure on the lateral femoral condyle.[28,50]

Therapy and Rehabilitation. Immediate therapy consists of ice, anti-inflammatory agents, and elimination of harmful training practices such as running on hills, banked tracks, and slanted roads. Using running shoes with enhanced shock absorption characteristics and which are free from lateral heel wear is also appropriate. Correction of leg-length imbalance with heel lifts and inhibition of overpronation of the foot with special shoes or orthotics to decrease internal tibial torsion may be warranted. Iliotibial

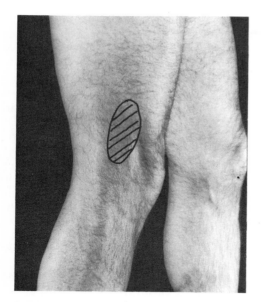

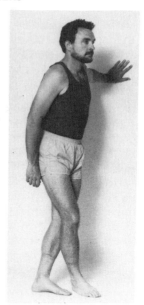

FIGURE 10.   Location of pain laterally in iliotibial band syndrome.

FIGURE 11.   Iliotibial band stretching. The subject is applying a varus stretch to the left iliotibial band by leaning gently into a wall.

band stretching (Fig. 11) should be emphasized, as well as encouragement of the patient to exercise only to the beginning of pain, as a means of preventing further inflammation. The use of corticosteroids applied by phonophoresis or iontophoresis often provides marked reduction in the inflammation. Some clinicians emphasize the use of injectable steroids for painful friction areas, but it has been found that conservative therapy short of injecting helps in more than 80% of cases of iliotibial band syndrome, with 50% of patients being improved in three weeks or less of conservative therapy.[36] After 12 months or more of conservative therapy without improvement, a surgical approach consisting of releasing posterior iliotibial band fibers concomitant with or releasing iliotibial band fibers from the lateral retinaculum of the knee and patella is recommended if the runner must continue in rigorous competition.[36]

LOWER LEG PAIN SYNDROMES[2,26,29,65]

Generically, lower leg pain syndrome (LLPS) describes a group of overuse syndromes consisting of pain distal to the knee and proximal to the ankle. Because of the great number of muscular, osseous, ligamental and tendinous structures involved in the lower leg, it would be impossible to describe all the potential overuse problems that arise. The majority of patients, however, will have one of a few distinct syndromes attributable to overuse in the lower leg. The main difficulty for the diagnostician is distinguishing benign conditions such as "shin splints" from the orthopedic emergency of acute compartment syndrome. LLPS also includes the most common source of osseous injury in the runner, i.e., tibial stress fracture. Each of the main components of LLPS will be described below.

Shin Splints.[2,5,17,29]   The term shin splints is a euphemism referring to a syndrome consisting of pain along the inner distal two thirds of the tibial shaft. The pathophysiology and biomechanical etiology of this syndrome cause some disagreement among authorities, with some believing that this syndrome is caused by excessive stress placed on the interosseous membrane between the tibia and fibula as a result of excessive activity of the posterior tibialis muscle, causing periostitis and periosteal stress reaction.[11] Others feel that the periostitis orginates from the area of the soleus muscle and excessive activity of the same.[17] Regardless of the muscle group involved, this syndrome usually presents with gradual increase in soreness and pain after running, then progresses to pain during activities such as walking. The pain has a dull, aching quality and typically is located over the posterior medial border of the tibia in the distal portion of the middle third.[3] The most common biomechanical abnormalities found on examination of the patient include escessive heel valgus and excessive forefoot pronation. Excessive pronation will cause increased internal tibial torsion that stresses the interosseous membrane and provokes increased activity of the tibialis posterior muscle.

Physical examination, discloses pain over the area described above.

Treatment and rehabilitation consist of relative or total rest, ice, anti-inflammatory medication, heel cord and hamstring stretching, and strengthening the dorsiflexion of the foot. As improvement of initial symptoms becomes evident, the patient may return to training with an emphasis on running on a soft flat surface with shoes of proper flexibility and shock absorption. If a biomechanical anomaly such as overpronation is noted, an orthotic, or in mild cases a simple arch support, should be utilized. Prophylaxis of shin splints mainly consists of the factors noted above plus careful attention to the detection of the recurrence of symptoms and immediate modification of training practices. A useful addition to training programs for runners bothered by chronic exacerbations of shin splints is to shift some of their training program to swimming and bicycling, which maintain aerobic conditioning without biomechanical overload.

Stress Fractures.[39] Stress fracture as a clinical entity may have been described as early as 1855, some 40 years before the first clinical use of radiographs, but perhaps more succinctly in 1939 when Roberts and Vogt defined pseudofracture of the tibia.[54] The tibia is the most common site of stress fractures in runners, but, since a stress fracture may occur in any lower extremity osseous structure, the diagnosis must be enter-

tained if the history or examination suggests pain from bone (Fig. 12). Pathophysiologically, they are due to repeated compression or impaction stress on bone or with excessive periosteal traction. As repetitive stress is applied to bone, remodeling and repair may be insufficient, and transition from microscopic to macroscopic fracture may occur. Careful serial analyses of bone stress reactions indicate that the bone initially at risk for stress fracture is on one cortical side of the diaphysis. With increasingly severe osseous inflammation, the stress becomes circumferential, but no frank displacement of bony cortex occurs. If bony stress continues, displaced fracture may occur through the diaphysis.[25]

Pathophysiologically, three fourths of lower extremity stress fractures probably result from training errors, most notably poor shock-absorbing shoes, excessive mileage, training with another type of lower extremity injury that changes normal biomechanics, or training with a known biomechanically abnormal gait.[12,39] The most common biomechanical abnormality found is hyperpronation with excessive varus alignment of the lower leg and foot.[65] Besides the obvious compressive forces that may cause microtrauma, another suggested etiology for stress fracture of the tibia is that which occurs when a bowing effect develops with forceful muscle contraction, i.e., in the gastrocnemius group.[14] Historically, the patient complains of pain initially after running, which progresses to pain while running progressively shorter distances.[8] As enough microtrauma

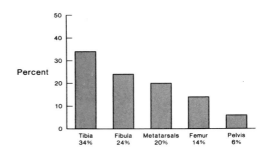

FIGURE 12. Most common bones involved with stress fractures in 1000 patients. (From McBryde AM: Clin Sports Med 4: Oct 1985.)

accumulates, pain occurs during nontraining activities and finally at rest. Most patients note unilateral tenderness and pain over the medial tibial diaphysis, but in neophyte runners accumulating high mileage without previous conditioning the pain may be bilateral.

Physical examination generally discloses point tenderness over the tibia, especially over the medial tibial diaphysis. In more dramatic cases evidence of periosteal reaction, such as swelling or increased warmth, may be noted, or a bony callus may be felt by palpation.[25] Ancillary testing such as plain radiographs and bone scans plays a prominent role in the early detection and diagnosis of stress fractures. Two to six weeks are generally required from the onset of pain to plain radiographic changes.[23] The earliest changes are periosteal reactions or small linear unilateral cortical defects perpendicular to the diaphysis. Many mild stress fractures occur without causing apparent changes on standard x-rays films. Technetium polyphosphate scanning of the tibia with multiple views is especially useful, since the agent will concentrate in an area of high blood flow and metabolic activity, such as that seen with bony remodeling in a stress fracture.[22] One of the main advantages of radionuclide bone scanning for stress fractures is its great sensitivity and specificity.[22,25] Although modalities such as ultrasound and thermography may play a role in delineation of stress fractures, radionuclide scanning provides the highest percentage of detection.[25] Within one week after development of symptoms, radionuclide scanning is usually positive for a stress fracture.[39] This capacity for early detection has clinical utility in that stress fractures detected early, before circumferential diaphyseal injury has taken place, heal in about one half the time required for a circumferential lesion.[8]

Therapy for stress fractures depend largely on the site of the fracture and the "criticalness" of the bone involved. For the uncomplicated tibial stress fracture with noncircumferential involvement of the diaphysis, healing may be expected in 4–6 weeks.[8,65] In a circumferential lesion, healing may be delayed for 8–14 weeks.[8] In general, it is prudent to advise the patient to take a relatively long period of rest from pounding exercise, because stress fractures tend to become recalcitrant or recurrent. Additionally, when stress fractures become complete fractures, there is a high rate of delayed union and nonunion. Treatment of tibial stress fractures other than those of the tibial plateau involves decreasing training mileage to a painfree level if the patient must continue to run. If the patient is agreeable, it might be best to switch to nonimpact aerobic sports such as swimming or bicycling. The patient should be placed in enhanced shock-absorbing footwear for both training and daily activities, and soft surfaces should be run upon, with no sprinting or banked surfaces.[39,65] Recalcitrant cases of stress fracture of the tibia should be carefully examined for pathologic fractures, tumor, or infection.[39] If no other complicating factors are noted, casting and non-weight-bearing management may be used for resolution of the fracture.

Compartment Syndrome. Compartment syndrome is one of the true orthopedic emergencies that may confront the primary care physician when dealing with overuse syndromes.[2] The most important entity is the acute anterior compartment syndrome, although any fascial compartment in the lower extremity may be involved in a potentially catastrophic event.[2] A compartment syndrome occurs when excessive muscle activity leads to an increased interstitial and muscle volume of as much as 20%.[13] The fascial compartments of the lower extremity are rigid containers; therefore, as muscle volume increases, compartment pressure rises, promoting first venous stasis then frank ischemia. The ischemic muscle tissue releases inflammatory mediators that cause further compartmental edema and increased tissue pressure. A vicious cycle of further tissue hypoxia and continued edema then occurs. When ischemia and hypoxia become insurmountable, tissue necrosis occurs.

In chronic compartment syndromes, the musculature of individual compartments may be overused, but the cascade of overuse to tissue swelling to ischemia may not occur to an extreme degree. In these individuals, symptoms may be noted during or immediately after exercise. In the acute compartment syndrome however, the tissue changes may be potentially irreversible unless immediate attention is given to releasing compartment pressure.

The history of acute compartment syndrome is of a patient who undergoes extreme exercise with progressive leg pain. In the anterior compartment syndrome, the pain is usually in the anterior tibial region secondary to overuse of the anterior tibialis group, but it also can occur laterally, representing overuse of the perinei muscles or, more rarely, as posterior calf pain implicating overuse of the posterior tibialis. Since the anterior compartment syndrome is the most common, the physician should be especially alert for acute anterior lower extremity pain.

Physical examination of the patient will show weakness in the involved musculature. The muscles are tender, swollen, and tense. For the anterior compartment syndrome, loss of foot dorsiflexion and decreased sensory appreciation in the toe web between the first and second toes are noted.[26,53] The dorsalis pedis pulse is usually normal, unless previous vascular disease has been present.[53] Increased compartment pressures can be recorded by catheterized measurements with a manometer.[44] In chronic anterior compartment syndrome, recurrent pain reproducible with activity will be noted in the anterior lower extremity. Diagnosis of this condition may be difficult unless anterior compartment pressures are measured during or after exercise.

Treatment for acute anterior compartment syndrome warrants immediate orthopedic consultation. Pending consultation the patient should be put at rest. The use of ice to the lower extremity is controversial, since the patient's sensation may be impaired and because tissue already under ischemic threat may be further injured. Prompt correction of any circulatory abnormality such as dehydration should be implemented. In acute cases where clinical examination or intracompartmental pressure analyses suggest impending tissue necrosis, fasciotomy should be done immediately.[53] In chronic compartment syndrome, after other diagnoses have been ruled out, surgical release of the anterior compartment accomplished by a 1–1½ inch incision over the mid-portion of the tibia medially may be required.[1]

Prophylaxis of future compartmental problems should be aimed at correcting any problems of biomechanics or training. Since compartment syndromes often arise after an episode of acute severe training or competition, the training and competitive goals may need to be redefined. Compartment syndrome of the anterior muscle group can also be provoked by toe or hill running. Such training practices may need to be eliminated.

OVERUSE SYNDROMES OF THE ANKLE AND FOOT

Overuse syndromes of the ankle and foot consist most commonly of Achilles tendinitis and plantar fasciitis. Although neither syndrome is as dramatic or as prominent as syndromes that occur more proximally, both are notable for their often disabling chronicity.

Achilles Tendinitis.[2,6,7] Achilles tendinitis presents as pain over the Achilles tendon and posterior heel (Fig. 13). The pain is usually most prominent 2–3 cm proximal to the insertion of the Achilles tendon on the calcaneus.[7] In early Achilles tendinitis, pain occurs at the onset of running, especially with hill running or sprinting. As inflammation becomes more chronic, the patient typically may note severe stiffness and pain of the Achilles tendon upon arising from bed. The pain may be particularly severe at the onset of a training period but will abate somewhat as the training session progresses. Physical examination discloses mild to excruciating pain over the Achilles tendon, usually at the base of the tendon and extending up to the level of the malleoli. The tendon and peritenon are often thickened. Severe cases may include visible swelling and inflammation as well as palpable crepitus.

Biomechanically, increased stress to the Achilles tendon results from a variety of factors, including excessive pronation, a cavus foot, or a short rigid Achilles tendon. Moderate to severe forefoot varus may be found in most runners with severe symptoms.[6] Up to 75% of runners with significant Achilles tendinitis will have training errors, usually involving hill running or excessive mileage, or interval training featuring sprinting bursts.[6,26]

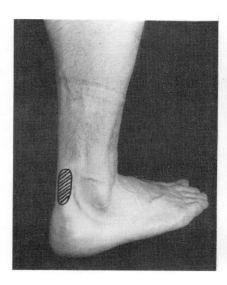 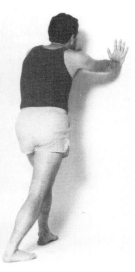

FIGURE 13. **Left,** Location of pain is directly over tendon, most notably at the level of the malleoli. **Right,** Achilles-gastrocnemius stretch. The subject is stretching the right gastroc-Achilles unit by leaning into a wall.

Some difficulty in differentiating Achilles tendinitis from retrocalcaneal bursitis may be noted. If tenderness is found more proximally on the tendon, the diagnosis is more apparent. Further diagnostic accuracy may also be achieved when the foot is plantar flexed forcibly against resistance or when having the patient perform toe walking. Ancillary testing such as radiographs is usually not needed, but in chronic cases it may show calcification in the body of the tendon or a spur at the insertion of the tendon into the calcaneus. These spurs are usually of no significance.[26] Further testing is useful if partial or complete rupture of the Achilles tendon is suspected. Such testing, including xeroradiography or nuclear magnetic resonance scanning of the tendon, may determine tendon integrity or rupture in difficult cases. Such rupture may be suspected in severe chronic overuse and a history of paroxysmal pain when exercising. Immediate physical examination in these cases, utilizing Thompson's test (forceful squeezing of the gasrocnemius muscle with the patient lying prone) may show no plantar flexion of the foot, thereby indicating complete tendon rupture.[26]

Therapy and rehabilitation of Achilles tendinitis consists of the measures usually employed for overuse syndromes. More specifically, ice before and after training may be especially useful. A heel lift of at least ½ inch should be present in the running shoe. Increased padding in the heel counter may decrease friction and provide better cushioning for the Achilles tendon. If excessive pronation is present, runner's orthotics may provide better control of the subtalar joint and reduce recurrent trauma. Because the Achilles tendon is not enclosed in a definitive tendon sheath, attempts to inject steroids into the peritenon region may be dangerous, since the injection may be directly into the tendon itself.[52] Injections into the tendon may weaken the tendon structure to the point that rupture may occur during further training. Prophylaxis of Achilles tendinitis is carried out by careful analysis of any biomechanical abnormalities, increasing soleus and gastrocnemius strength and flexibility, and revising the training schedule until symptoms are minimal.[63]

Plantar Fasciitis.[2,26] Plantar fasciitis presents as sharp, shooting pain in the arch and medial aspect of the foot (Fig. 14). The patient usually first notices pain with activity or upon arising. This syndrome may progress to pain during walking or any maneuver that involves stretching of the plantar fascia. Biomechanically, this syndrome results from repetitive microtrauma to the plantar fascia secondary to increased traction at the insertion of the fascia on the calcaneus. Such in-

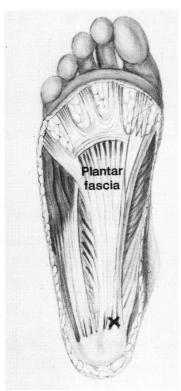

FIGURE 14. Plantar fascia, plantar fasciitis. The plantar's fascia serves as a stabilizer of the arch. The pain of plantar fasciitis may occur along the fascia but especially over its insertion into the calcaneus (x). (Reprinted from *Mayo Clinic Health Letter* with permission of Mayo Clinic, Rochester, Minnesota 55905.)

creased tension occurs most commonly in the high arch or cavus foot, creating a bowstring effect upon the fascia.

Physical examination discloses point tenderness of the fascia at its origin at the middle of the distal edge of the plantar surface of the culcaneus. The pain can usually be easily reproduced in the office by the examiner stretching the plantar fascia or by having the patient walk on his toes.[26] Specific treatment involves decreasing arch stretch with the use of an orthotic or arch support. Steroid injection at the origin of the plantar fascia may be effective although occasionally painful. One theory is that it works mainly by weakening the plantar fascia, leading to its disruption.

Ancillary testing is usually not necessary but radiographs of the foot may disclose a calcaneal spur.[18] It is controversial whether

removal of a calcaneal spur is appropriate for treatment of uncomplicated plantar fasciitis. Prophylaxis of plantar fasciitis involves conscientious use of appropriate orthotics, stretching of the plantar fascia prior to training or competition, using shoes with a firm heel counter, and employing a soft heel cup (such as Tuli's heel cup) in the running shoe. In the young runner, calcaneal pain similar to that noted in plantar fasciitis may occur idiopathically or with Sever's disease in which inflammation of the calcaneal epiphysis occurs. Heel cord stretching generally is therapeutic. Persistent calcaneal pain that does not respond to treatment directed at plantar fasciitis may be suspicious for stress fracture of the calcaneus, and investigation should be directed toward this possibility.

Less common overuse syndromes of the foot should also be considered in the differential diagnosis of plantars fasciitis. Most important among these are stress fracture of the calcaneus or the metatarsal. Pain over the lateral mid-foot just anterior to the calcaneus could represent cuboid syndrome, peroneus longus tendinitis, or plantar nerve entrapment.[38,18] Pain between the proximal phalanges of the toes suggests interdigital, or Morton's, neuromas.

SUMMARY

Although any anatomic structure of the lower extremity can be affected by overuse related to running, the primary care physician can generally provide an accurate diagnosis and appropriate treatment by being knowledgeable about a relatively few specific syndromes. Because of the biomechanical chain of shock absorption and torque, the knee will be the most common area afflicted by overuse syndromes in runners. Patellar pain syndrome will be the most likely diagnosis if the knee pain is anterior. Discomfort, euphemistically described as shin splints, may encompass a variety of syndromes, the most critical of which is anterior compartment syndrome. This syndrome should always be ruled out before initiating treatment directed toward a less critical diagnosis. Overuse syndromes of the ankle and foot, although less dramatic and prominent epidemiologically, can be particularly frustrating for the patient to overcome. In all the overuse syndromes mentioned above, the basics of treatment always include correction of biomechanical abnormalities, the search for training errors, and encouragement of the patient to adopt aerobic fitness practices that do not substitute pain for progress.

REFERENCES

1. Apple DF: End Stage Running Problems. Clin Sports Med 4:657, 1985.
2. Brody DM: Running injuries. Clinical Symposia 32:2, 1980.
3. Calabrese LH, Rooney TW: The use of nonsteroidal anti-inflammatory drugs in sports. Phys Sportsmed 14:89, 1986.
4. Chrisman OD, Snook GA, Wilson TC: Aspirin against degeneration of human cartilage. Clin Orthop 84:193, 1972.
5. Clancy WG: Runners injuries, Part 1. Am J Sports Med 8:138, 1980.
6. Clement DB, Taunton JE, et al: A survey of overuse running injuries. Phys Sportsmed 9:47, 1981.
7. Clement DB, Taunton JE, Smart GW: Achilles tendonitis and peritendonitis: etiology and treatment. Am J Sports Med 12:179, 1984.
8. Collier BD, Johnson RP, et al: Scintigraphic diagnosis of stress-induced incomplete fractures of the proximal tibia. J Trauma 24:156, 1984.
9. Cook SD, Kester MA, et al: Biomechanics of running shoe performance. Clin Sports Med 4:619, 1985.
10. Cox JS: Patellofemoral problems in runners. Clin Sports Med 4:669, 1985.
11. D'Ambrosia R: Orthotic devices in running injuries. Clin Sports Med 4:611, 1985.
12. Daffner RH, Martinez S, et al: Stress fractures of the proximal tibia in runners. Diag Radiol 142: 63, 1982.
13. Detmer DE: Chronic leg pain. Am J Sports Med 8:141, 1980.
14. Devas MV: Stress fractures of the tibia in athletes or "shin soreness." J Bone Joint Surg 40B:227, 1958.
15. Devereaux M, Parr G, et al: The diagnosis of stress fractures in athletes. JAMA 252:531, 1984.
16. Drez D: Running footwear. Am J Sports Med 8:140, 1980.
17. Dumont M, Lamourex F, et al: Diagnosis and followup of shin splint syndrome with Tc 99M MDP bone scintigraphy. J Trauma 24:156, 1984.
18. Eggold JF: Orthotics in the prevention of runners's overuse injuries. Phys Sportsmed 9:125, 1981.
19. Falkel J: Methods of training. Clin Phys Ther 10:1986.
20. Festa S, Schuster R: Ask the experts what the doctor says. The Runner 9:61, 1986.
21. Franklin BA, Rubenfire M: Losing weight through exercise. JAMA 244:377, 1980.
22. Geslien, CE, Thrall JH, et al: Early detection of stress fractures using 99M Tc polyphosphate. Radiology 121:683, 1976.
23. Giladi M, Ziv Y, et al: Comparison between radiography, bone scan, and ultrasound in the diagnosis of stress fractures. Milit Med 149:459, 1984.
24. Grana W, Kriegshauser LA: Scientific basis of extensor mechanism disorder. Clin Sports Med 4:247, 1985.
25. Hallel T, Amit S, Seycl D: Fatigue fractures of tibial and femoral shaft in soldiers. Clin Orthop 118:35, 1976.
26. Harvey JS: Overuse syndromes in young athletes. Pediat Clin North Am 29:1369, 1982.
27. Hastings AW: The fitness boom. Medical World News, 1984, p. 44.
28. Hoppenfeld S: Physical Examination of the Spine and Extremities. Norwalk, CT, Appleton-Century-Crofts, 1976.
29. James SL, Bates BT, Osternig LR: Injuries to Runners. Am Sports Med 6:40, 1978.
30. James SL, Brubaker CE: Biomechanics of running. Orthop Clin North Am 4:605, 1973.
31. Knight KL: I.C.E. Phys Sportsmed 10:137, 1982.
32. Koplan JP, Powell KE, Sikes RK, et al: An epidemiologic study of the benefits and risks of running. JAMA 248:3118, 1982.
33. LaPorte RE, Dearwater MS, et al: Cardiovascular fitness: is it really necessary. Phys Sportsmed 13:145, 1985.
34. Leard JS, Guifogle JE: Physiologic basis of warm up and cool down. Clin Phys Ther 10:81, 1986.
35. Levine J: Chondromalacia patella. Phys Sportsmed 7:41, 1979.
36. Lindenberg G, Rinshaw R, Noakes T: Iliotibial band function syndrome in runners. Phys Sportsmed 12:118, 1984.
37. Lutter LD: The knee and running. Clin Sports Med 4:685, 1985.
38. Mann RA, Hagy J: Biomechanics of walking, running, and sprinting. Am J Sports Med 8:345, 1980.
39. McBryde AM: Stress fractures in runners. Clin Sportsmed 4:737, 1985.
40. McKeag DB: The concept of overuse. Primary Care 11:43, 1984.
41. McMaster W: Cryotherapy. Phys Sportsmed 10: 112, 1982.
42. Mindess RC, Kramer D: Chondromalacia patella: diagnosis and treatment Fam Prac Recert 8:26, 1986.
43. Monahan T: Exercise and depression: swapping sweat for serenity. Phys Sportsmed 14:192, 1986.
44. Mubarah SJ, Haryens AR, Owne CA, et al: The wick catheter technique for measurement of intramuscular pressure. J Bone Joint Surg 58A:1016, 1976.
45. Murphy P: Warming up before stretching advised. Phys Sportsmed 14:45, 1986.
46. Nash H: Can exercise made us immune to disease. Phys Sportsmed 14:250, 1986.
47. Newell SG, Brainvell ST: Overuse injuries to the knee in runners. Phys Sportsmed 12:12, 1984.
48. Newell AG, Woodle A: Cuboid syndrome. Phys Sportsmed 9:71, 1981.
49. Paffenbarger RS, Hyde RT, et al: Physical activity

all-cause mortality and longevity of college alumni. N Engl J Med 314:605, 1986.

50. Polley HF, Hinder GG: Rheumatologic Interviewing and Physical Examination of the Joints, 2nd ed, Philadelphia, W. B. Saunders, 1978.

51. Powell KE, Kohl HW, et al: An epidemiological perspective on the causes of running injuries. Phys Sportsmed 14:100, 1986.

52. Reilly DT, Martens M: Experimental analysis of the quadriceps muscle force and patello-femoral joint reaction force for various activities. OCTA Orthop Scand 43:126, 1972.

53. Reneman RS: The anterior and lateral compartment syndrome of the leg due to intensive use of muscles. Clin Orthop 113:69, 1975.

54. Roberts SM, Vogt EC: Pseudofracture of the tibia. J Bone Joint Surg 21:891, 1939.

55. Roy S, Irvin R: Injuries to the running athlete. Sports med 1983, p. 412.

56. Rubin BD, Collins HR: Runner's knee. Phys Sportsmed 8:49, 1980.

57. Sady SP, Wortman M, Blanke D: Proprioceptive neuromuscular facilitation. Arch Phys Med Rehab 63:261, 1982.

58. Scott S: Current concepts in the rehabilitation of the injured athlete. Mayo Clinic Proc 59:77, 1984.

59. Shyne K: To stretch or not to stretch. Phys Sportsmed 10:1982.

60. Simon HB: Current topics in medicine I. Scientific American Medicine, 1984.

61. Smith WB: Environmental factors in running. Am J Sports Med 8:138, 1980.

62. Stamford B: Training distance and injury in runners. Phys Sportsmed 12:160, 1984.

63. Stanish WD, Curwin S, Rubinovich M: Tendinitis: the analysis and treatment for running. Clin Sports Med 4:593, 1985.

64. Subotnick SI, Newell SG: Podiatric Sports Medicine. Mount Kisco, NY, Futura Publishing Co., 1975.

65. Taunton JE, Clement DB, Webber D: Lower extremity stress fractures in athletes. Phys Sportsmed 9:77, 1981.

Index